POLYMER YEARBOOK 16

POLYMER YEARBOOK

An annual desk reference featuring pertinent data, mini-reviews and useful information for polymer scientists.

Edited by Richard A. Pethrick

This book is part of a series. The publisher will accept continuation orders which may be cancelled at any time and which provide for automatic billing and shipping of each title in the series upon publication. Please write for details.

POLYMER YEARBOOK 16

Edited by
RICHARD A. PETHRICK
University of Strathclyde, UK

Associate Editors
GENNADI E. ZAIKOV
Institute of Chemical Physics
Russian Academy of Sciences, Moscow

TEIJI TSURUTA
NAOYUKI KOIDE
Science University of Tokyo, Japan

harwood academic publishers
Australia • Canada • China • France • Germany • India • Japan • Luxembourg
Malaysia • The Netherlands • Russia • Singapore • Switzerland

Amsteldijk 166
1st Floor
1079 LH Amsterdam
The Netherlands

Library of Congress Cataloging-in-Publication Data

Polymer yearbook.—1st ed.—Chur.:
Harwood Academic Publishers, 1984–
v.: ill.; 24 cm
Annual.
ISSN 0738-1743 = Polymer yearbook.

1. Polymers and polymerization-Collected works.
QD380.P654 547.7dc19 84-648226
AACR2 MARC-S
Library of Congress [8508]

ISBN: 90-5702-473-X

Contents

Preface

Because of changes in the accessibility of information the contents of Polymer Yearbook have changed over the years. The current issue contains a mixture of indepth reviews and current awareness material. This year the dissertation abstracts have been reduced to being collated under subject headings and their access codes. The titles of the theses to which the reference relates have been omitted since this is readily available from the source. We propose to continue with this policy in the future. We are reviewing the extent to which the volume should contain current awareness information and would be interested in receiving comments on this topic.

This volume contains a broad spectrum of articles which cover topics that range from synthesis to theory, and from biodegradation to inhibition of aging. The article on the constitutive equations for undiluted linear polymers summarises the controversy on the applicability of the reptation model. It considers the validity of this approach and presents an alternative way of approaching the problem. This article is controversial and brings some interesting views to this very important topic. Another article considers the problem of prediction of the physical properties of the solid state and proposes a topographic based theory that is different from that usually used to approach this problem. There are also articles on thermal and biodegradation and related issues and the problems of synthesis of siloxane based polymers.

This year Professor Teiji Tsuruta has retired from the Editorial Board and the Japanese activity will be continuing through Professor Naoyuki Koide. I would like to take this opportunity to acknowledge Professor Tsuruta's support of Polymer Yearbook over almost twelve years. It has been through his efforts and those of Professor Koide that the very valuable insight into Japanese polymer science has been provided. Professor Zaikov has continued to actively seek valuable contributions from authors in his geographic area and help maintain the broad spectrum of interest reflected in the articles contributed.

Contributions from conference organisers should be sent to the Chief Editor, Professor R.A. Pethrick, for consideration for publication in future volumes of Polymer Yearbook. The editors welcome suggestions from readers on topics to be included in future volumes. The editors gratefully acknowledge the continuing help and meticulous devotion to Polymer Yearbook by Helen Paton who sustains the project at the University of Strathclyde.

Contributors

Yu.A. Altukhov	Altai State Technical University, Barnaul, Russia
M.S. Arzhakov	Moscow State University, Moscow, Russia
S.A. Arzhakov	Moscow State University, Moscow, Russia
E.Ya. Davydov	Institute of Biochemical Physics RAN, Moscow, Russia
N.M. Emanuel	Russian Academy of Sciences, Moscow, Russia
K.Z. Gumargalieva	Russian Academy of Sciences, Moscow, Russia
T. Hashimoto	Fukui University, Fukui, Japan
K. Hatanaka	Tokyo Institute of Technology, Yokohama, Japan
A. Higuchi	Seikei University, Tokyo, Japan
D. Horak	Academy of Sciences of the Czech Republic, Prague, Czech Republic
A. Imamura	Hiroshima University, Higashi-hiroshima, Japan
R.K. Jensen	Ford Motor Company, Dearborn, USA
T. Kajiyama	Kyushu University, Fukuoka, Japan
O.N. Karpukhin	Russian Academy of Sciences, Moscow, Russia
V.M. Kopylov	Russian Federation State Scientific Research Institute, Moscow, Russia
S. Korcek	Institute of Biochemical Physics RAN, Moscow, Russia
V.A. Kovjazin	Russian Federation State Scientific Research Institute, Moscow, Russia
S.M. Lomakin	Russian Academy of Sciences, Moscow, Russia
Yu.V. Moiseev	Russian Academy of Sciences, Moscow, Russia
T. Nakano	Nagoya University, Nagoya, Japan
N. Nemoto	Kyushu University, Fukuoka, Japan
T.V. Pokholok	Russian Academy of Sciences, Moscow, Russia
V.N. Pokrovskii	Russian Academy of Sciences, Moscow, Russia
V.P. Pustoshny	Institute of Biochemical Physics RAN, Moscow, Russia
G.V. Pyshnograi	Altai State Technical University, Barnaul, Russia

T. Sato	Osaka University, Osaka, Japan
E.L. Shanina	Russian Academy of Sciences, Moscow, Russia
V.Ya. Shlyapintokh	Russian Academy of Sciences, Moscow, Russia
Yu.A. Shlyapnikov	United Institute of Chemical Physics, Moscow, Russia
A. Takahara	Kyushu University, Fukuoka, Japan
K. Tanaka	Kyoto Institute of Technology, Kyoto, Japan
L.S. Troitskaya	Russian Academy of Sciences, Nizhny Novgorod, Russia
B.B. Troitskii	Russian Academy of Sciences, Nizhny Novgorod, Russia
M. Tsunooka	Osaka Prefecture University, Osaka, Japan
K. Ueda	Yokohama National University, Yokohama, Japan
A.P. Vorotnikov	Institute of Biochemical Physics RAN, Moscow, Russia
H. Yamane	Kyoto Institute of Technology, Kyoto, Japan
Yu.G. Yanovsky	Russian Academy of Sciences, Moscow, Russia
G.E. Zaikov	Institute of Biochemical Physics RAN, Moscow, Russia

Review Section

Kinetics and Mechanism of the Product Conversions in Reaction of 2,4,6-Tri-*t*-Butylphenol with NO_2

E.Ya. DAVYDOV, S. KORCEK, R.K. JENSEN and G.E. ZAIKOV

Ford Motor Company, SRL-3083, P.O. Box 2053, Dearborn, MI 48121, USA
Institute of Biochemical Physics RAN, 117977, Moscow, Russia

Kinetics of the thermal decay and NO_2 interaction with *o*-quinolide hydroperoxides (*o*-QHP) have been studied in hexadecane. The formation of *o*-QHP was initiated by bubbling of NO_2 and air mixtures through 2,4,6-Tri-*t*-butylphenol solution in a batch reactor. The rate constant of the *o*-QHP thermal decay with the *o*-quinone formation is $k_d = 10^{15} \exp(-114 \pm 4\,\text{kJ/RT}), \text{s}^{-1}$. The kinetics of the *o*-QHP consumption at 295 K for the reaction with NO_2 are described by the second order equation relative to hydroperoxide. The mechanism of this process is discussed. The effective values of the activation energy and preexponent of the thermal decomposition of 2,4,6-Tri-*t*-butylnitrocyclohexadienone are 60 kJ/mol and $3.5 \cdot 10^6, \text{s}^{-1}$.

It was shown previously[1,2] that the nitrocyclohexadienone (NCHD) formation is a characteristic feature of hindered phenol nitration by nitrogen dioxide in the liquid phase. This reaction for 2,4,6-Tri-*t*-butylphenol (TTBP) can be depicted by the following scheme:

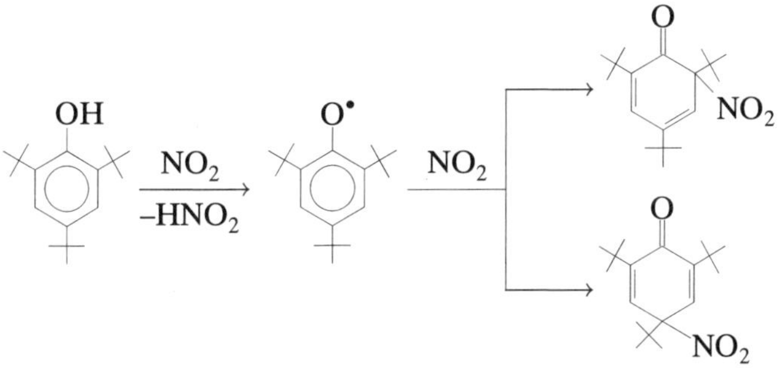

(1)

The products of this reaction are easily identified by an absorbance band in UV spectrum with $\lambda_{max} \approx 240$ nm. But NCHD is a rather unstable compound.[1] In this report the results of investigation of the NCHD conversion kinetics and mechanism are presented.

NCHD were obtained by bubbling (–) through a TTBP solution in hexadecane (HD) in a batch reactor by a gas mixture containing NO_2 (750 ppm) and the balance air? This technique has been described before.[3] The initial concentration of TTBP in

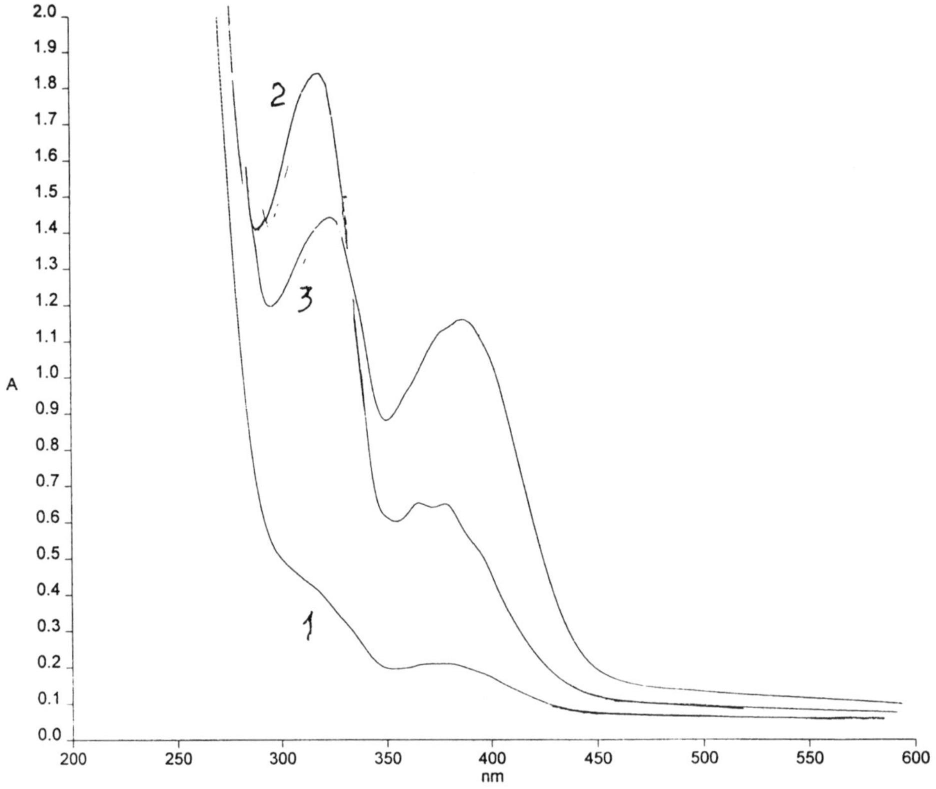

Figure 1 UV spectra of TTBP solution in the course of NO_2 bubbling (1), after 15 hours of the bubbling completion (2), after 10 min of heating at 333 K (3).

HD was $2 \cdot 10^{-3}$ M. The solution (50 ml) was bubbled at a flow rate (FR) of gas mixture from 50 ml/min to 300 ml/min. The kinetic measurements were performed in UV/VIS spectrophotometer, Perkin Elmer Lambda 18 using 0.1 and 1 cm optical cells. The kinetics of NO_2 solubility in HD at different FR was also determined by spectrophotometer. In these experiments HD, saturated for a different time, was inserted in 10 cm cell and NO_2 concentration was measured by the optical density at 410 nm.[4]

Among NCHD, the formation of other products was registered at 295 K. Their UV spectrum are shown in Figure 1 in which two absorbance bands at 320 nm and 380 nm are observed. The 320 nm band is substantially increased if the solution is kept after complete decay of TTBP in reactions (1) for time 15–20 hours outside of reactor (Figure 2). In these conditions the decrease of the NCHD band intensity is also exhibited. These facts indicate that 320 nm and 380 nm bands belong to different compounds produced as a result of the reaction (1) main product transformation.

It would appear natural that the 320 nm band corresponds to *o*-quinolide peroxy groups which have the absorbance peak just in this spectral region.[5] The formation

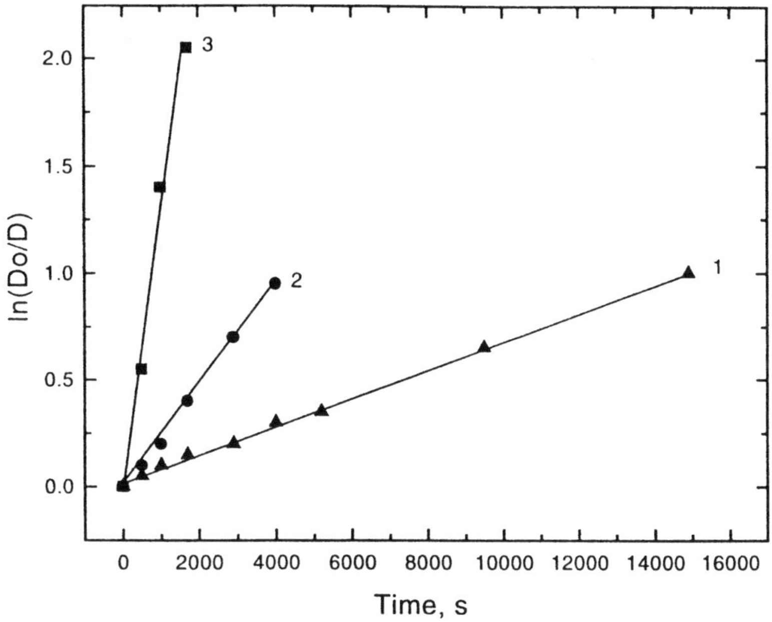

(a)

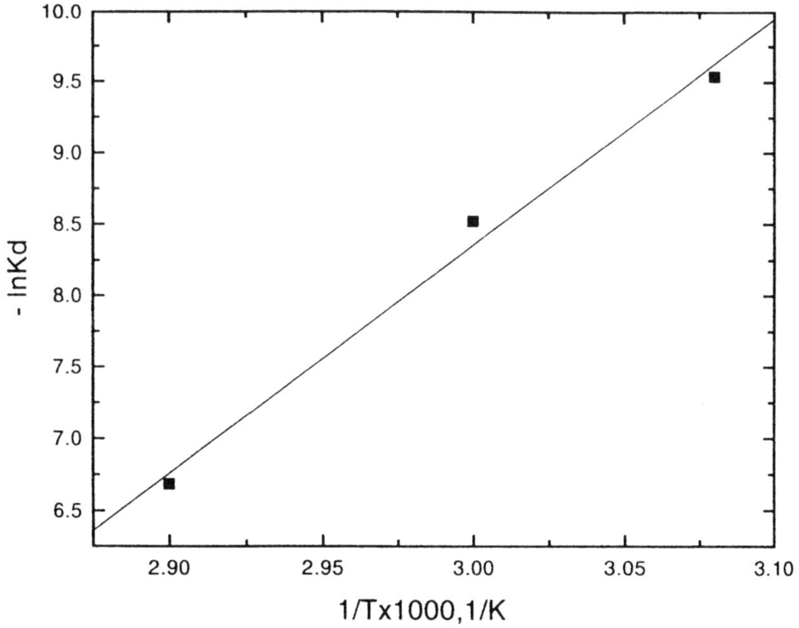

(b)

Figure 2 Kinetics of the 320 nm band decrease (a) at 323 K (1), 333 K (2), 346 K (3) and Arrhenius plot of k_d.

of these substances by TTBP nitration can be attributed to reactions of the intermediate phenoxy radical oxidation.

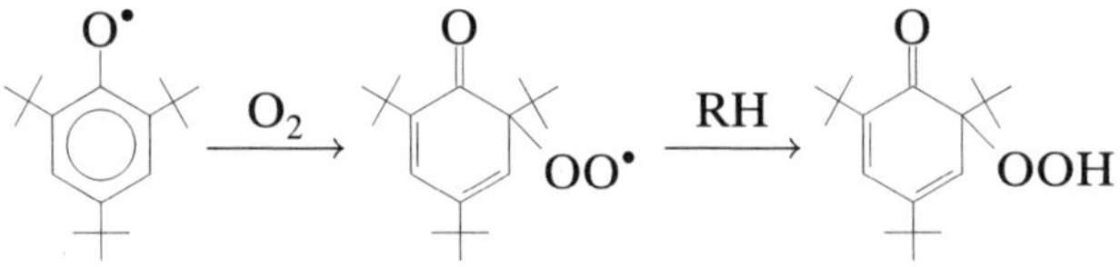

(2)

In support of the assignment of the 320 nm band to *o*-quinolide hydroperoxides (*o*-QHP) the kinetics of these compound thermal decay have been studied. It is well known that this process for quinolide peroxides is characterized by distinct values of kinetic parameters. Thermal decay at not very high concentrations ($< 10^{-2}$ M) is unimolecular reaction with activation energy of ≈ 120 kJ/mol and preexponential factor of 10^{14}–10^{15} s^{-1}.[6]

After treatment of TTBP in HD by a gas mixture in the course of 3 hours at FR = 300 ml/min, the solution was held outside the reactor for 20 hours until the attainment of the maximum band intensity at 320 nm. An estimation on a basis of known extinction coefficients[5] of hydroperoxide concentration is not over $8 \cdot 10^{-4}$ M. Then the kinetics of this band decrease were measured in the temperature range of 323 K to 346 K. The kinetic curves obtained was found to be straightened out in co-ordinates of the first order equation (Figure 2a). The Arrhenius plot corresponding to the rate constant values is shown in Figure 2b. From this plot it was determined: $k_d = 10^{15} \exp(-114 \pm 4\,\text{kJ/RT}), s^{-1}$. As is clear, the activation energy and preexponent values are closely to those reported in literature[6] and serve as verification of the 320 nm band assignment to *o*-QHP.

The mechanism of the thermal *o*-QHP decay involves apparently two consecutive reactions. The primary step is the breaking of O—O bond

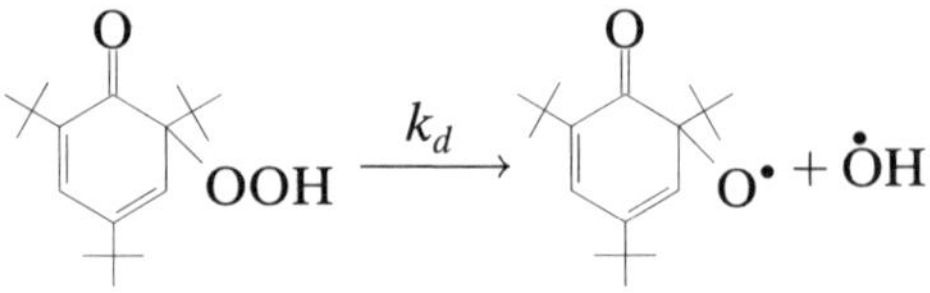

(3)

The resulting cyclohexadienone alcoxy radical, as is shown by the chemical nuclear polarization study,[7] is capable to dissociate rapidly (10^{-10} s) with *o*-quinone formation

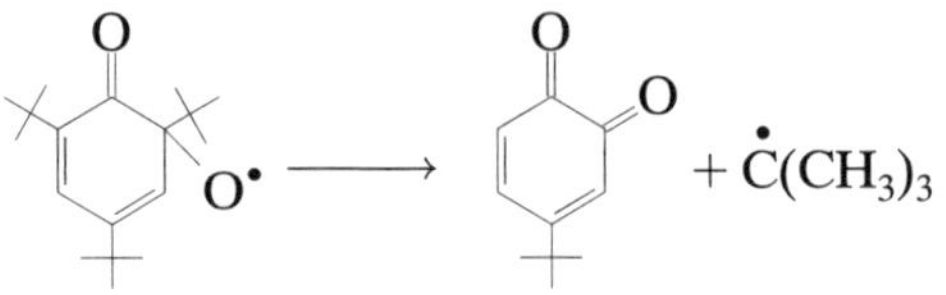

(4)

UV spectrum of *o*-quinone has an intense absorbance band in the region of 380–390 nm.[8,9] Actually, an increase of absorbance at 380 nm is observed in the course of *o*-QHP thermal decomposition (Figure 3).

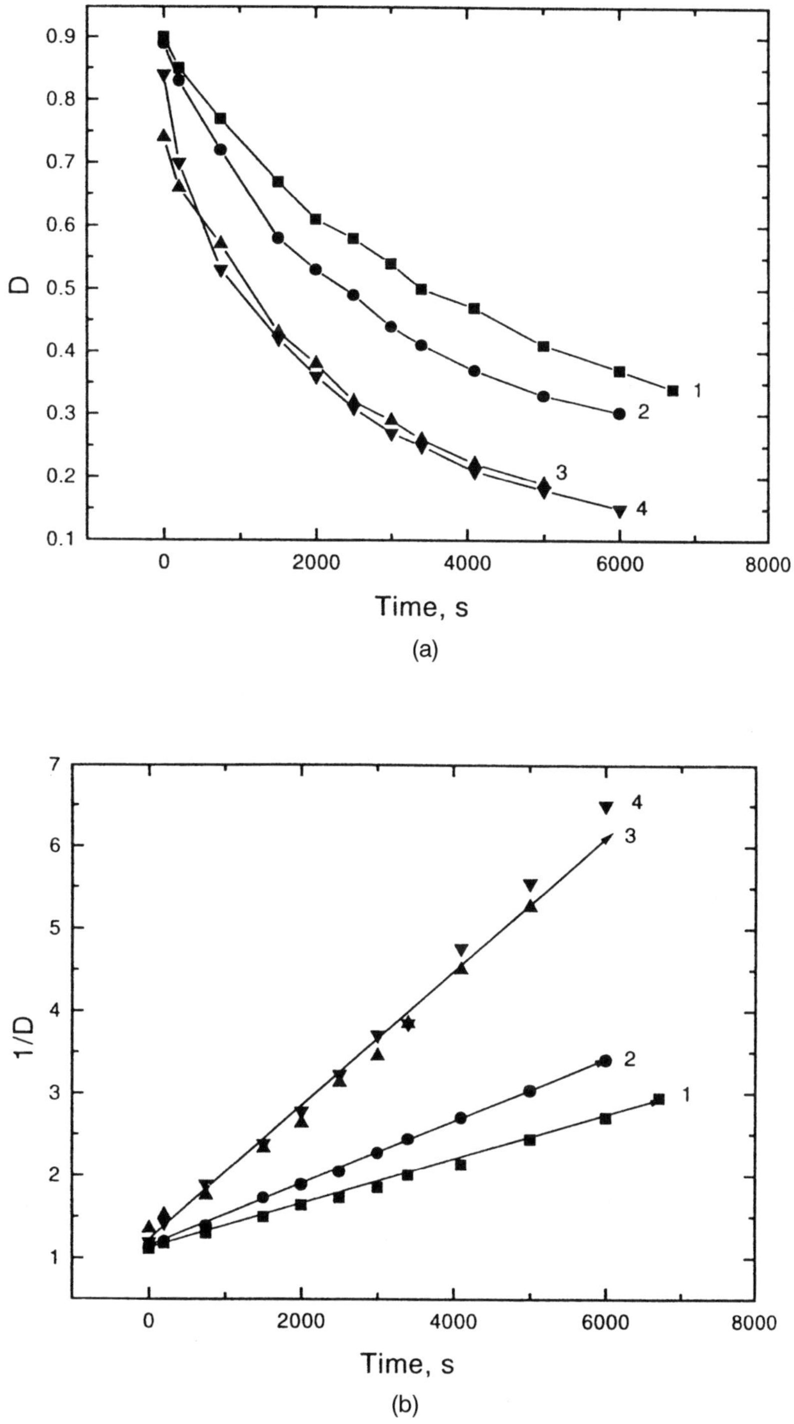

Figure 3 Kinetics of the 320 nm band decrease (a) and their straightening (b) during bubbling at NO_2 with a FR of 50 ml/min (1), 100 ml/min (2), 200 ml/min (3) and 300 ml/min (4).

The 320 nm band belonging to *o*-QHP is also confirmed by other facts. This band disappears during the bubbling of NO_2 in the reactor. As was shown previously with different peroxy compounds,[10] just hydroperoxides decay in the liquid phase reaction with NO_2. In contrast, diaryl and dialkyl peroxides do not show significant interaction.

The TTBP solution tentative treatment was carried out similarly above for the thermal decay of QHP to study the kinetics of QHP with NO_2 reaction. The solution at 295 K was bubbled at different FR. The change of optical density at 320 nm in these conditions are shown in Figure 3a. As illustrated in the figure, the kinetics are essentially the same for highest FR but for 100 ml/min and 50 ml/min they are significantly distinguished. It turns out that the kinetic curves obtained are well described by the second order equation relative to optical density of 320 nm band (Figure 3b). These data testify that QHP decay is not associated with simple bimolecular reaction with NO_2 and the concentration of soluble NO_2 in HD depends on FR. To account for kinetic regularities of QHP consumption the solubility of NO_2 was studied at 295 K in the batch reactor conditions. The plots obtained at different FR are exhibited in Figure 4a. The kinetics match almost exactly at FR = 200 ml/min and 300 ml/min, while they are differed both by rate and limiting value of solubility at lesser FR. The experimental dependencies are satisfactorily described by the equation

$$[NO_2] = [NO_2]_{lim}[1 - \exp(-k_s t)] \qquad (5)$$

where $[NO_2]_{lim}$ is the limiting concentration, k_s is constant depending on FR. The corresponding straightening confirming this conclusion are given in Figure 4b.

One can assume the following scheme to provide the explanation for the kinetics of QHP decay in reactions with NO_2

$$\mathrm{QHP} + \mathrm{NO_2} \underset{k_{-1}}{\overset{k_1}{\rightleftarrows}} \mathrm{QHP^{\bullet}NO_2} \qquad (6)$$

$$\mathrm{QHP^{\bullet}NO_2} + \mathrm{QHP} \xrightarrow[\mathrm{RH}]{k_2} \text{products} \qquad (7)$$

In the primary reversible step, QHP forms the intermediate with NO_2 which is subsequently transformed into resulting products by reaction with other QHP molecule. We could not measure the NO_2 solubility in TTBP solution by spectrophotometer because it is disguised by the intense absorbance of phenol. But $[NO_2]_{lim}$ may be thought of the same at the rather small TTBP concentrations.

Assuming that $QHP^{\bullet}NO_2$ and soluble NO_2 concentrations are at steady-state we obtain from (5)–(7) the following equation of the QHP decay rate

$$\frac{d[\mathrm{QHP}]}{dt} = -\frac{k_1 k_2 [\mathrm{QHP}]^2 k_s [\mathrm{NO_2}]_{lim}}{k_1 k_2 [\mathrm{QHP}]^2 + k_s k_2 [\mathrm{QHP}] + k_s k_{-1}} \qquad (8)$$

If $k_1[\mathrm{QHP}]^2 \ll k_2[\mathrm{QHP}] \ll k_{-1}$, then (8) is rearranged to equation which is in agreement with the experimental kinetic plots

$$\frac{d[\mathrm{QHP}]}{dt} \approx -\frac{k_1 k_2}{k_{-1}} [\mathrm{NO_2}]_{lim} [\mathrm{QHP}]^2 \qquad (9)$$

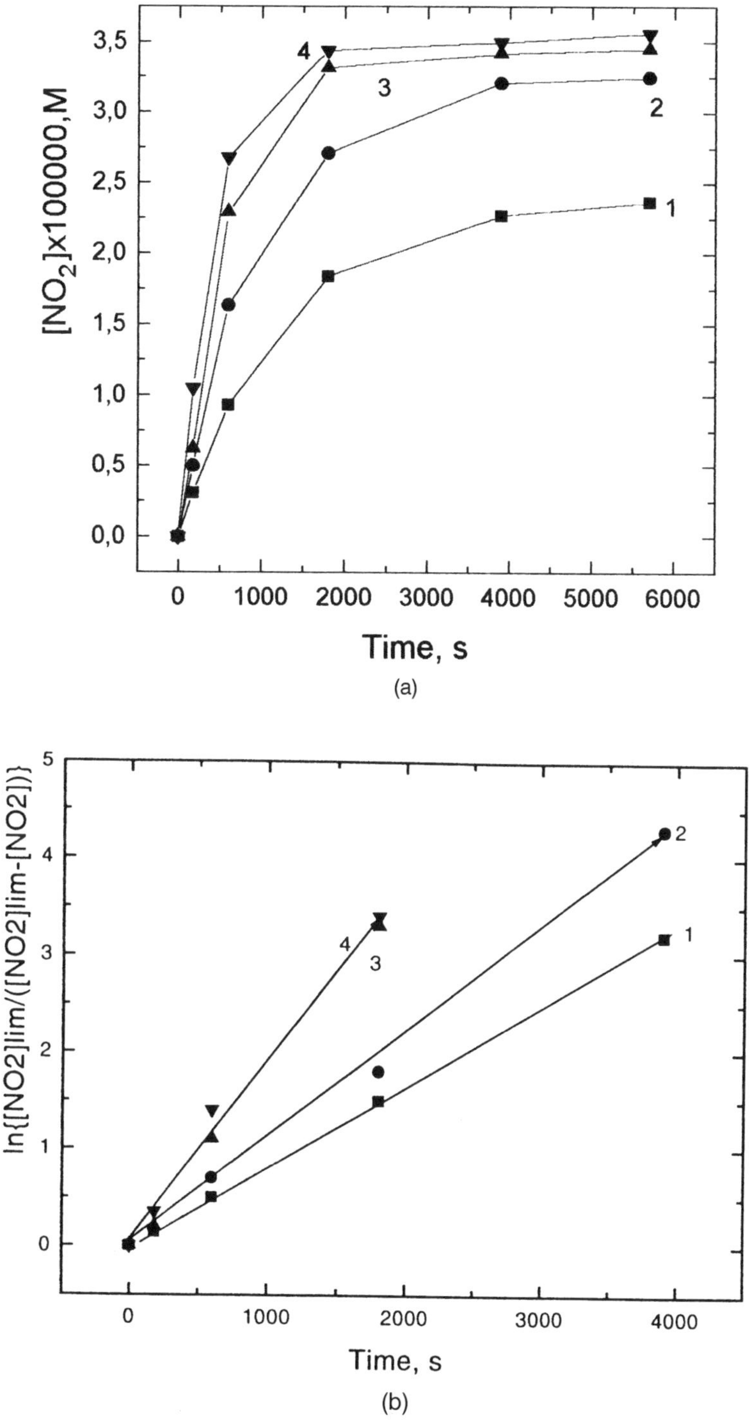

Figure 4 Kinetics of NO_2 solubility in HD (a) and their straightening (b) at FR of 50 ml/min (1), 100 ml/min (2), 200 ml/min (3) and 300 ml/min (4).

It seems reasonable that the specific mechanism of reaction (7) includes formation and decomposition of a highly ordered cyclic hydrogen bonded transition state

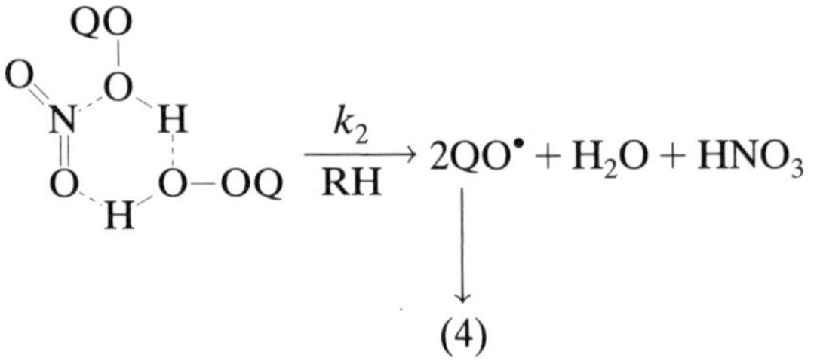

(10)

It should be noted that a similar conversion can also take place for *p*-QHP, but these compounds have high absorbance only at 240 nm.[5] At a relative small concentration of *p*-QHP, this band is overlapped by the intense absorbance of the main product (NCHD).

The formation and conversion reactions of QHP are initiated by decomposition of NCHD in intermediate phenoxy radicals

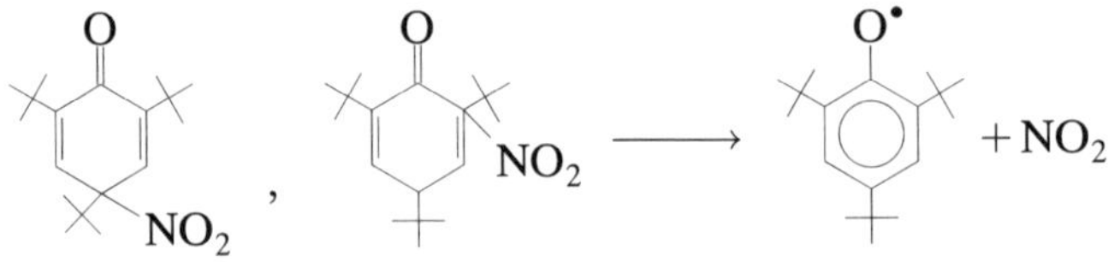

(11)

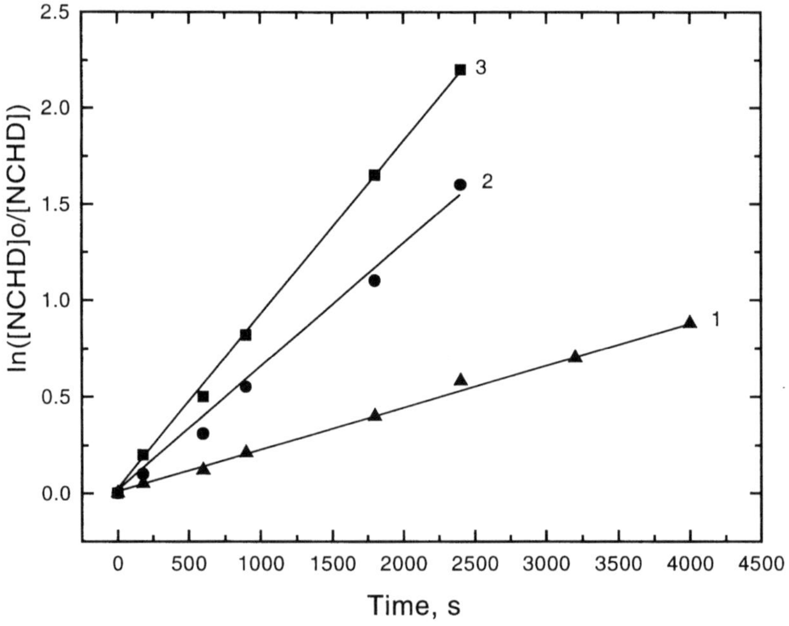

Figure 5 Kinetics of the NCHD thermal decay at 323 K (1), 333 K (2) and 343 K (3).

In this work the kinetic parameters of this process were determined. For this purpose TTBP solution at $[TTBP]_0 = 2\cdot 10^{-3}$ M was bubbled (FR = 300 ml/min) at 295 K for three hours until the complete transformation of TTBP into NCHD. Thereafter the kinetics of NCHD thermal decay were measured at 323–343 K by the optical density change of 240 nm band. This reaction is formally described by the first order law (Figure 5). The effective values of activation energy and preexponent determined from Arrhenius plot are 60 kJ/mol and $3.5\cdot 10^6, s^{-1}$ respectively. An approximate estimation, taking into consideration these values, shows that NCHD half conversion time is about seven hours at room temperature. This fact correlates with noted nonstability of these compounds.[2]

Thus, the liquid phase reaction of TTBP with NO_2 in the presence of balance air produces a variety of products of nitration and oxidation. These products are chemically active and are controlled by a free radical mechanism in the subsequent thermal reactions and reactions with NO_2 in the end quinones. QHP has the capability to decompose even at ordinary temperatures by interaction with NO_2. The function of NO_2 in this process lies in the organization of the molecular transition complex for the subsequent re-distribution of chemical bonds.

REFERENCES

1. G. Brunton, H.W. Cruse, K.M. Riches and A. Whittle, *Tetrahedron Letters*, 1979, **12**, pp. 1093–1094.
2. C.D. Cook and R.C.J. Woodworth, *Amer. Chem. Soc.*, 1953, **75**, pp. 6242–6244.
3. R.K. Jensen, S. Korcek, L.R. Mahoney and M.J. Zinbo, *Amer. Chem. Soc.*, 1979, **101**, pp. 7574–7584.
4. T.C. Hall and F.E.J. Blacet, *Chem. Phys.*, 1952, **20**, pp. 1745–1749.
5. A.F. Bickel and E.C.J. Kooyman, *Chem. Soc.*, 1953, pp. 3211–3218.
6. V.A. Roginskii, V.Z. Dubinskii, I.A. Shlyapnikova and V.B. Miller, *Eur. Polymer J.*, 1977, **13**, pp. 1043–1051.
7. A.L. Buchachenko, *Khimicheskaya Polarizatsiya Yader i Elektronov*, 1974, Nauka, Moscow.
8. S. Nagakura and A.J. Kuboyama, *Amer. Chem. Soc.*, 1954, **76**, pp. 1003–1005.
9. H.S.J. Mason, *Amer. Chem. Soc.*, 1948, **70**, pp. 138–140.
10. W.A. Pryor, L. Castle and D.F.J. Church, *Amer. Chem. Soc.*, 1985, **107**, pp. 211–217.

Physical and Mechanical Behavior of Polymer Glasses. IV. Cross-Linked Poly(Methyl Methacrylate)

M.S. ARZHAKOV and S.A. ARZHAKOV

Polymer Department, Faculty of Chemistry, Lomonosov Moscow State University, Vorob'evy Gory, Moscow, 119899 Russia

Temperature-induced relaxation of plastic deformation in cross-linked PMMA samples was studied. For cross-linked PMMA with a low concentration of cross-linking agent (less, than 5.2 mol.%), relaxation curves involve a low-temperature component at temperatures well below the glass transition temperature and high-temperature component at temperatures close to glass transition. Increasing the concentration of cross-linked agents in the polymer samples to 11.2 mol.% is accompanied by degeneration of the high-temperature component of the relaxation, and complete relaxation of the plastic deformation proceeds via the low-temperature component. The effect of cross-linking on the temperature-induced relaxation of plastic deformation was discussed in terms of restriction of segmental mobility within certain structural regions in the polymer sample.

INTRODUCTION

Temperature-induced relaxation of the plastic deformation of polymer glasses is known to involve the low-temperature component at temperatures well below the glass transition temperature and high-temperature component in the vicinity of glass transition.[1–4] Earlier,[5,6] the two-stage character of the relaxation was discussed in terms of the structural inhomogeneity of glassy polymers, that is, the existence of structural sublevels with different packing densities and degrees of ordering. The existence of a set of the above structural sublevels is responsible for the gradual involvement of segmental mobility in the temperature-induced relaxation of plastically deformed polymer sample.

Decreasing contribution from low-temperature component to total relaxation of residual deformation was observed as a result of increasing deformation temperature of PMMA, plasticization of PMMA, and copolymerization of methyl methacrylate with methacrylic monomers.[5,7] This experimental evidence was attributed to enhancement of local segmental mobility in certain structural sublevels. From this standpoint, the ratio between the low-temperature and high-temperature components of temperature-induced relaxation of plastic deformation provides important information concerning structural pattern of development of segmental mobility in glassy polymer. Generally speaking, this ratio may be treated as a physical parameter describing plastic deformation of polymer glasses, and their physical and mechanical behavior.[5,6]

In the present work, temperature-induced relaxation of plastic deformation of cross-linked PMMA was studied to gain a deeper insight in physical and mechanical behavior of glassy polymers.

EXPERIMENTAL

The copolymers of methyl methacrylate (MMA) with bifunctional monomers ethylene glycol dimethacrylate (EGDM) and triethylene glycol dimethacrylate (TGDM) were used as cross-linked PMMA. The content of bifunctional monomer in polymerization system was 2.5, 5.2, and 11.2 mol.%. The development of a network took place immediately during bulk polymerization.

Glass transition temperatures of copolymers studied were estimated by differential scanning calorimetry using a "Mettler TA-4000". Heating rate was 20 K/min.

The test samples were cylinders with a height of 30 mm and a diameter of 15 mm. Prior to testing, polymer samples were annealed at temperatures, which exceeded glass transition temperature by 10–15 K. Then, they were cooled down to room temperature. The height of the as-prepared samples was denoted as h_0.

The samples of initial PMMA and PMMA, cross-linked with EGDM and TGDM, were uniaxially compressed at 293 K with strain rate of 0.1 mm/min using an UTS-100 tensile machine (Germany). After that, they were unloaded at this temperature with the same rate. The height of deformed samples was denoted as h_{def}.

In the deformed polymer samples, temperature-induced relaxation of residual deformation was studied by measuring the changes in their height on heating from 293 K at a heating rate of 1 K/min. The height of the samples at a given temperature was denoted as h_T. Residual deformation at a given temperature was estimated as $\varepsilon_{\text{res}} = (h_0 - h_T)/(h_0 - h_{\text{def}})$ with an accuracy of $\pm$ 2%.

RESULTS AND DISCUSSION

For initial PMMA and PMMA, cross-linked with EGDM and TGDM, Figure 1 shows stress–strain diagrams, corresponding to uniaxial compression of polymer samples. Note, that all samples show well-pronounced plastic deformation and storing residual deformation after their unloading. Let us emphasize, that for cross-linked samples their elastic modulus and yield stress seem to be independent of the concentration of cross-linking agent (EGDM and TGDM), and are equal to those for initial PMMA.

For initial PMMA and cross-linked PMMA, Figures 2 and 3 show temperature dependences of residual deformation ε_{res}. For the lack of space, relaxation curves are presented only for polymer samples with 20 and 30% strains. As follows from Figures 2 and 3, for PMMA samples (curves 1), temperature-induced relaxation of plastic deformation takes place in two well-defined temperature regions below glass transition temperature T_g and close to T_g via low-temperature component ε_1 and high-temperature component ε_2, respectively. These components of relaxation are shown in Figure 2a.

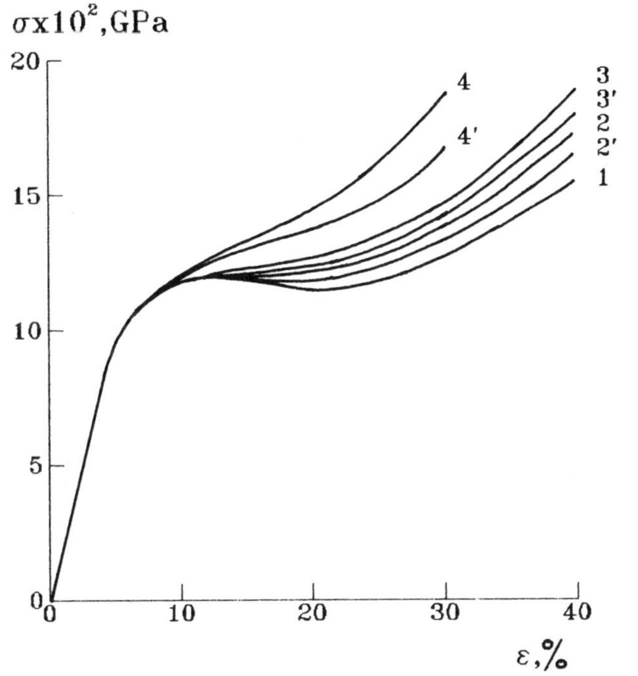

Figure 1 Stress–strain diagrams of PMMA (1) and PMMA, cross-linked with EGDM (2–4) and TGDM (2′–4′). Concentration of cross-linking agents: 2.5 (2, 2′), 5.2 (3, 3′) and 11.2 mol.% (4, 4′). Uniaxial compression at 293 K.

Earlier,[5,6] the two-stage character of the temperature-induced relaxation of the residual deformation of polymer glasses was interpreted in terms of their structural inhomogeneity, that is, coexistence of structural sublevels with different packing densities and degrees of ordering. Each of these sublevels is characterized by its own relaxation time and activation energy of segmental mobility. Hence, at each temperature below the glass transition temperature, local segmental mobility in certain structural sublevels is allowed. With increasing temperature, structural sublevels with higher packing densities become involved in segmental mobility, and finally, at the glass transition temperature, segmental mobility is observed in the whole polymer sample. In other words, the existence of a set of structural sublevels with different packing densities is responsible for the spectrum of segmental mobility in polymer glasses.

Low-temperature relaxation of the residual deformation is controlled by the low-temperature fraction of the spectrum of segmental mobility because of temperature-induced segmental mobility within structural sublevels with lower packing densities at temperatures well below T_g. Evidently, a certain part of the low-temperature fraction of the spectrum of the segmental mobility is able to relax during polymer loading. From this standpoint, the low-temperature component ε_1 of relaxation is likely to be associated with the stored plastic deformation, which remained unrelaxed during loading.

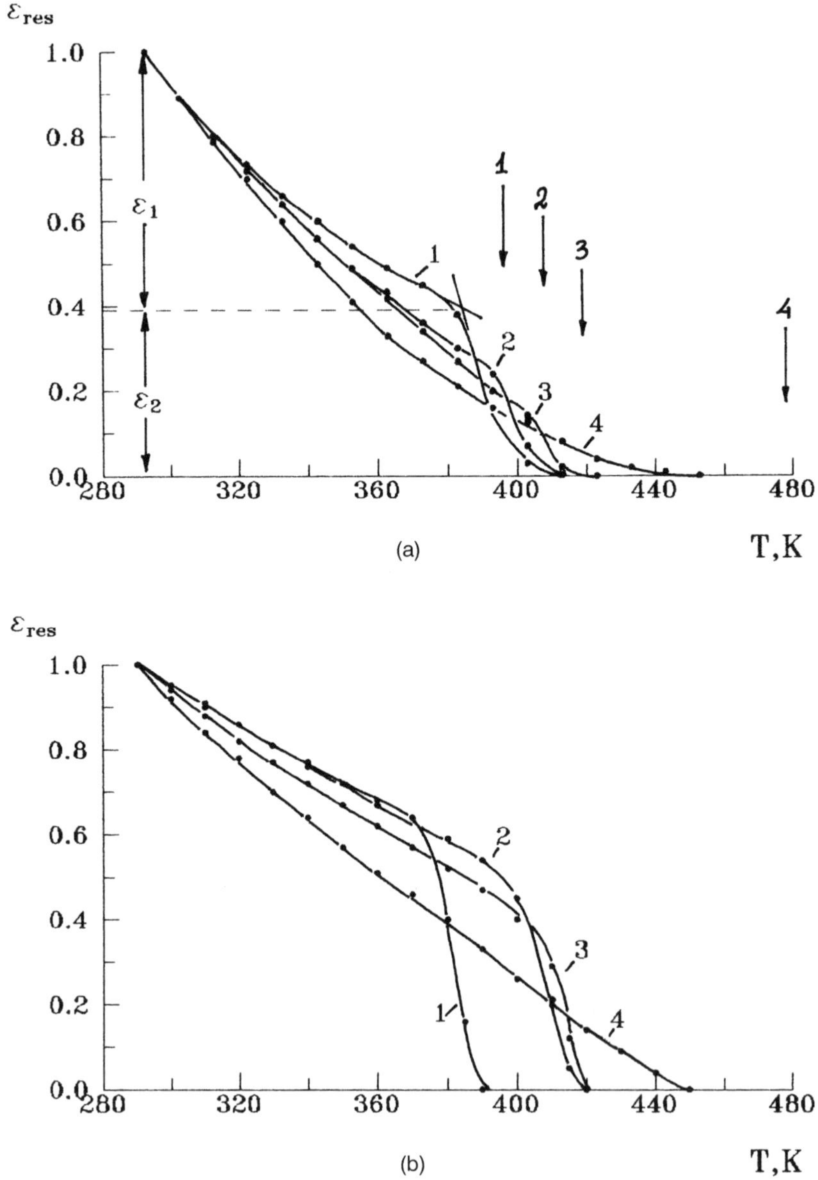

Figure 2 Temperature dependences of residual deformation ε_{res} of PMMA (1) and PMMA, cross-linked with 2.5 (2), 5.2 (3) and 11.2 mol.% EGDM (4). Strain: 20 (a) and 30% (b). The arrows show T_g of the corresponding polymer samples.

High-temperature fraction of the spectrum of segmental mobility is responsible for high-temperature component ε_2 of the relaxation. This component is accumulated in the polymer during loading, and is able to relax only at temperatures close to T_g via temperature-induced segmental mobility within structural sublevels with higher packing densities.

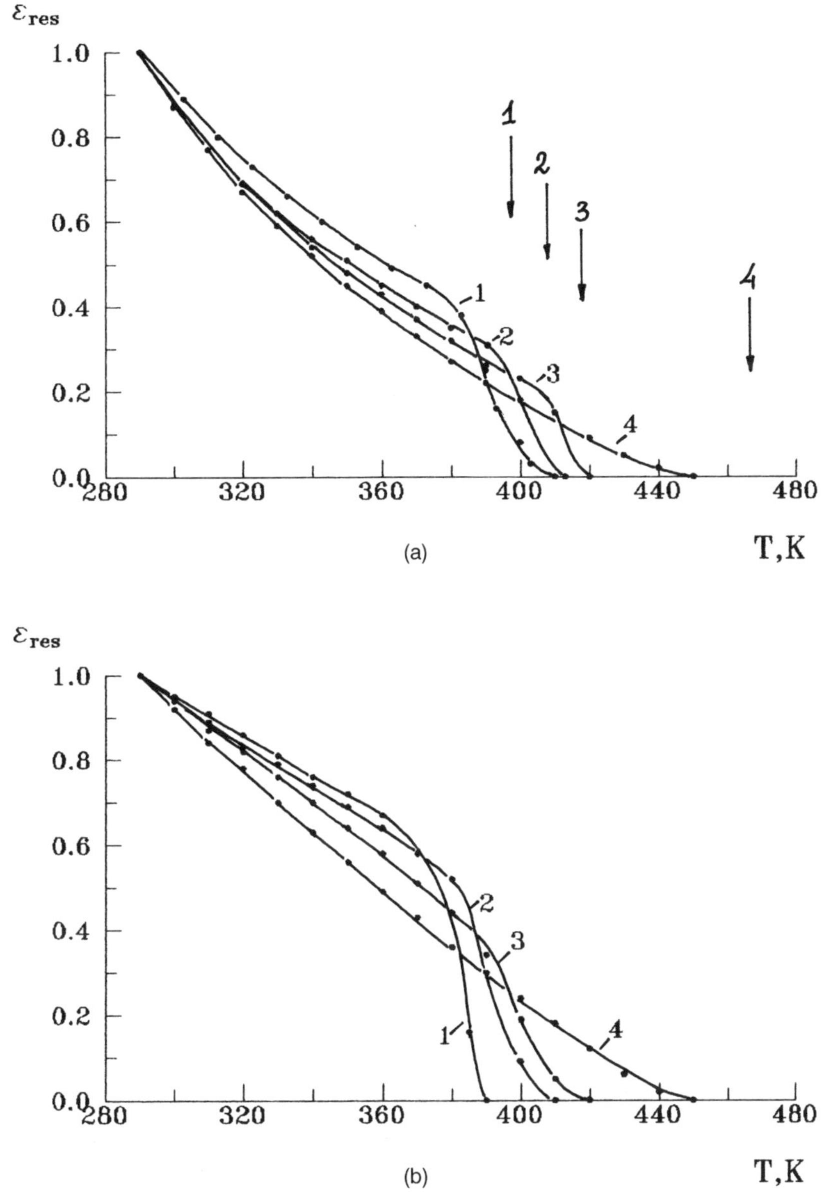

Figure 3 Temperature dependences of residual deformation εres of PMMA (1) and PMMA, cross-linked with 2.5 (2), 5.2 (3) and 11.2 mol.% TGDM (4). Strain: 20 (a) and 30% (b). The arrows show T_g of the corresponding polymer samples.

Hence, the ratio between the low-temperature and high-temperature components of the relaxation provides important information concerning the structural pattern of the development of temperature-induced segmental mobility in plastically deformed glassy polymers.

The effect of strain on the ratio between the low-temperature and high-temperature components of the relaxation[5,6] in combination with direct structural studies in deformation using positron annihilation lifetime spectroscopy[8,9] allowed us to advance the structural pattern of the plastic deformation. Polymer deformation to strains below or equal to yield strain is associated with stress-induced local segmental mobility within structural sublevels with lower packing densities. With increasing strain above the yield point, segmental mobility within structural sublevels with higher packing densities comes in to play. In other words, for polymer glasses plastic deformation is controlled by the gradual involvement of segmental mobility within structural sublevels characterized by different packing densities in deformation and relaxation processes.

Earlier,[5,7] increasing deformation temperature, plasticization of PMMA, or copolymerization of methyl methacrylate with methacrylic monomers was shown to be accompanied with decrease in contribution from the low-temperature component ε_1 to the total temperature-induced relaxation of residual deformation. This fact is likely to be associated with enhancement in local segmental mobility in certain structural sublevels. As a result, the higher fraction of low-temperature mode of the whole spectrum of segmental mobility is able to relax during deformation, and decrease in low-temperature component ε_1 is observed.

This experimental evidence allows one to suggest that restriction of segmental mobility in polymer should result in the growth in a contribution from the low-temperature component ε_1 to the relaxation. Restriction of segmental mobility in polymer samples may be achieved by cross-linking of polymers.[10] For PMMA samples, cross-linked with EGDM and TGDM, restriction of segmental mobility is evidenced by increasing T_g with increase in concentration of cross-linking agents in polymer samples. To verify the effect of cross-linking on the ratio between low-temperature and high-temperature components of relaxation, temperature-induced relaxation of cross-linked PMMA samples was studied.

For PMMA samples, cross-linked with 2.5 and 5.2 mol% of cross-linking agents (Figures 2 and 3, curves 2 and 3), temperature dependences of the residual deformation are also characterized by the low-temperature and high-temperature components. A well-pronounced two-stage character of temperature-induced relaxation of residual deformation allows one to suggest that, for cross-linked samples, relaxation is controlled by temperature-induced segmental mobility within structural sublevels with different packing densities as for the initial PMMA. In other words, cross-linked PMMA samples are likely to be characterized by structural inhomogeneity. Note, that, at low concentration of cross-linking agents, morphology of cross-linked polymer is known to be similar to that for linear polymer.[10] This experimental evidence allows one to suggest, that, in these cases, cross-links are localized in both loosely and densely packed structural sublevels.

Cross-linking of structural sublevels with lower packing densities is responsible for the increase in the low-temperature component ε_1 of relaxation because of restriction of segmental mobility within these structural regions.

Cross-linking of structural sublevels with higher packing densities is evidenced by stress-strain diagrams of the cross-linked polymer samples (Figure 1). As was mentioned above, post-yield behavior of polymer glasses is controlled by stress-induced segmental mobility in structural sublevels with higher packing densities. As follows from Figure 1, for cross-linked PMMA samples, post-yield deformation proceeds at higher stress as compared with the initial polymer. This fact may be attributed to the restriction of segmental mobility within these structural regions because of cross-linking.

With increasing concentration of EGDM and TGDM to 11.2 mol.% (Figures 2 and 3, curves 4), the high-temperature component ε_2 is degenerated, and temperature-induced relaxation of residual deformation proceeds via low-temperature component ε_1. Complete relaxation is observed at temperatures well below T_g within the glassy state.

Such relaxation behavior may be explained from two standpoints. At first, the increasing concentration of cross-linking agent in PMMA is likely to be responsible for the further cross-linking of structural sublevels with lower packing densities. As a result, a noticeable restriction of segmental mobility within these structural sublevels is observed, and total temperature-induced relaxation of the residual deformation is primarily controlled by the low-temperature component ε_1. Secondly, increasing the concentration of cross-linking agent in the polymerization system is known[10] to present severe difficulties for formation of morphological structures with a high degree of ordering. Finally, the degeneration of these structures is observed. In this case, one could expect one-stage recovery of residual deformation.

Hence, cross-linking of PMMA is accompanied by restriction of the segmental mobility within certain structural sublevels in polymer samples. As a result, the lower fraction of the low-temperature mode of the whole spectrum of segmental mobility is able to relax during deformation, and increase in contribution from a low-temperature component ε_1 to total temperature-induced relaxation of residual deformation is observed. Obviously, restriction of segmental mobility should be controlled by the length of the molecule of cross-linking agent.

Figure 4 shows the temperature dependences of the residual deformation ε_{res} for cross-linked PMMA samples with the similar concentrations of EGDM and TGDM. When passing from EGDM to TGDM (curves 2 and 3, respectively), increasing the length of cross-links results in decrease in the low-temperature component ε_1. Note, that, for the samples cross-linked with EGDM, post-yield deformation proceeds at higher stress as compared with the samples cross-linked with TGDM (Figure 1). This behavior may be attributed to the fact, that the higher restriction of segmental mobility is observed for the samples cross-linked with the shorter cross-linking agent.

CONCLUSION

The effect of cross-linking on the temperature-induced relaxation of plastic deformation of PMMA was studied. Increasing the concentration of cross-linking agent in the polymerization system to 5.2 mol.% is responsible for an increase in the low-temperature component of the relaxation. For polymer samples with 11.2 mol.% of cross-linking agent, complete relaxation is observed at temperatures well below the glass transition temperature via only the low-temperature component. Increasing contribution from the low-temperature component to the total relaxation of plastic deformation, and, finally, degeneration of the high-temperature component is likely

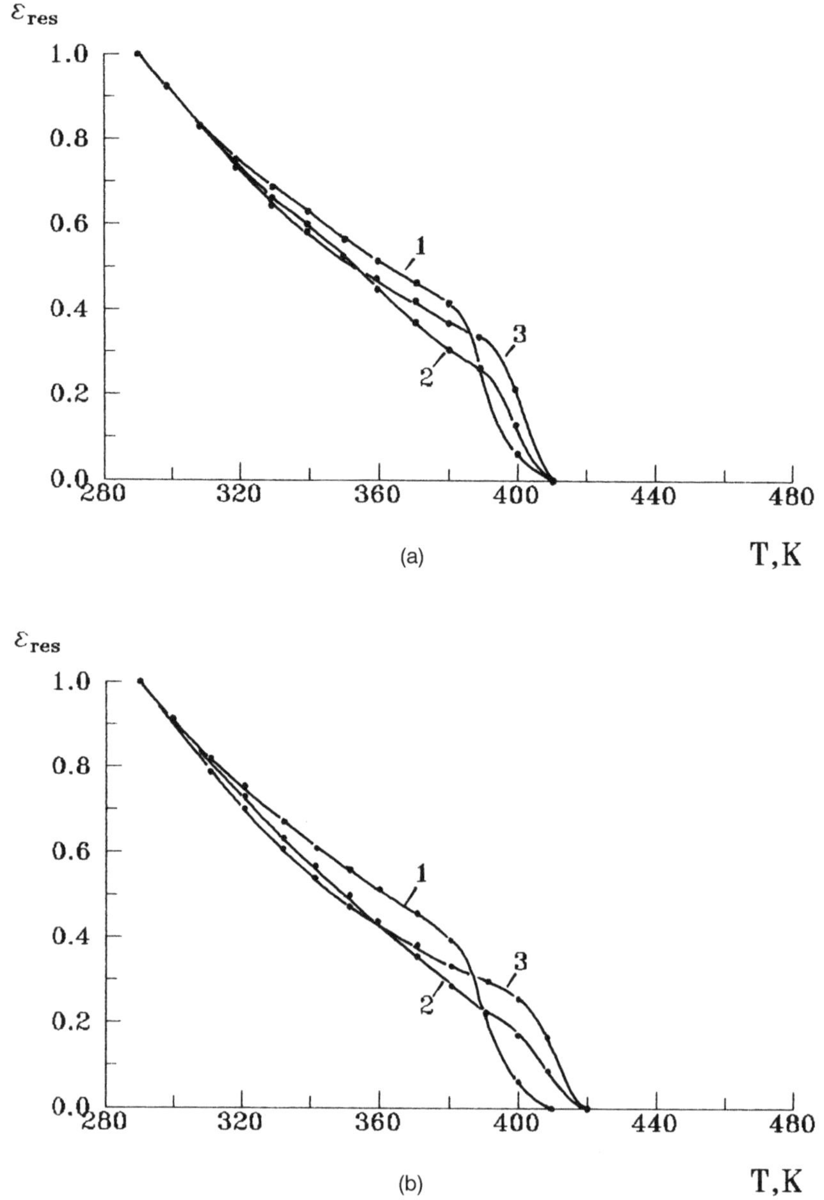

Figure 4 Temperature dependences of residual deformation ε_{res} of PMMA (1) and PMMA, cross-linked with EGDM (2) and TGDM (3). Concentration of cross-linking agents: 2.5 (a) and 5.2 mol.% (b). Strain: 20%.

to be controlled by restriction of segmental mobility within certain structural sub-levels.

Increasing the length of the cross-links results in decrease in the low-temperature component of the relaxation. This behavior may be explained by the fact, that the higher restriction of segmental mobility is observed for the samples cross-linked with the shorter cross-linking agent.

This experimental evidence suggests the possibilities to control the low-temperature reversibility of strain in polymer glasses at temperatures well below the glass transition temperature via their cross-linking.

REFERENCES

1. S.A. Arzhakov, Doctorate (Chem.) Dissertation, Moscow: Karpov Institute of Physical Chemistry, 1975 (in Russian).
2. S.A. Arzhakov, N.F. Bakeev and V.A. Kabanov, *Vysokomol. Soedin. A*, 1973, **15**, p. 1154 (in Russian).
3. E. Oleynik, *Progr. Colloid & Polym. Sci.*, 1989, **80**, p. 140.
4. E.F. Oleinik, O.B. Salamatina, S.N. Rudnev and S.V. Shenogin, *Polym. Sci.*, 1993, **35**, p. 1532.
5. M.S. Arzhakov and S.A. Arzhakov, *Intern. J. Polymeric Mater.*, 1995, **29**, p. 249.
6. M.S. Arzhakov and S.A. Arzhakov, in: *Fizikokhimiya polimerov (Physics and Chemistry of Polymers), Tver'*, 1996, **2**, p. 64 (in Russian).
7. M.S. Arzhakov, S.A. Arzhakov, M.B. Lachinov, E.V. Nechaeva and D.V. Trachenko, *Intern. J. Polymeric Mater.*, 1996 (in press).
8. V.P. Shantarovich, M.S. Arzhakov and I.B. Kevdina, *Polym. Sci., B*, 1995, **37**, p. 171.
9. M.S. Arzhakov, S.A. Arzhakov, I.B. Kevdina and V.P. Shantarovich, in: *Fizikokhimiya polimerov (Physics and Chemistry of Polymers), Tver'*, 1996, **2**, p. 59 (in Russian).
10. V.I. Irzhak, B.A. Rozenberg and N.S. Enikolopyan, *Setchatye polimery (Polymer Networks)*, 1979 Moscow: Nauka (in Russian).

Effect of Polymer Matrix on Kinetics and Mechanism of Carbene Reactions

E.Ya. DAVYDOV, A.P. VOROTNIKOV, V.P. PUSTOSHNY and G.E. ZAIKOV

Institute of Biochemical Physics RAN, Moscow, Russia

The features of the kinetics and mechanism of the cage radical reactions initiated by carbenes in solid polymers has been considered. The low temperature reaction of arylcarbenes is their interaction in clusters with formation of biradicals (BR). The yield of BR is a measure of the distribution non-homogeneity of the carbene precursors in polymers. The reaction of BR formation is a probe to study the molecular dynamics at cryogenic temperatures. The main factor determining the kinetic non-equivalence of triplet carbenes in the low temperature reaction of the hydrogen atom abstraction is the dispersion of the cage distances between carbenes and C—H bonds of macromolecules. The strong effect of structural modifications in filled polymers on the thermal decay of carbenes has been established. The matrix effect on the mechanism of the product formation in the carbene reactions, associated with the relaxation processes, has been recognised by the polyvinylalcohol cross-linkage. The advantage of polyisoprene stabilisation against thermoxidation by the phenol grafting in carbene synthesis has been shown.

INTRODUCTION

At the present time the applications of the carbene reactions are developed to modify polymers with the aim of the advent of materials with required mechanical, chemical, ecological purposes.[1–3] The most general-purpose techniques of the carbene generation are thermal, thermocatalytic and photodecompositions of diazocompounds. The thermal decomposition of diazocompounds is conducted at moderate temperatures of 80–100°C. Without question the advantage of the carbene photochemical generation is the possibility to use low (cryogenic) temperatures for stabilising in matrix and studying of conversions by direct spectral methods. It has been found that the mechanism of the carbene reactions in frozen organic compounds differs essentially from that in liquids and gases. These features are due to the fundamental property of the solid phase reactions that lies in the dependence of reactivity on the physical structure of matrix.[4]

In spite of the substantial amount of data on the gas and liquid phase carbene reactions, the quantitative kinetic data of these processes in solid polymers are very limited. The question of the polymer matrix effect on the carbene reactivity requires closer examination. The distinctive characteristic of solid polymers is the structural-physical non-homogeneity that must probably effect the composition of products and kinetics of the carbene reactions. So the structural non-homogeneity can rise to the nonuniform distribution of the low molecular additives. Diazocompounds consequently can have an effect on the efficiency of the competitive carbene reactions:

recombination or reaction with macromolecules. Another possible manifestation of the structural non-homogeneity of polymers is the wide distribution by frequencies and amplitudes of molecular motions[5] and by the mutual space configurations of reacting carbenes and chemical bonds of macromolecules.

By this mean the predetermined influence of the polymer phase on the kinetics and the mechanism of the carbene reactions should be forthcoming. In turn the peculiarities of the mechanism of these reactions contain information relating to the molecular organisation of polymers on the cage surrounding level. In this connection, the investigation of the carbene reaction mechanism and the composition of resulting products represents the topical problem in two aspects. The researches of this kind are required to develop subsequently the method of the solid polymer modification by grafting of different functional groups on macromolecules. This research is of interest to solve the questions of the influence mechanism of polymer medium on the reactivity in the cage reactions, the nature of kinetic non-equivalence in the elementary reactions of the hydrogen atom transfer and reactions involving the radical pairs (RP).

In this paper, the structural effect of polymer matrix on the kinetics of this kind are required to develop subsequently the method of the solid polymer modification by grafting of different functional groups on macromolecules. This research is of interest to solve the questions of the influence on the mechanism of the polymer medium on the reactivity in the cage reactions, the nature of kinetic non-equivalence in the elementary reactions of the hydrogen atom transfer and reactions involving the radical pairs (RP).

In this paper, the structural effect of polymer matrix on the kinetics, the possibility of application of the carbenes to stabilise rubbers against thermoxidation.

The Solid Phase Effect on the Mechanism of the Carbene Reactions

The carbene reactivity is determined by the spin state.[6] The singlet carbene can be inserted into ordinary chemical bonds by the one-step process and stereospecifically added to alkenes with the cyclopropane formation

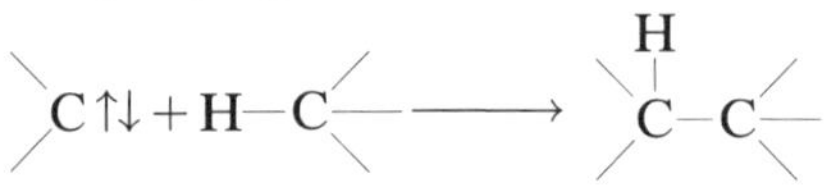

(1)

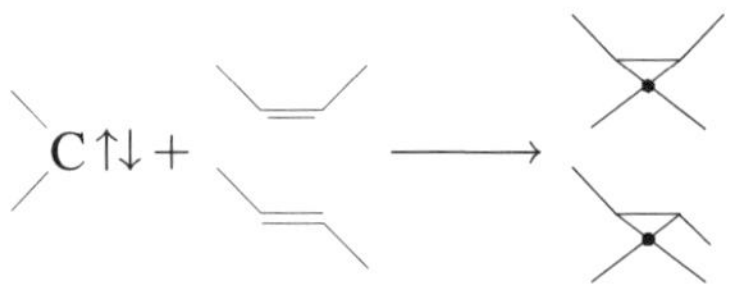

(2)

The spin retention rule for triplet carbene forbids the one-step interaction. The addition of triplet carbenes to alkenes takes place nonstereospecifically because of rotation around C—C bond is faster than intersystem conversion.[7]

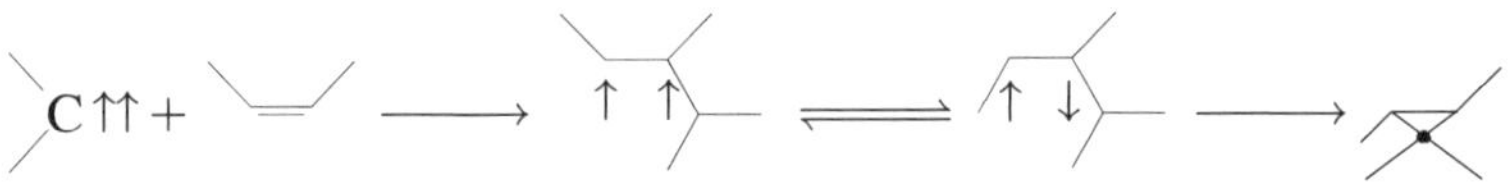

(3)

The reaction of triplet carbenes with C—H bonds results in the RP formation that can recombine by conversion in the singlet state.

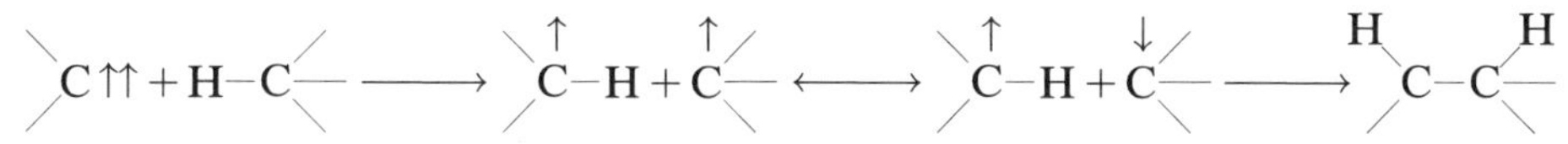

(4)

Formally in the general view the carbene conversions can be presented as follows:[8]

$$>C{=}N{=}N \xrightarrow[-\mathbf{N_2}]{\mathbf{h\nu,\ kT}} $$

$$\text{products} \xleftarrow{k_1} >C\uparrow\downarrow \underset{k_{TS}}{\overset{k_{ST}}{\rightleftharpoons}} >C\uparrow\uparrow \xrightarrow{k_2} \text{products} \tag{5}$$

The transition from gas and liquids to frozen organic matrices must provide the relaxation of carbenes from the excited singlet state into the ground triplet state and consequently the increase of the carbene conversion efficiency by the abstract—recombination mechanism (4). The matrix effect was observed for reactions of carbenes with alkenes[9] and alcohols.[10] By the change of the phase state not only the spin state of carbenes, but the structural-physical characteristics (volume, form of the matrix molecules and carbene precursors) can exhibit effect on the kinetics and product composition. In this connection the investigations directed to the elucidation of the role of the mutual spatial arrangement of the carbene centre and its surroundings are of most interest for the carbene reactions in the rigid matrix.

The dramatic example of the space-orientation effect on the carbene chemistry is the dependence of selectivity for reactions of the diphenylcarbene (DPC) insertion into different C—H bonds of isopropanol at 77 K on the nature of the carbene precursor.[11] The reason of distinctions in relation of products is evident from the space—configuration correspondence of the carbene precursor and the matrix molecules of alcohol, from their relative sizes.

The characteristic feature of the cage reaction of the thermal decay of triplet carbenes in solids connected with the hydrogen atom transfer from surrounding molecules to carbenes is the kinetic non-equivalence of particles. Because of this the kinetics of DPC decay in frozen glasses (77 K) depends on the duration of their photochemical production stage.[12] The effective rate constant of the carbene decay decreases as the photolysis time increases. The explanation must be invoked to account for this result within the limits of concepts about the structural non-homogeneity of the reaction cages of the matrix. The reactivity of carbenes depends on the located orientations in cages, in so doing each orientation corresponds to the distinct rate constant k_t. In the reacting system, the distribution by the rate constants is steadily changed as the disappearance of the most favourable orientations for reaction takes place. Because of the strong hindering of molecular movements at low temperatures the favourable carbene orientations are not regenerated and the distribution is concentrated by less and less active.

The special feature of the environmental influence results from a two-step mechanism of the carbene conversion (4). In this case the structural peculiarities of cages can have an effect both on the kinetics of the hydrogen atom transfer and the RP reactions. The dynamics of these steps of one process can undergo the influence of local surroundings by different way. Actually, the approaching to 0.3–0.4 nm of carbene and C—H bond is required for hydrogen atom transfer. As a result of this step, the primary triplet RP is formed which can recombine only with the singlet state conversion. The frequency of singlet-triplet transforms in RP[13] is $10^8\,s^{-1}$. It is known that the small scale molecular motions connected with the rotational oscillations of small groups have frequencies of the such order.[14] By this means the RP spin dynamics is in the same time scale with the molecular dynamics capable of providing transfers and minor turnings of radicals for recombination. At the same time the experimentally determined rate constants of the triplet carbene decay at 77 K in different organic matrices are very small[15] (10^{-3}–$10^{-4}\,s^{-1}$). In so doing the effective kinetic parameters have very low values of $E \cong 12$ kJ/mol and $\lg k_0 = 5.4$. Such values of the Arrhenius parameters are markers of tunnel transfer of the hydrogen atom.[16]

It must be emphasised that there are principal distinctions between RP resulting as active intermediates during the carbene decay and RP stabilised in organic glasses[17] and polymers[18] registered by the ESR characteristic spectra. The first type represents short-lived RP with the life time in the cage compared with the spin evolution time ($\equiv 10^{-8}$ s). The high recombination rate of such RP is conditioned probably by two reasons: the small distance between radicals (0.3 nm) and the time delay of the chemical bond rearrangements relative to the hydrogen atom transfer.[19] RP of second type is compared with isolated free radicals by their thermal stability. For them the distances between radicals are 0.5–0.8 nm. Their formation in the carbene reactions can be connected with molecular relaxation of the first type RP.

Thus, the reactions in the ground triplet state are typical by mechanism (4) for carbenes in glasses. In some systems this peculiarity can be explained in the context of the singlet-triplet equilibrium (5) and the increase of population of the carbene triplet state at low temperatures. A number of literature data can be explained by action of the space-orientation and molecular-dynamic factors on the source side of the nearest cage surroundings.

Kinetics of the Low-temperature Carbene Decay in Polymers

The experiments were performed on carbenes of two types: DPC and cyclohexadienone carbene (CHC) as well as its 2,6-di-*t*-butylsubstituted analogue (DTBCHC). As precursors of DPC, CHC and DTBCHC diphenyldiazomethane (DDM), quinonediazide (QDA) and 2,6-di-*t*-butylquinonediazide (DTBQDA) were used. The kinetics of the carbene decay was studied in glass polymers and oligomer: polymethylmethacrylate (PMMA, $M_w = 124000$), fully deuterated PMMA (PMMA-D_8, $M_w = 230000$) polystyrene (PS, $M_w = 300000$), (PS-D_8, $M_w = 300000$), acetylcellulose (AC, $M_w = 330000$), oligopiperylene (OP, $M_w = 1200$). The concentrations of DDM, QDA, DTBQDA in polymer films accounted for about 10^{-3} mol/kg. QDA and DDM were added in PMMA, PS, AC from solutions in CH_2Cl_2 and in OP from the diethylether solution. All polymer and oligomer samples placed in tubes were pumped by pressure of 10^{-4} torr. The samples were irradiated by filtered light of the mercury lamp at 77 K until the complete decomposition of diazocompounds was achieved. The photolysis of DDM in polymers was carried out by light with $\lambda > 500$ nm at 77 K. CHC and DTBCHC were generated by light with $\lambda > 300$ nm at 77 K. Kinetics of the carbenes decay was measured by signals of ESR spectra at 110 G for DPC and 4600 G for CHC (DTBCHC).

a. *The non-exponential kinetics of the triplet carbene decay*

The series of studies concerning the low-temperature carbene decay was carried out in glass and polycrystalline solids.[12,20,21] In any single case the non-exponential kinetics was observed which can be described well by equation

$$N(t) = N_0 \exp(-Bt^{0.5}) \tag{6}$$

where B is the temperature-dependent parameter. The kinetic curves of the CHC decay in PMMA at 77–160 K are shown in Figure 1.[22] The kinetic analysis of reactions, controlled by equation (6), was developed in detail.[23] The explanation of non-exponential kinetics is made taking account of the spread in the rate constants. In general, the time dependence of the particle concentrations is

$$N(t) = N_0 \int \rho(k) \exp(-kt)\,\mathrm{d}k \tag{7}$$

where $\rho(k)$ is the distribution of the rate constants. The function

$$\rho(k) = \frac{b}{k^{1.5}} \exp\left(-\frac{b^2}{4k}\right) \tag{8}$$

satisfy the equation (6). This function has an extreme at $k = b^2/6$ that is the most probable value of the rate constant.

The other pattern appears when decays of DPC and DTBCHC proceed in PMMA.[24,25] The equation (6) does not work well in the wide temperature range of 77–183 K but the kinetic curves are straightened in co-ordinates $N/N_0 - \ln t$ (Figure 2). Such description is characteristic of processes with the so-called kinetic stop.[26] In this case the distribution function is evaluated by the following equation

$$\rho(k) = \frac{1}{k \ln(k_{max}/k_{min})} \tag{9}$$

where k_{max}, k_{min} are limiting values of the rate constants. The function $\rho(k)$ as (9) is consistent with the wide spread of particles by their reactivity, such as $\ln(k_{max}/k_{min}) = 13$ for DPC in PMMA at 77 K. The kinetic relationship for (9) is

$$\frac{N}{N_0} = \frac{-\ln k_{min}t}{\ln(k_{max}/k_{min})} \tag{10}$$

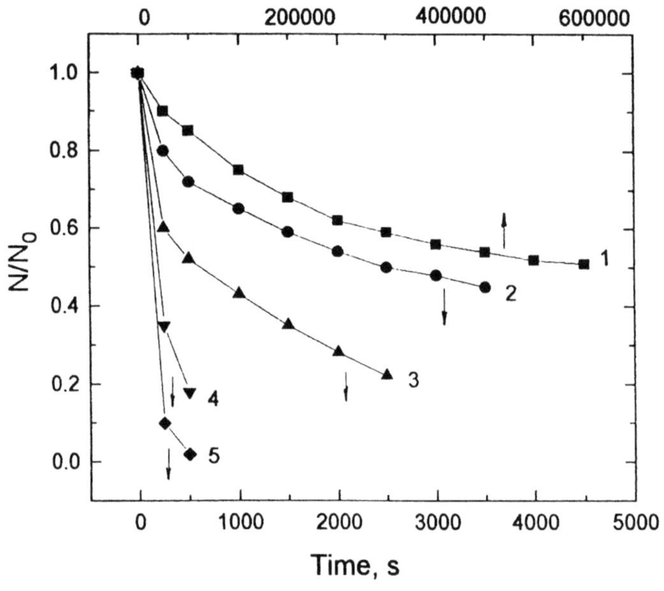

(a)

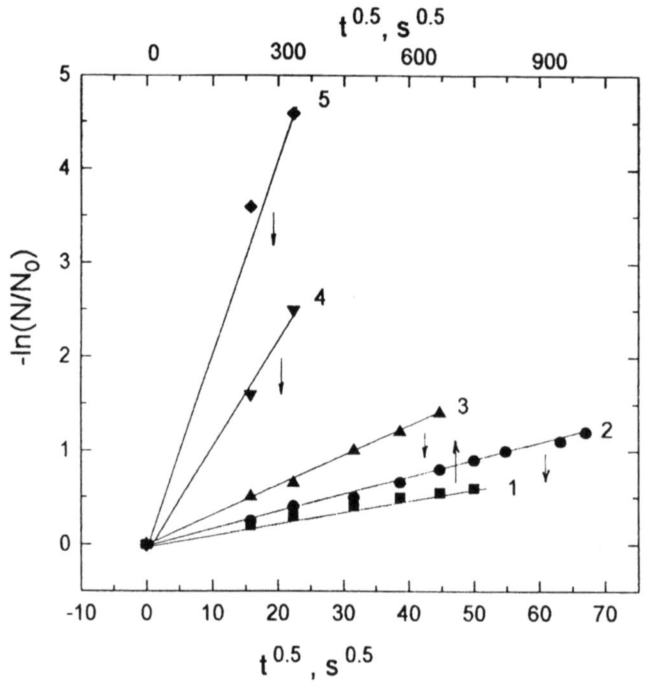

(b)

Figure 1 Kinetics of CHC decay in PMMA (a) and straightenings (b) in co-ordinates of (6): 1—77 K, 2—113 K, 3—128 K, 4—148 K, 5—161 K.

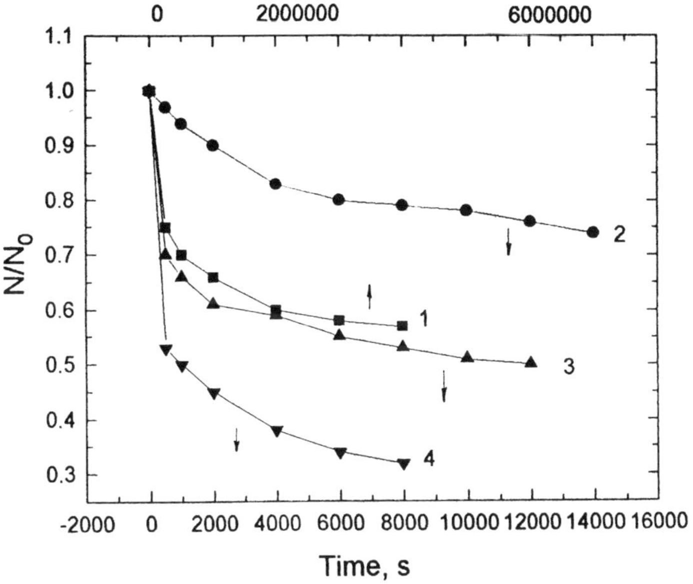

(a)

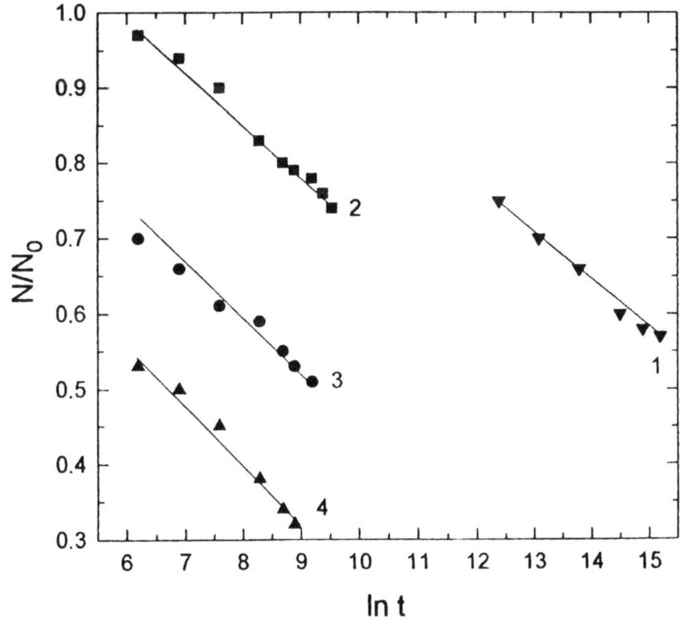

(b)

Figure 2 Kinetics of DTBCHC decay in PMMA (a) and straightenings (b): 1—77 K, 2—100 K, 3—115 K, 4—131 K.

It should be noted that the function (8) is approximated easily by (9) when $k > k$. This approximation is quite realistic for the narrow distribution of the rate constants: $\ln(k_{max}/k_{min}) < 10$. The K value is in agreement with k_{min}. The value of k_{max} can be evaluated from initial rates of the carbene decay. In this manner values of k_{min} and k_{max} for kinetics presented by equation (6) can be estimated thanks to the closeness of (8) and (9) for narrow distribution.

The definite influence of space-orientation factors on the kinetic nonequivalence of triplet carbenes follows from the comparison of CHC and DTBCHC reactivities in PMMA. The width of distribution of the rate constants of CHC decay $\ln(k_{max}/k_{min})$ turned out to be 5 at 77 K. In the same conditions $\ln(k_{max}/k_{min})$ of DTBCHC is 13. Apparently the volume tert-butyl groups are responsible for large variety of the carbene centre and C—H bond orientations.

b. The temperature dependence of the carbene decay rates in polymers

The temperature dependencies of the rate constants during the carbene decay in polymers show appreciable deviations from Arrhenius law (Figure 3). The effective activation energy drops from 12–16 to 5 kJ/mol with the temperature decrease from 180 to 77 K.[22,24,25,27,28] As observed, the kinetic peculiarities in polymers are co-ordinated with those of the hydrogen atom abstraction by free radicals in the course of tunneling. A number of works[29] indicated that the temperature dependencies can be described by the equation

$$k(T) = \alpha \exp(\beta T) \tag{11}$$

where α and β are experimental constants. The equation (11) presents as well the temperature dependence in polymers, as exhibited in Figure 3. It is important to

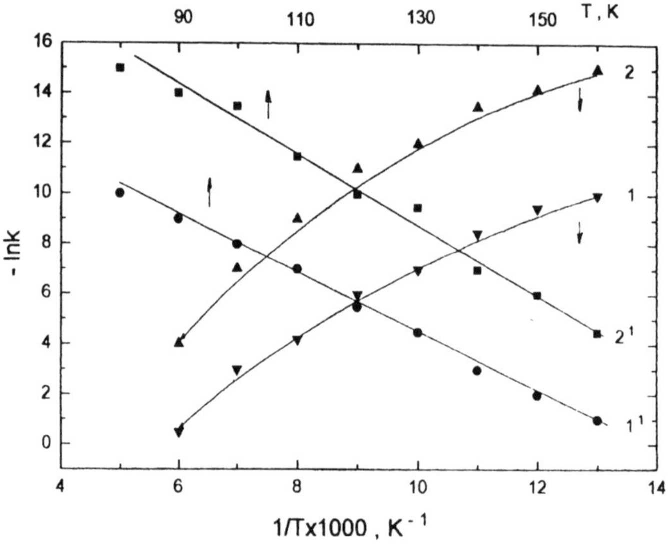

Figure 3 Temperature dependencies of k_{max} (1, 1′) and k_{min} (2, 2′) of CHC decay in PMMA.

note that $k(T)$ is in agreement with the tunneling of H atom by the reaction (4) for all numbers of triplet carbenes due to the likeness of the k_{max} and k_{min} temperature plots. This result is essential to understand a reason of non-exponential kinetics. It is likely the rate constant distribution is called forth by the same cause such as a scattering of parameters of the hydrogen atom tunneling.

There are two models to explain the exponential temperature dependence (11). One model accounts for this dependence by the thermal population of the highest oscillation levels of the hydrogen atom in potential well.[29] Such being the case the tunneling probability is increased in the atom transfer from higher levels as the potential barrier becomes lower.

The another model is based on intermolecular oscillations inducing the height and width of the potential barrier.[30] It was shown that the excitation of the C—H bond highest levels can be neglected when the tunneling should prevail over the atom transfer by activation. The bonding of hydrogenous type is assumed to arise between C—H bonds of the matrix molecules and radicals (or carbenes): ≡C—H$\cdots$:C<. Then the rate constant of the tunneling are expressible by the equation

$$k(T) = \omega_{\text{C—H}} W_0 \exp(\beta \text{T}) \tag{12}$$

where $\omega_{\text{C—H}}$ is the oscillation frequency of C—H bond ($\omega_{\text{C—H}} \cong 3000\,\text{cm}^{-1}$), W_0 is the tunneling probability obtained by extrapolation of $k(T)$ at $T \to 0$

$$W_0 = \exp\left(-\frac{2}{\text{h}}\int_{x_1}^{x_2} \{2m[U(x, A) - E]\}^{0.5} \text{d}x\right) \tag{13}$$

where m is the hydrogen atom mass, $U(x, A)$ is the potential energy, E is the hydrogen atom energy on the zero oscillation level, x_1 and x_2 are the potential barrier limits, A is the distance between carbon atoms in the complex of "carbene-molecule".

The estimation of U, x and the equilibrium A_0 was carried out at different temperatures.[27] The potential barrier was represented for simplicity by the superposition of two potential curves[31] of C—H bond of molecules and radicals resulting from the H atom transfer to carbenes

$$U(r, A_0) = -D\exp\left\{\left[-\frac{\gamma(r - r_0)^2}{2r}\right] + \exp\left[-\frac{\gamma(A_0 - r - r_0)^2}{2(A_0 - r)}\right]\right\} \tag{14}$$

In (14) r_0 is the C—H bond length, D is the dissociation energy of C—H bonds. This energy is assumed to be the same in molecules and radicals. The parameter γ is defined as follows

$$\gamma = \frac{m\omega_{\text{C—H}}^2 r_0}{D} \tag{15}$$

The probabilities of tunneling for given A_0 were estimated by equations (13–15) and these ones were compared with experimental W_0.[27] In this manner A_0 values were determined. Table 1 lists results obtained for DPC and CHC in OP. As is seen, the limit values of width and height are decreased with the temperature increasing.

TABLE 1
Parameters of hydrogen atom tunneling to CHC and DPC in OP.

Carbene	T, K	U_{min}, kJ/mol	U_{max}, kJ/mol	χ_{min}, nm	χ_{max}, nm	$A_{0\,min}$, nm	$A_{0\,max}$, nm
CHC	→0	150	208	0.115	0.140	0.375	0.400
	77	125	150	0.100	0.115	0.375	0.400
	133	108	121	0.094	0.100	0.375	0.400
DPC	→0	167	188	0.120	0.130	0.360	0.370
	77	138	159	0.110	0.118	0.360	0.370
	133	121	138	0.103	0.110	0.360	0.370

c. *The kinetic isotope effect on the carbene decay in polymers*

For tunnel reactions the considerable excess of the kinetic isotope effect (KIE) should be expected over the one attributed to the difference of the oscillation zero energies of C—H and C—D bonds.[32] The literature data show however that this condition is not accomplished in low-molecular glasses. The kinetic analysis of DPC and DTBCHC decay in PMMA, PMMA-D_8 and PS, PS-D_8 has brought to light the characteristic properties of KIE. A complex relationship of KIE relative to the temperature and the degree of conversion was established. The kinetic curves of DTBCHC decay in PS and PS-D_8 are shown in Figure 4.[25] At higher temperatures the initial rates of decay in these polymers coincide but they are characteristically different at long-term conversion. It follows from these results there is evident dependence of KIE on the triplet carbene reactivity. The ensembles of carbenes with higher rate constants are of smaller KIE at constant temperatures. KIE disappears

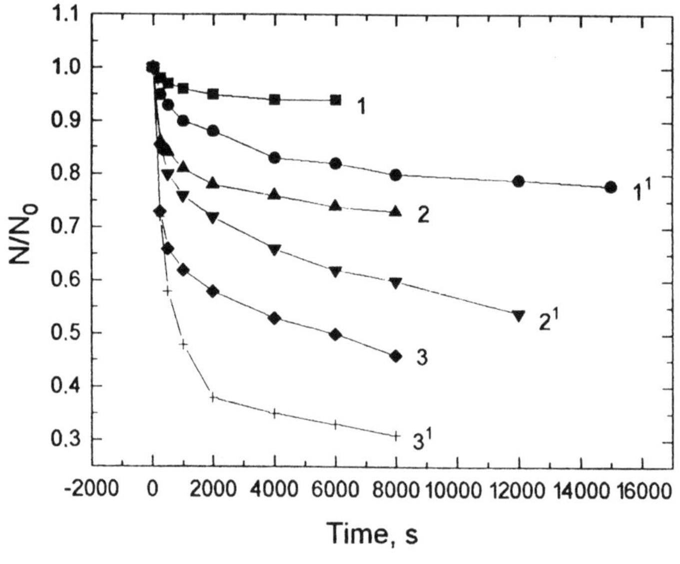

Figure 4 Kinetics of DTBCHC decay in PS and PS-D_8 at 100 K—1, 1′, 115 K—2, 2′ and 136 K—3, 3′.

practically at $T > 100$–115 K. The explanation of KIE observed was given on base of H atom tunneling through oscillating barrier.[33] KIE was shown to fall off linearly at

$$\frac{h\Omega}{4k} < T < \frac{hM\Omega^2}{m\Omega_{C—H}k} \quad \text{by equation}$$

$$\ln\frac{k_H}{k_D} = \frac{\theta^{0.5}R_0^2}{2h}\left(m_D^{0.5} - m_H^{0.5}\right) - \frac{\theta R_0^2}{2h}(m_D - m_H)\frac{kT}{hM\Omega^2} \tag{16}$$

where $\theta = m_H\omega_{C—H}^2 = m_D\omega_{C—D}^2$ is the parameter characterizing the rigidity of C—H and C—D bonds, R_0 is spacing between potential wells, M is the effective mass of carbene—C—H bond complex, Ω is the intermolecular oscillation frequency in polymer matrix. At higher temperatures

$$T > \frac{hM\Omega^2}{m\omega_{C—H}} \text{KIE varies as } T^{-2}$$

$$\ln\frac{k_H}{k_D} = \frac{h}{2\theta^{0.5}}\left(\frac{1}{m_H^{0.5}} - \frac{1}{m_D^{0.5}}\right)\left(\frac{M\Omega^2 R_0}{kT}\right)^2 \tag{17}$$

The analysis of KIE was carried out making use of equations (16) and (17). The temperature dependencies of $\ln(k_H/k_D)$ was plotted for different ensembles of carbenes defined by conversion degree $\Psi = N/N_0$ at given temperature including the KIE of the maximal rate constants. These ones were found by extrapolation of straightening in co-ordinates $\Psi - \ln t$ at $\Psi \to 1$.[25] The corresponding graphs for DTBCHC in PMMA and PMMA-D_8 are shown in Figure 5. Two regions of the temperature plots can be resolved: the linear region from 77 to 100 K (Figure 5a) and the region aligned in co-ordinates of equation (17) at $T > 100$ K (Figure 5b). This behaviour of KIE enables to form an estimation of the intermolecular oscillation frequency in PMMA activating the hydrogen atom transfer to triplet carbene. From the condition of the linear interval going to the plot of T^2 the frequency was calculated as

$$\left(T = \frac{hM\Omega^2}{m\omega_{C—H}k}\right)$$

$\Omega \equiv 52\,\text{cm}^{-1} = 10^{13}\,\text{s}^{-1}$. The value obtained correlates with Debye frequencies of molecular crystals.[30]

The difference in distances between potential wells for transfer reactions of the carbene ensembles was determined through experimental temperature dependencies of KIE. It was interesting to compare this value and the rate constants of the carbene decay of the same kinetic ensembles. The results obtained are listed in Table 2. As can be seen the decrease of the rate constant by an order is consistent with the increase of distance between potential wells of 0.006 nm. This fact confirms the tunnel mechanism of the hydrogen atom transfer.[30]

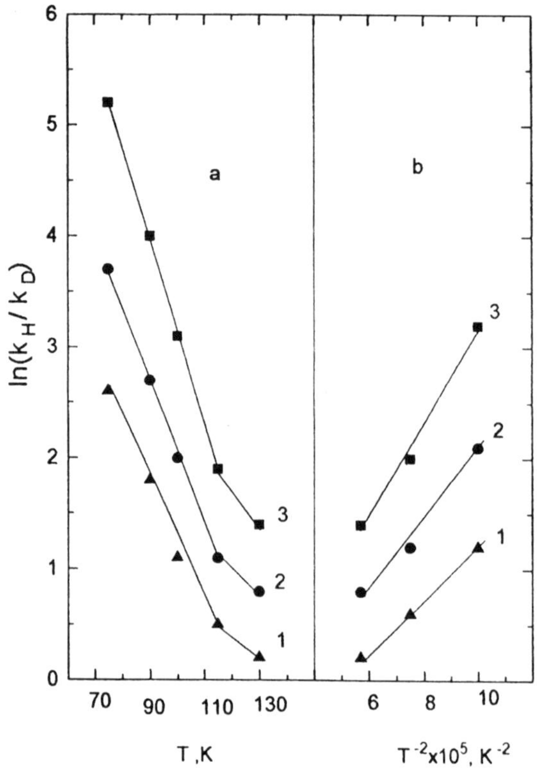

Figure 5 Temperature dependencies of KIE on DTBCHC decay in PMMA according to (16a) and (17b): N/N_0 1(1), 0.8(2), 0.6(3).

d. The magnetic field effect (MFE) on the rate of the carbene decay in low-molecular glasses and polymers

MFE is of interest first of all as a tool for the understanding of the mechanism of radical reactions. This research method can provide unique information about the nature of kinetic non-equivalence in the solid phase radical reactions owing to the determination of the cage structural-physical parameters.

The kinetic curves of DTBCHC decay in ethylacetate (EA) and hexaethylsiloxane (ES) in the magnetic field of different strength are shown in Figure 6.[34] As far as the highest degree of conversion had not exceeded 20% at 77 K the initial rates (W_0) were chosen as experimental parameter undergoing the magnetic field influence. The dependencies obtained are given in Figure 7. It is seen these rates are changed as a function of field with extremes in both glasses.

The rate is also affected by magnetic field in polymers (Figure 8).[35] In this case magnetic dependencies are varied monotonically, namely the abrupt changes take place within fairly narrow ranges of field (2000–3000 G) by 40% in PMMA and 50% in AC. The fact of MFE on the triplet carbene decay at 77 K resulting from the hydrogen atom transfer as such, makes it possible to conclude that this process is reversible. To explain MFE the following mechanism can be suggested:

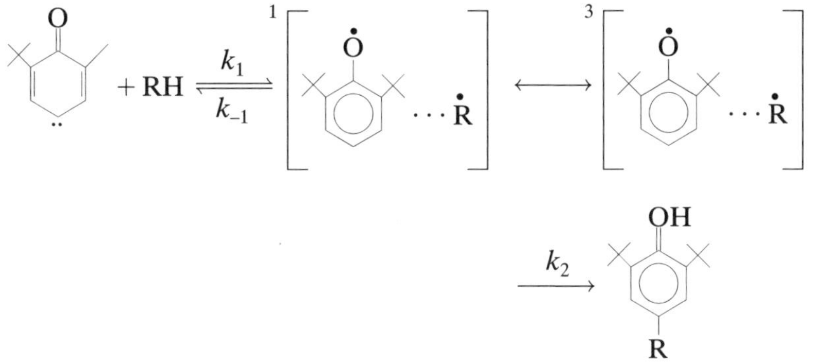

(18)

The triplet RP is formed in the primary act. This RP undergoes the singlet-triplet evolution. RP in the triplet state is converted into original triplet carbene by the back hydrogen atom transfer but in the singlet state RP is recombined. The efficiency of recombination is dependent on the relative population of triplet and singlet levels of RP (P_T/P_S). From (18) it follows that effective rate constants of DTBCHC decay in zero field expressed as

$$k_{\rm ef} = \frac{k_1}{(k_{-1}P_T/k_2P_S)+1} \tag{19}$$

TABLE 2
The dependence of rate constants of DTBCHC and DPC decay in PMMA and PMMA-D_8 on change of equilibrium distances in complex "carbene—C—H bond"

Carbene	T, K	ψ	$\Delta R_0 = R_0^{\psi} - R_0^{\psi=1}$, nm	$-\lg k_{\rm H}$	$-\lg k_{\rm D}$
DTBCHC	77	1.0	0	4.0	5.0
	100			2.7	3.3
	115			1.7	1.8
	131			0.6	0.6
	77	0.8	$6\cdot10^{-3}$	5.0	6.4
	100			3.6	4.4
	115			2.6	2.9
	131			1.4	1.6
	77	0.6	$1.3\cdot10^{-2}$	6.2	7.9
	100			4.6	5.6
	115			3.4	3.9
	131			2.3	2.6
DPC	77	1.0	0	4.0	4.9
	148			0.9	1.3
	183			−0.9	−0.9
	77	0.8	$1.2\cdot10^{-2}$	5.0	6.3
	148			1.7	2.3
	183			0.4	0.5
	77	0.5	$2.7\cdot10^{-2}$	6.7	8.6
	148			2.9	3.9
	183			1.3	1.6

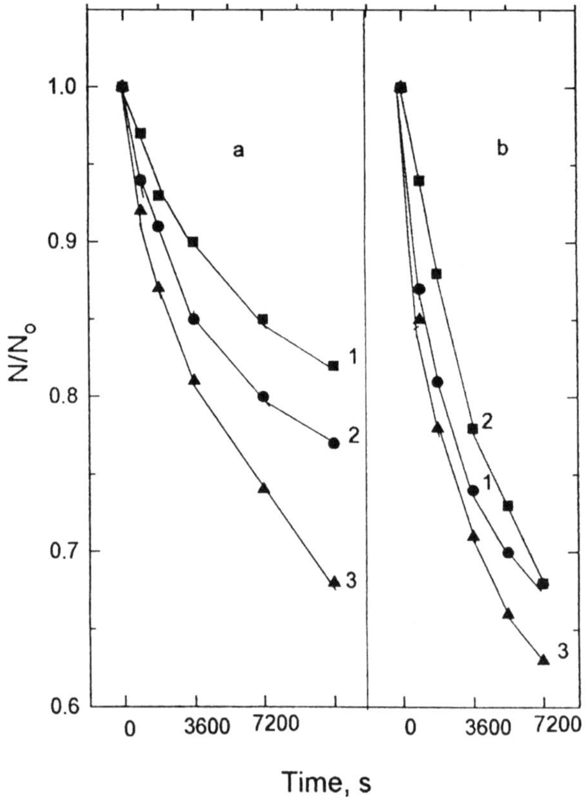

Figure 6 Kinetics of DTBCHC decay (77 K) at magnetic fields 1—0 mT, 2—300 mT, 3—160 mT in EA (a) and 1—0 mT, 2—300 mT, 3—30 mT in ES (b).

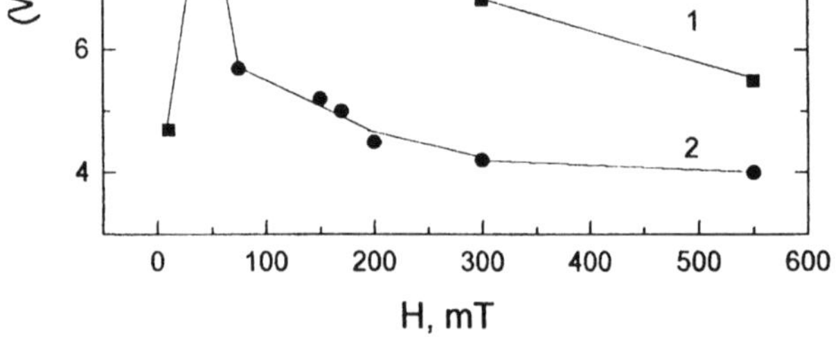

Figure 7 MFE on DTBCHC rate decay (77 K) in EA (1) and ES (2).

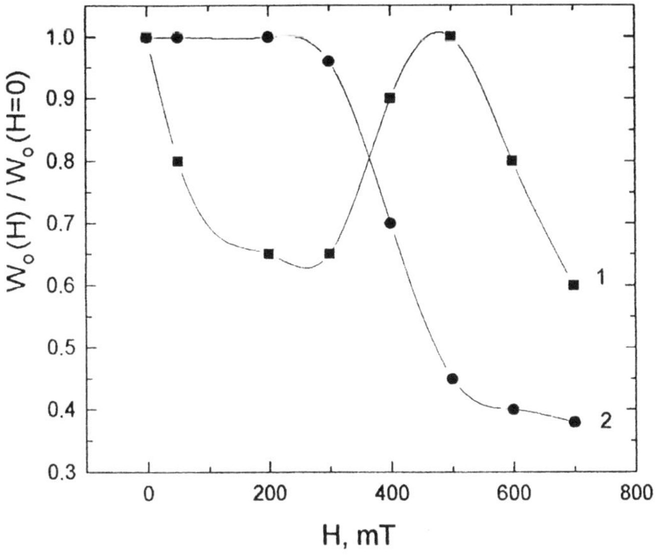

Figure 8 MFE on DTBCHC rate decay (77 K)in PMMA (1) and AC (2).

It will be noted that k_{ef} at 77 K is about $10^{-4}\,s^{-1}$ whereas the characteristic time for the spin dynamics is 10^{-8} s. For the MFE initiation k_2 and k_1 should be comparable to the spin evolution frequency. In this connection one can conclude that the limiting step of the low-temperature decay of carbenes is the formation of the primary triplet RP. This stage defined by k_1 includes the cage reorganisation for favourable mutual orientations of C—H bonds and carbenes to create as well as the tunnel transfer of H atom. The slow process of the cage reorganisation ($\approx 10^4$ s) seems to lie in the leveling of two potential wells in energy needed to occur the forward and the back atom tunneling. The fluctuation of the polarisation forces as a result of the polar group motions can induce changes of the potential well configurations with time. In so doing two levels are varied by energy and can coincide for a while with the subsequent atom transfer.

The magnetic field splits the triplet level of RP into three levels T_0, T_+ and T_- with the result that the probability of the triplet-singlet conversions is decreased. In sufficiently high field the mixture of T_0 and T_+ by the HFI mechanism may be neglected. Then the effective rate constant is averaged over the rate constants of RP arising in the primary act on all T_0, T_+ and T_- levels. The equation (19) is turned to $k_{ef} = k_1\varphi(H)$ where

$$\varphi(H) = \frac{1}{3}\left[\frac{1}{(k_{-1}P_{T_0}/k_2P_s)+1} + \frac{1}{(k_{-1}P_{T_+}/k_2P_s)+1} + \frac{1}{(k_{-1}P_{T_-}/k_2P_s)+1}\right] \tag{20}$$

In (20) the relative populations P_{T_+}/P_s and P_{T_-}/P_s are functions of magnetic field. On account of the Figure 6 plots MFE observed can be believed to result from the exchange interactions J of non-pair electrons in intermediate short-lived RP.

The exchange interaction, splitting triplet and singlet levels of RP, can lower the probability of the spin evolution in the zero field. Within some interval of the magnetic field the mixture of T_- and S levels makes it possible to increase abruptly the population of the RP singlet level. As a consequence, the part of primary RP, disappearing in the triplet state by the back transfer of H atom with the formation of the starting carbene, is reduced and accordingly the fraction of RP decaying by the recombination is increased. Thus the rate of DTBCHC decay is built up to a maximum at the field strength complying with the resonance condition

$$2J = -\frac{a}{8} \pm \frac{g\beta H}{h} \tag{21}$$

The question of the J significance in magnetic effects is dealt within the literature in some detail.[36] It follows from the available data that MFE with the dependence observed of kinetic constants on the field strength can occur under specific conditions. The exchange interaction as a function of distance takes usually the form of exponential law.[37] The average spacing in RP must be consistent with J, exceeding by energy other interactions mixing S and T levels (spin-orbital, dipole-dipole, HFI). The lifetime of radicals in field of the S and $T_\pm$ intersections must be sufficient for the intersystem crossing to occur. The low-temperature decay seems to fit these requirements. In such reactions RP are formed by small distances (≈ 0.35 nm) and the strong restriction of the molecular mobility increases essentially the lifetime of RP in certain configurations to (10^{-7}–10^{-8} s).

All points in the experimental plots (Figure 6) were obtained under conditions when the theory of the RP spin dynamics in high magnetic fields may be used to analyse MFE. It should be pointed out equation (20) was derived, assuming that triplet RPs are formed equally probably in T_0, T_+ and T_- without transitions between triplet levels, that is different channels of singlet-triplet transitions are displayed by the additive manner.

The complete analysis of MFE was accomplished for RP with one magnetic nucleus of 1/2 spin. The approximations can be applied for a more complex case when RP contains several protons. Then the root-mean-square constant of HFI with all protons may be introduced into the treatment:

$a = \left(\sum a_{1k}^2 + \sum a_{2n}^2\right)^{0.5}$, a_{1k} and a_{2n} are HFI constants of RP. The Kaptein's model,[38] in which the radical distances are fixed, was used to deal with the spin evolution of RP. By this model the singlet state population of RP is deduced

$$P_{S(T_0)} = \frac{a^2\tau^2/8}{1 + (a^2/4 + 4J^2)\tau^2} \tag{22}$$

$$P_{S(T\pm)} = \frac{a^2\tau^2/4}{1 + [a^2/2 + (2J + a/4 \pm g\beta H/4)^2]\tau^2} \tag{23}$$

where τ is the lifetime of RP, a is HFI, RP is formed in primary act in T_0, T_+ and T_-. The relative populations of singlet and triplet levels in magnetic field

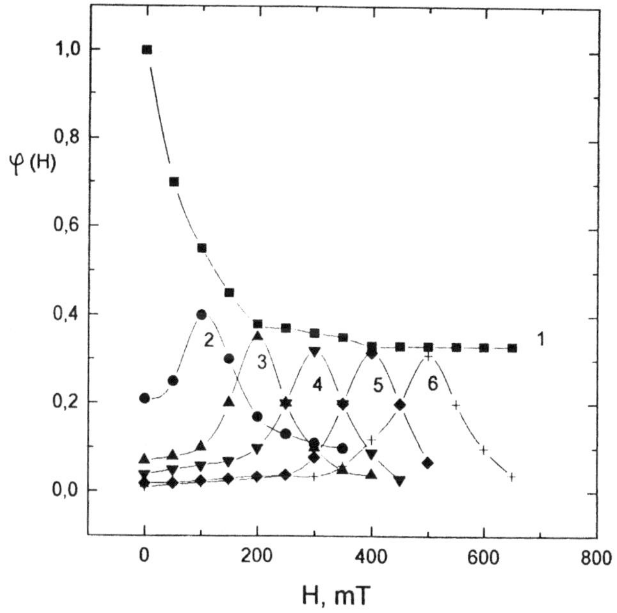

Figure 9 Probabilities of RP recombination in magnetic field at $2J = 0$ (1), $1.7 \cdot 10^{10}$ (2), $3.5 \cdot 10^{10}$ (3), $5.2 \cdot 10^{10}$ (4), $7 \cdot 10^{10}$ (5), $8.8 \cdot 10^{10}$ rad/sec (6); $k_{-1}/k_2 = 1.8 \cdot 10^{-3}$.

$P_T/P_S = (1 - P_S)/P_S$ are estimated by (22) and (23). In all studied systems the HFI effective constants amount to 30–40 G (5.2–$6.9 \cdot 10^8$ rad/s). If $\tau \approx 10^{-8}$ s and $a^2\tau^2 \gg 1$ then

$$\frac{P_{T_0}}{P_S} \approx \frac{8}{a^2}(2J)^2 + 1 \tag{24}$$

$$\frac{P_{T_+}}{P_S} \approx \frac{4}{a^2}(2J + a/4 \pm g\beta H/h)^2 + 1 \tag{25}$$

The dependencies of probabilities of the RP recombination on magnetic field can be plotted by relations (20, 24, 25).[35] The form of $\varphi(H)$ is determined by J and k_{-1}/k_2 (Figure 9). At J comparable to the effective HFI constants $\varphi(H)$ decreases steadily to a plateau while $\varphi(H = 0) \approx 3\varphi(H_\infty)$ in accordance with numbers of the inter-system crossing channels working effectively in the zero and high magnetic fields. The dependence has a maximum at $H = (2Jh)/g\beta$.

The comparison of estimated plots of Figure 9 with the experimental ones shows that MFE observed in PMMA and AC is approximated by the set of $\varphi(H)$ with different values of J. So in PMMA two types of BR can be resolved with $J = 0$ and $J = 4.4 \cdot 10^{10}$ rad/s. The availability of the RP five types in AC with $J = 0$; 0.87; 1.7; 2.62; $3.50 \cdot 10^{10}$ rad/s can account for MFE.

The distribution of J corresponding to the MFE scale cannot be due to the spacing of radicals. The fact is that calculations[36] by $J = J_0 e(-\sigma r)$ must give Δr of the order of 0.05 nm for the J distribution in AC. At 77 K the increase of equilibrium distances in the complex of carbene—C—H bond by 0.006 nm gives rise to the tenfold decrease of the rate constant of DTBCHC decay (Table 2) whereas the magnetic field affects the rate by 40–50%. The orientation factor, connected with angles of rotation of the orbital axes of non-pair electrons about one another, seems to be responsible for the exchange energy spread.

For example, calculations performed for the model RP[39] show the change J to a great extent in angles of rotation.

The results obtained show that MFE at cryogenic temperatures is qualitatively like in the solid phase. The degree of distinctions is defined by the nature of the matrix. The reaction cages are more homogeneous relative to J in low-molecular glasses of EA and ES as compared with polymers in view of pronounced changes of rates in magnetic field.

The Mechanism of the Carbene Reaction Product Formation in Polymers

There is a need to study both the ultimate molecular products and the intermediate radicals to establish the carbene reaction mechanism in polymers. But, in spite of the wide use of the different spectral techniques (UV, IR, ESR) and the flash photolysis to determine such characteristics of carbenes as the geometrical parameters, the oscillation frequencies, the electron transitions, the products of the primary reaction of carbenes with the environment are poorly known. The data about the free radical products with the low-molecular organic solids are no more than in the several works.[40–43]

a. The structure of RP resulting by the low temperature reactions of CHC and DPC in polymers

The ESR spectra of the insulated triplet CHC[44] and the spectrum at $g \approx 2$ were observed at 77 K in the PMMA films with QDA during irradiation by light. The spectrum shown in Figure 10a was obtained under action of the light with $\lambda > 380$ nm.[22] It is the characteristic signal of RP.[17] The average distance (r) between radicals in RP can be determined from parameters of dipole-dipole interaction $D_\perp = 114$ G, $D_\parallel = 228$ G by the equation

$$D_\perp = \frac{27.8}{r^3} \tag{26}$$

The estimation gives the value of $r = 0.6$ nm. The signals of isolated radicals are observed in the central region of spectrum. It was established that the RP and isolated radical proportion in PMMA is about 10% of triplet CHC, but in so doing this value does not change during QDA photolysis. From this fact it transpires that all three products of the QDA photolysis at 77 K are formed in parallel. The thermal decay of the stabilised triplet CHC in a time of irradiation can be ignored, that is, the thermal reaction of carbenes with PMMA cannot give the PR and radical formation with detectable rate. The effect observed is explained by the excess of the absorbed energy of 200 kJ/mol in comparison with the dissociation energy of the quinonediazide

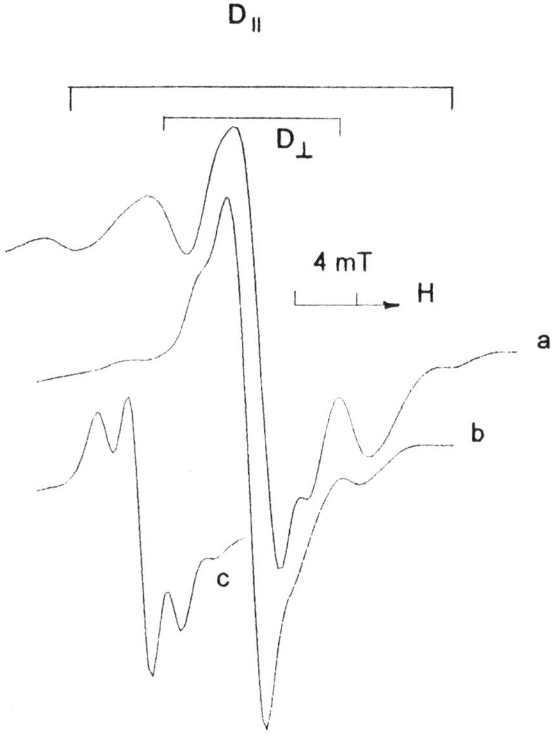

Figure 10 ESR spectra of PMMA with QDA irradiated at 77 K by light $\lambda > 380$ nm (a), $\lambda > 300$ nm (b) and after heating of (a) at 183 K (c).

C—N bonds. The concentration of the excess energy in cages leads to the essential increase of the carbene reaction rate with C—H bonds of macromolecules.

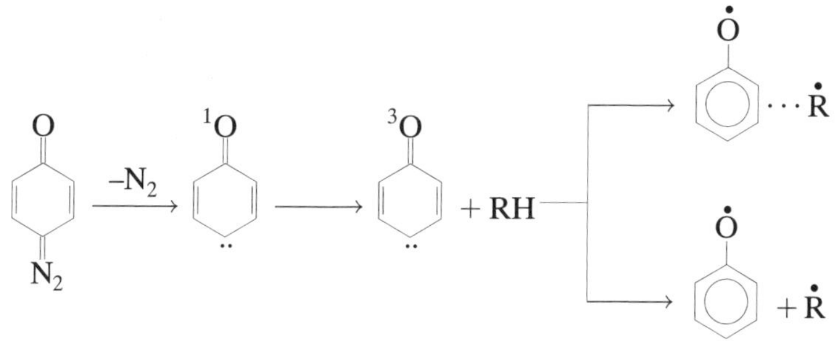

(27)

The main part of triplet CHC ($\approx$ 90%) is stabilised at 77 K as a result of this energy dissipation in the polymer matrix. The phenoxy radical formation by the reaction (27) is exhibited by UV spectrum. It contains the bands with a maximum at 390 nm and 405 nm.[45]

The absence of the thin structure in ESR spectrum (Figure 10a) does not permit immediately to establish the nature of PMMA radicals involved in RP. To identify these radicals the typical reactions of thermal and photochemical conversions[46,47] were used. The signal of RP in ESR spectrum disappears during the shorter wave light irradiation ($\lambda > 300$ nm, Figure 10b). The PMMA macroradicals sensitive to the light with $\lambda > 300$ nm have the structure $\sim CH_2C(CH_3)(COOCH_2)CH_2\sim$ (I). These radicals are decomposed in the following manner

$$\sim CH_2C(CH_3)(COOCH_2)CH_2\sim \xrightarrow[\lambda > 300\,\text{nm}]{h\nu} \sim CH_2C(CH_3)CH_2\sim (II) + CO + CH_2O \quad (28)$$

As a result of the macroradical photodissociation the distance between the unpair electrons in RP must be increased by at least 0.3 nm and RPs are transformed into isolated radicals.

The radicals II dissociate with the breaking of macrochain.

$$\sim CH_2C(CH_3)CH_2\sim \longrightarrow \sim CH_2C(CH_3)(COOCH_3)(III) + \sim CH_2C(CH_3)(COOCH_3)CH_2\sim \quad (29)$$

Actually, the nine components ESR spectrum, belonging to radicals (III), was observed by the sample heating to the room temperature. The ESR spectrum of radicals (I) was detected at 183 K in pure form (Figure 10c). By this mean RPs and isolated radicals are formed at 77 K by the hydrogen atom abstraction from the PMMA ester groups.

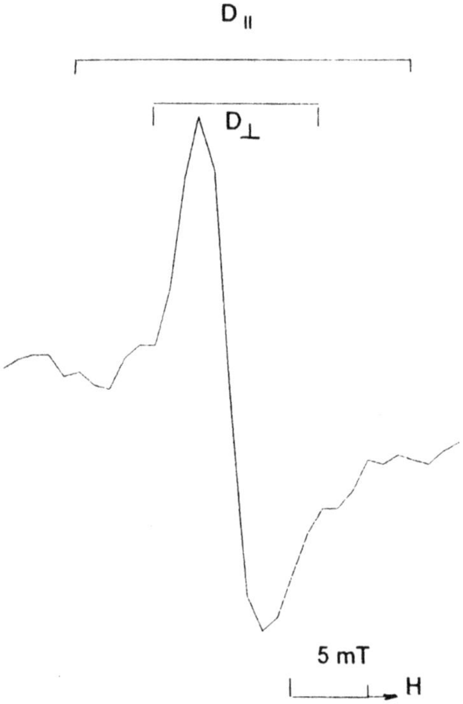

Figure 11 ESR spectrum of OP with QDA irradiated by light $\lambda > 370$ nm at 77 K.

The ESR spectrum in the $g \approx 2$ region Figure 11, was observed during the irradiation of OP with QDA by light with $\lambda > 370$ nm among the signal of triplet CHC.[27] This spectrum involves the unresolved central component of at the extremes of which further components are seen. From the spectrum shape analysis it follows that the photodecomposition of QDA in OP at 77 K brings into existence isolated radicals and RP in the ratio of 3:2. The values of splitting in the zero field $D_{\perp} = 100$ G and $D_{\|} = 200$ G show that the average distance between unpair electrons is 0.64 nm. The process going on in the low temperature irradiation of QDA in OP can be represented by scheme similarly to (27). For lack of the rather resolved ESR spectrum the nature of the OP radicals constituent of RP along with phenoxy radicals can be established by the circumstantial evidence obtained in the spectral investigation.[48] The macroradicals of OP are formed as a result of the hydrogen atom transfer to carbenes from allylic C—H bonds of 1.4 and 1.2 links. Based on the ESR data it was concluded that in RP allylic radicals $\sim CH_2CH{=}CHC(CH_3)CH_2\sim$ (IV) and $\sim CH_2C(CH{=}CHCH_3)CH_2\sim$ (V) are present.

The several kinds of paramagnetic particles are formed in samples of OP with DDM irradiated at 77 K by light with $\lambda > 500$ nm. The triplet DPC is identified by the characteristic ESR spectrum[49] and also by the absorbance band at 465 nm in UV spectrum.[50] Hand in hand with the appearance of ^{3}DPC signal the ESR spectrum

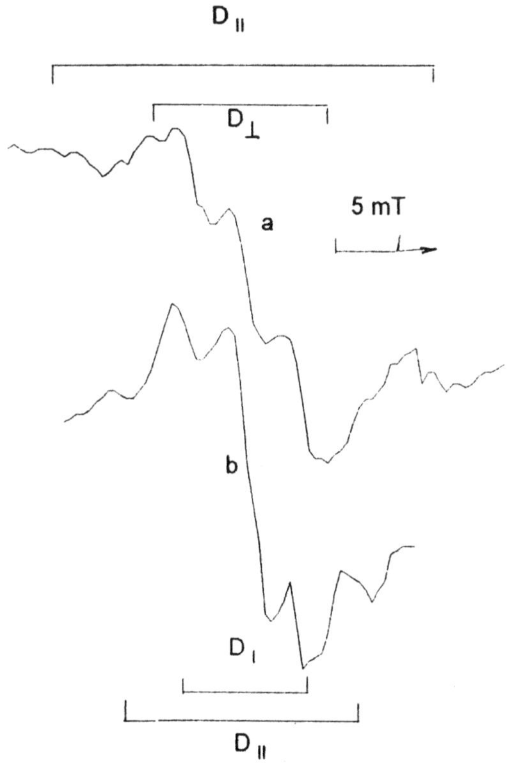

Figure 12 ESR spectra of OP with DDM irradiated by light $\lambda > 500$ nm at 77 K (a) and after heating of (a) at 145 K (b).

with $g \approx 2$ is registered (Figure 12a). The anisotropic doublet signal of triplet RP with poor resolution is observed. In this system OP macroradicals and diphenylmethyl radicals Ph_2CH (VI) can be formed. The dipole-dipole interaction of unpaired electrons in RP is characterised by $D_{\perp} = 195\,G$ and $D_{\parallel} = 390\,G$. These values show that the average distance between electrons in such pairs is 0.52 nm that is significantly less than in RP discussed above in PMMA and OP with CHC. In spite of the poor resolution the splitting of 10–15 G typical of radicals (IV), (V), (VI) can be observed. The heating of samples leads to the RP spectrum change (Figure 12b). The initial signal with $D_{\perp} = 195\,G$ disappears and the signal with $D_{\perp} = 110\,G$ is remained which corresponds to RP with the average distance between radicals of 0.63 nm. In addition the severe narrowing of the spectrum components from 70 to 15 G takes place.

b. Kinetics of the biradical formation by the low temperature conversions of DPC in polymers

The formation of new biradical (BR) product in OP indicates some distinctive features of the triplet DPC reactions in comparison with CHC. To establish the BR nature and the formation mechanism the DPC conversions in different polymers were studied. The appearance of identical ESR spectrum was discovered for DPC by photolysis of DDM in PMMA, PS, PMMA-D_8, PS-D_8 and polycarbonate (PC).[51,52] One can assert that they are not RP because of the same parameters of ESR spectra characterising distances between radicals.

As molecules of low molecular substances are in defects of polymer packing, this corresponds to parts with decreased density because of the relative arrangement disturbance of macromolecules,[53] one can suppose carbenes are accumulated both in isolated states and in clusters of two or more DPC. Therefore the carbene dimer conversion products can be presented as follows

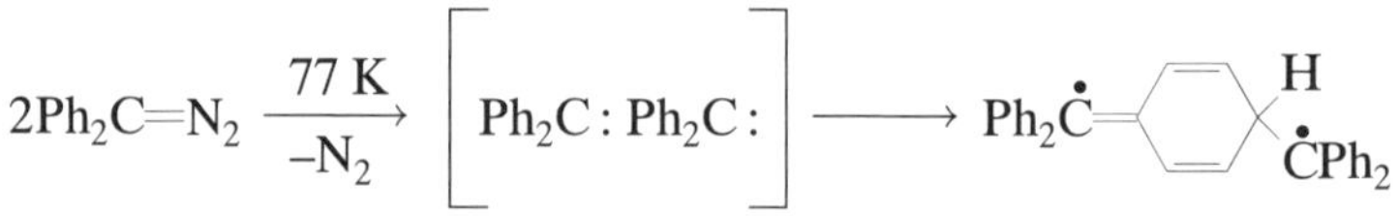

(29)

The reaction of carbenes localised in micropores is interesting in two aspects. The BR yield must reflect apparently the non-homogeneity of DDM distribution and can be used to estimate the distribution by concentrations of other low-molecular additives in solid polymers. The kinetics of this process must depend on the intensity of small-scale molecular mobility of the micropore surrounding. The BR formation by the reaction (29) is confirmed by the increase of their yields, determined by the ratio of initial rates of the BR and isolated DPC formation, with the DDM concentration increase (Figure 13).

The dependence of BR yield on DDM concentration is described satisfactorily by an empirical equation

$$\mu = \frac{\mu_{\infty}[DDM]}{C + [DDM]} \tag{30}$$

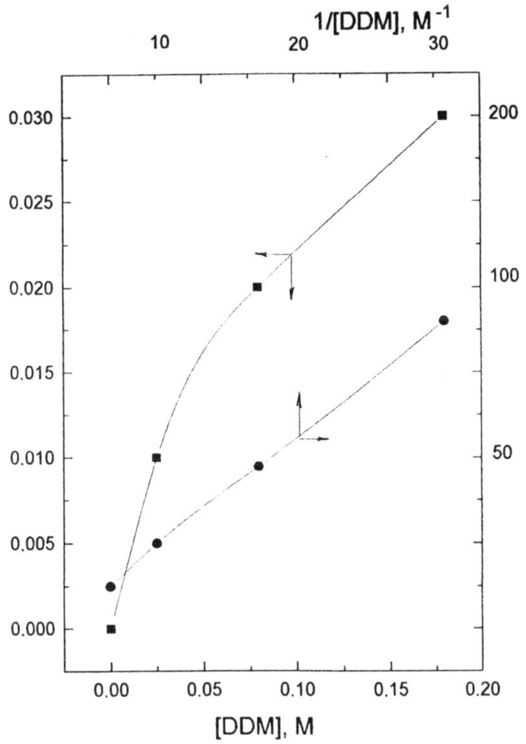

Figure 13 The dependence of BR yield in PC on DDM concentration.

where μ_∞ and C are empirical constants. The deviation of $\mu([DDM])$ from linearity is connected evidently with the high filling of polymer micropores at [DDM] > C. The intense line belonging to BRs with distances between spins of 0.9–1.0 nm and more appeared at the centre of the ESR spectrum at deep stages of DDM photolysis. Such particles are formed if three DPC will react

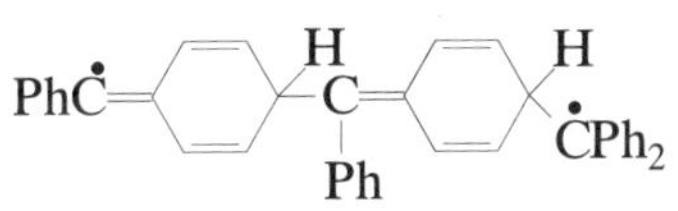

These BRs are produced in bigger clusters. The ESR spectrum shows that the portion of "polymeric" BR in PC and PMMA does not exceed 20% relatively to the all quantity of BR.

The results obtained can be used to evaluate the non-homogeneity of low molecular additives like DDM by chemical structure. For example, the analogous distribution of bimolecular, threemolecular and polymolecular clusters must be in glass polymers for some photostabilisers, antioxidants, photosensibilisers (salicilates, benzophenones, bisphenols).

The peculiarities of the BR formation in the course of the thermal reaction are expressed by the annealing of samples irradiated at 77 K (Figure 14). These curves were obtained by the annealing of samples in isothermal conditions. The annealing

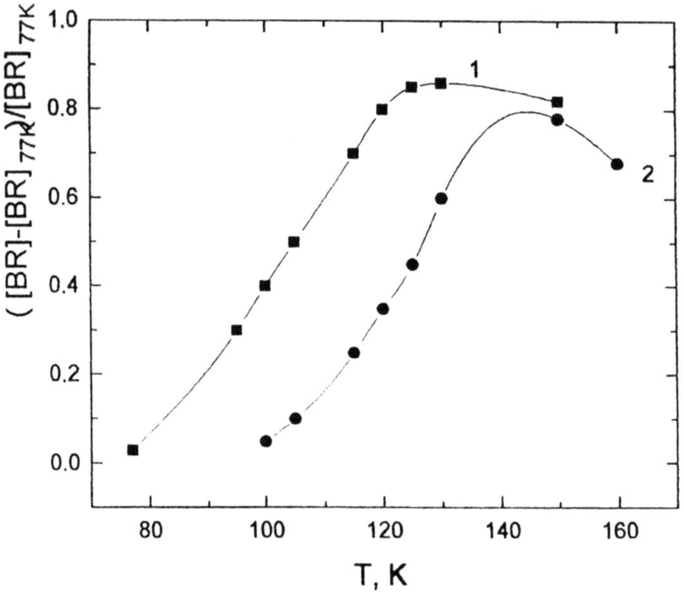

Figure 14 Annealing curves for BR formation in PC (1) and PMMA (2); the exposure time is 4 min in isothermal conditions.

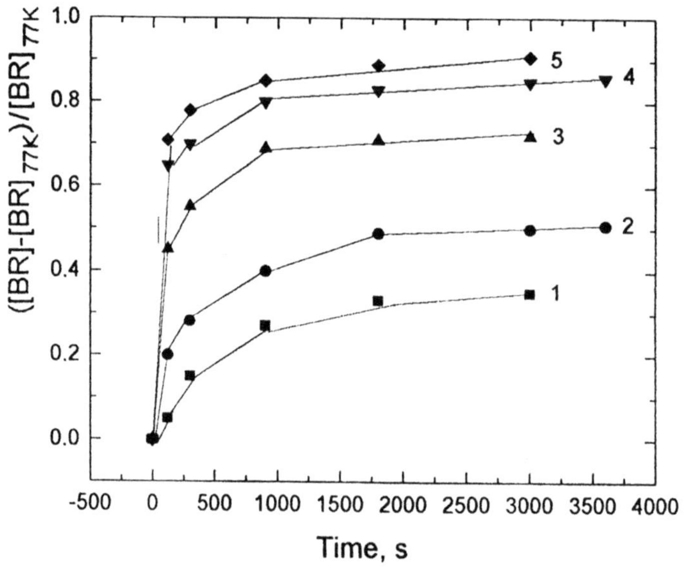

Figure 15 Kinetics of BR formation in PC at 1—94 K, 2—100 K, 3—107 K, 4—115 K, 5—120 K.

curves are displaced relatively to one another at 15–20 K showing that the reactivity of carbenes in clusters depends on the nature of polymer. It was established that annealing curves may be considered as the characteristics of the distribution of the particle reactivity.[26] The kinetics of the BR formation in PC (Figure 15). These kinetics are straightlhened in co-ordinates of "concentration – lg t". This fact suggests that the distribution function of carbenes has the straight-angle type[26] by the activation energy of the BR formation

$$\rho(E) = \frac{1}{E_{\max} - E_{\min}}, \quad E_{\min} < E < E_{\max} \tag{31}$$

The gradual annealing of mobility of the kinetic nonequivalent carbenes in clusters determines the temperature dependence of the BR formation rate. The rate constant dispersion in PC permits to define the Arrhenius parameter distribution which in the general case is connected with distributions both by activation energy and by preexponential factor. The method stated in work[54] may be used to be determine the distribution by these parameters. The kinetic curves set $\theta(t, T)$ (Figure 15) was cut by horizontal straight lines and the values of the rate constants $k(\theta, T) = t^{-1}(\theta, T)$, determining the reactivity of given kinetic ensembles, were found. Then the temperature dependencies of $k(\theta, T)$ values were constructed in Arrhenius co-ordinates and activation energies and pre-exponents were determined. The $\theta(E)$ and $\theta(k_0)$ plots are the distribution integral functions by corresponding parameters. These plots are essentially linear (Figure 16) and the distribution functions of carbenes in clusters by Arrhenius parameters may be considered as a straight angle type. The extrapolation of linear relationships of $\theta(E, k_0)$ to 1 and 0 gives the values of $E_{\max}$, $E_{\min}$, $\lg k_{0\max}$ and $\lg k_{0\min}$. These values in PC are $E_{\max} = 38$ kJ/mol, $E_{\min} = 26$ kJ/mol, $\lg k_{0\max} = 14.4$, $\lg k_{0\min} = 12.8$.

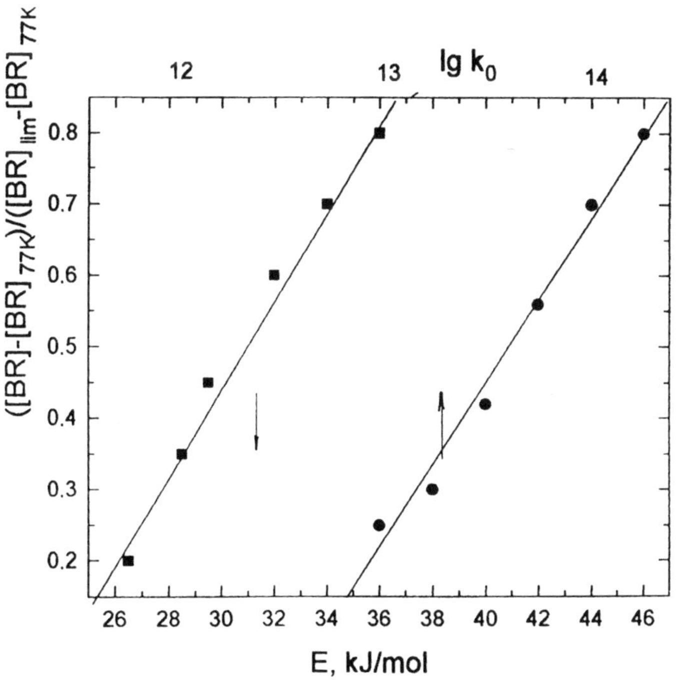

Figure 16 Distribution functions of DPC by Arrhenius parameters of BR formation in PC.

The activation energy values obtained are typical of the relaxation processes in PC (40 kJ/mol) caused by the motions of monomer links and side groups of macrochains. These values are adjusted with the activation energy of the spin probe rotation.[55,56] The reaction of the BR formation in PC is controlled by rotary motions of carbenes. In fact, the values of $k_0 = 10^{13}$–$10^{14}\ s^{-1}$ are compared with the frequencies of the orientational motions of the low molecular particles in polymers. One can note the small dispersion of the Arrhenius parameters: $\Delta \lg k_0 = 1.6$, $\Delta E = 12$ kJ/mol.

In PMMA the limiting values are $E_{max} = 50$ kJ/mol, $E_{min} = 22$ kJ/mol, $\lg k_{0\,max} = 16.0$, $\lg k_{0\,min} = 10.5$. The average Arrhenius parameters of the BR formation are $\lg k_{0\,av} = 13.25$, $E_{av} = 36$ kJ/mol. These values correlate satisfactorily with the activation energy and the rotation time of spin probes in PMMA: $E = 38$–42 kJ/mol, $\lg \tau = -13.2$.[55] But the high dispersion of Arrhenius parameters attracts attention: $\lg k_0 = 6.5$, $E = 28$ kJ/mol.

The results obtained may be explained by the existence of wider scattering of hindered molecular motions in PMMA that are annealed with the temperature increase. The calculations[57] shows that the activation energy of the side ester group rotations combined with relative vibrations of a main chain near equilibrium positions is 21.6 kJ/mol. This value coincides with the minimum activation energy for the BR formation. But the activation barrier of the ester group rotation is increased with the declination of rotational angles from equilibrium values. The calculation gives maximum potential barrier of 68 kJ/mol for torsional oscillations around the C—C bonds of a main chain. Therefore, the increase of activation energy to 50 kJ/mol can be considered as the transition of the carbene orientational dynamics into regime controlled mainly by the macrochain mobility. In this way manner the differences observed in kinetic regularities of the BR formation for two polymers are caused by molecular organisation of environments. In the temperature region studied the distribution width of the rate constants determined by $\lg (k_{max}/k_{min})$ is 1.5–2 times more in PMMA than in PC. On the basis of the rate constant dispersion one can conclude that the structural non-homogeneity of the micropore surrounding in PMMA is higher as compared with PC.

The BR thermal decay prevails at $T > 130$–150 K over their formation (Figure 14). The kinetics of the BR decay expresses molecular dynamics defining the reaction rate for bigger particles relative to carbenes. The kinetic data show that BRs are unequal in the reaction of decay too. The kinetic curves of this process in PMMA are straightened in co-ordinates $[BR]/[BR]_0 - \lg t$ at 183–218 K (Figure 17). One can see that the slope angle of the plots do not change with the temperature, therefore the BR non-equivalence observed in a given temperature interval does not connect with the activation energy distribution. The rate dependence of the BR decay is submitted to Arrhenius law. The limiting constants are $k_{max} = 5 \cdot 10^{12} \exp(-46 \pm 4\,\text{kJ/RT})\ s^{-1}$, $k_{min} = 10^9 \exp(-46 \pm 4\,\text{kJ/RT}) s^{-1}$. It is followed from limiting values that in PMMA the activation energy of the BR decay corresponds to the maximum activation energy of the BR formation. The distributions by frequency factors are overlapped too. Thus the conversion limiting steps of BRs and carbenes with the lowest reactivity are controlled in micropores by the same molecular dynamics: torsional movements of main chains.

The results obtained reveal the determining role of the carbene rotational motions concentrated in micropores of polymers to generate BR. In this regard, such reaction

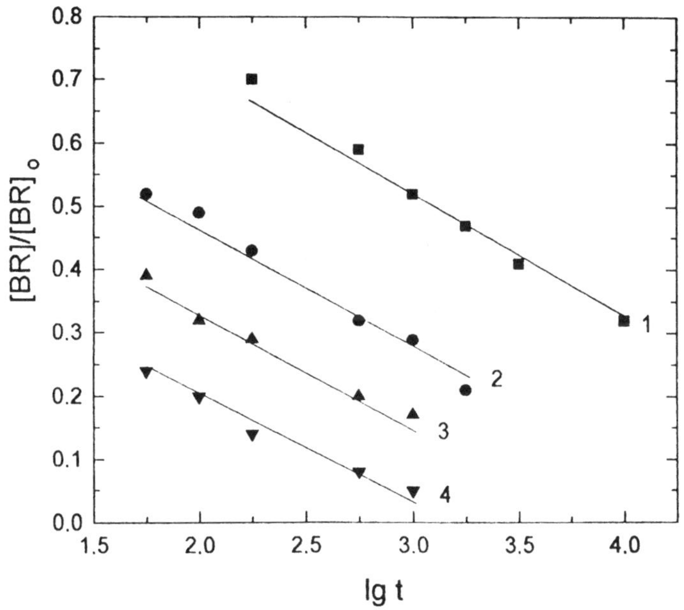

Figure 17 Kinetics of BR decay in PMMA at 1—183 K, 2—193 K, 3—203 K and 4—218 K.

may be considered as a special probe to study the molecular dynamics at low temperatures. It is known that the traditional spin probe method is intended to obtain the information about molecular motions at a temperature near and above the glass temperature. At temperatures lower than T_g, the wide distribution of paramagnetic probes by rotational frequencies appeared as the ESR method assimilates, the high frequency part only. The development of ESR with the transfer of saturation allows the extent of the interval of reliable determinations of the spin probe correlation times to the region of slow motions ($\tau = 10^4$ s) at $T < T_g$. The technique based on kinetic measurements of the BR formation due to DPC conversions extends significantly the temperature region to investigate the small scale dynamics of macromolecules. This method with the combination of the BR decay kinetics permits direct examination of the distribution of particles by reactivity connected with the non-homogeneity of the physical structure of polymers when the use of other techniques is difficult.

c. *The molecular products of the carbene reactions in polymers*

The analysis of the molecular product composition is one of the main instrument for study of the mechanism of the carbene reactions in solid polymers. But a set of methods applied for this purpose is bounded by the low solubility of the carbene precursors. UV and IR methods have the most importance for the identification of groups grafted on macromolecules in the carbene reactions in conditions that molecular extinctions are reasonably high. Apart from spectral techniques, the mechanism of the carbene reaction product formation in polymers can be established by the measurement of the insoluble gel fraction resulting during the cross-linkage of

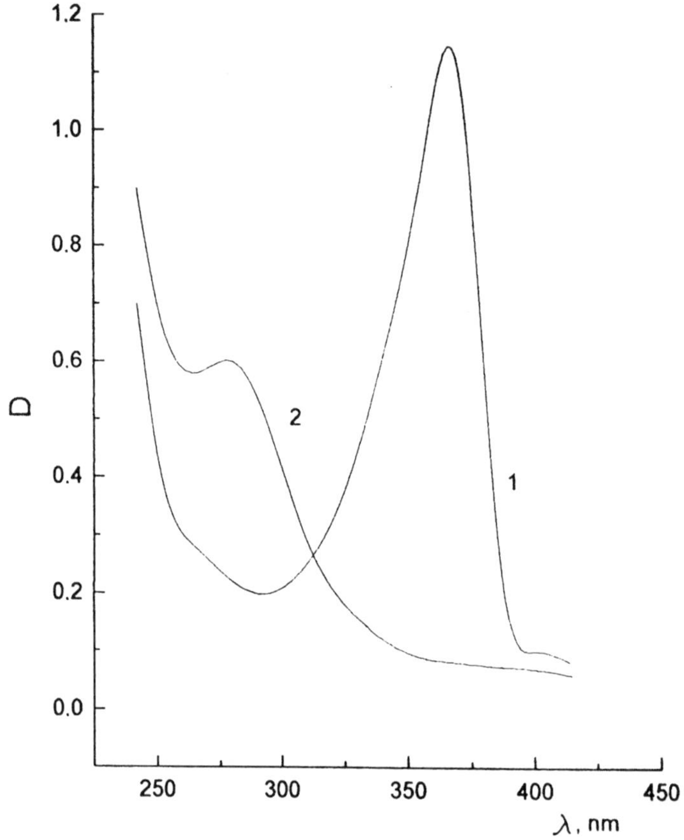

Figure 18 UV spectra of PMMA with QDA (1) and after irradiation by light $\lambda \sim 363$ nm at 295 K (2).

macromolecules by biscarbenes. In this case the conversions of diazocompounds into products are directly exhibited by the gel fraction yield.

The irradiation of PMMA films with QDA by light with $\lambda \approx 365$ nm at 295 K results in the appearance of new UV absorption band at 275 nm[22] (Figure 18) which is typical of phenols. The bands of the hydroxyl groups (3440 cm^{-1}), C—H bonds (1596 cm^{-1}) and C=C (1500 cm^{-1}) of the phenol aromatic ring arise in the IR spectrum. The phenol formation is also observed in PMMA films as a result of the CHC decay at $T > 77$ K. The detectable decrease of the phenol absorption band was not detected in the course of the reprecipitation of samples irradiated at 295 K and 77 K by ethanol, suggesting that these phenol groups are chemically bonded with macromolecules.

As discussed above the low temperature reactions of ^{3}CHC involve the RP and isolated radical formations by the hydrogen atom abstraction from C—H bonds of the PMMA ester groups. The subsequent recombination of RP must give rise to the respective product $\sim CH_2C(CH_3)(COOCH_2C_6H_4OH)CH_2\sim$. At 295 K CHC, resulting in the singlet state in primary reaction of the QDA photodecomposition, either can immediately react with macromolecules with the formation of the insertion product or transform to the ground triplet state in time of 10^{-10} s with the following reaction by scheme (4). A comparison between the UV intensities of initial and irradiated samples it is found that the CHC conversion occurs quantitatively in the insertion product at 295 K and 77 K in the range of [QDA] = 10^{-3}–10^{-1} M and is not followed by formation of other compounds, for example, diphenoquinone or *p*-benzoquinone as result of two CHC recombinations or CHC oxidation.

The similar product was observed in OP with QDA during irradiation by light with $\lambda \approx 365$ nm. The absorption band with $\lambda_{max} \approx 280$ nm results in UV spectrum. The same band was detected in OP irradiated by light at 77 K after warming to room temperature. The phenol groups are chemically bonded with macromolecules since repeated extracting by ethanol did not rise to the disappearance of 280 nm band. The reaction product has the following structure $\sim CH_2CH{=}CHC(C_6H_4OH)(CH_3)\sim$. We emphasise that in this system the products of CHC attaching to double bonds are not exhibited.[59] The formation of these products must not be excluded. But, as was shown in work,[60] such spirocyclohexadienones are extraordinary sensitive to impurities of acids and bases and can be easily isomerised at room temperature with the cycle decomposition into phenols.

Consider now the results of the investigation of the thermal and photochemical transformation of BQDA in PVA. The currently available evidence[59] suggests that cyclohexadienone carbenes are able to react with alcohols giving hydroquinone esters $(OH)C_6H_4(OR)$. The band of BQDA with $\lambda_{max} \approx 360$ nm disappears during the film irradiation by light with $\lambda > 300$ nm and the heating from 320 K to 363 K. As this takes place, the films partly lose the water solubility and the band with $\lambda_{max} = 290$ nm belonging to the hydroquinone ester[61] makes their appearance in the UV spectrum of insoluble fraction. On the strength of these results the assumption was made that the cross-linkage takes place owing to the BCHC insertion into PVA hydroxy groups. For simplicity the cross-linkage process can be presented in the following manner

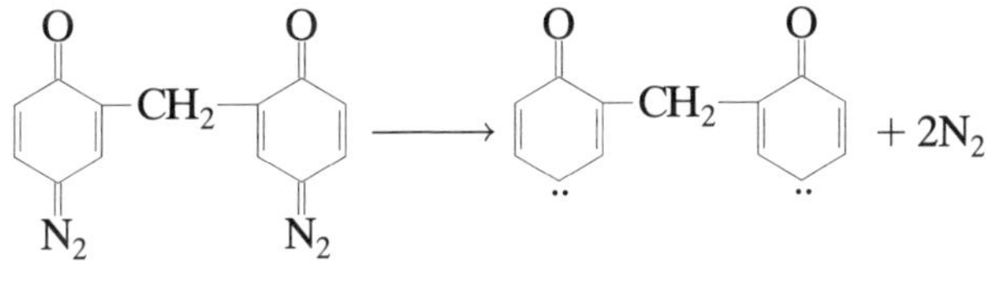

(32)

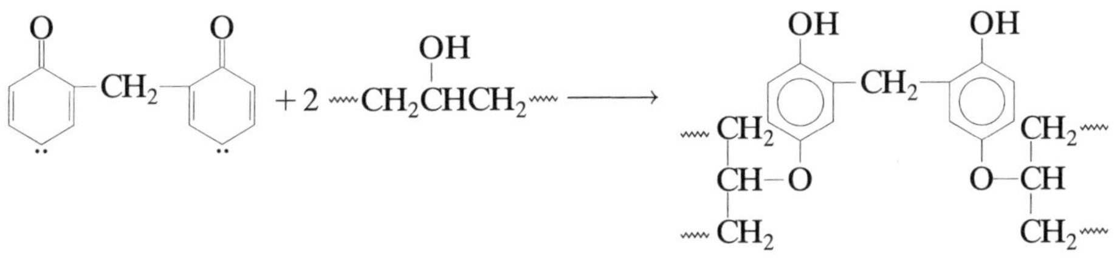

(33)

An alternative mechanics of the cross-linkage connected with the recombination of PVA macroradicals and phenoxy radicals is also possible

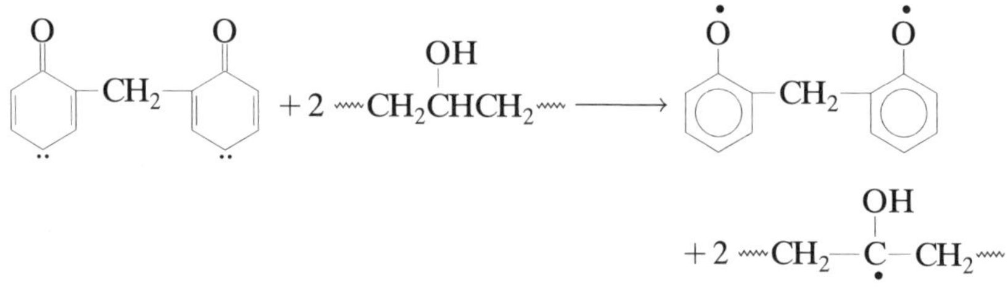

(34)

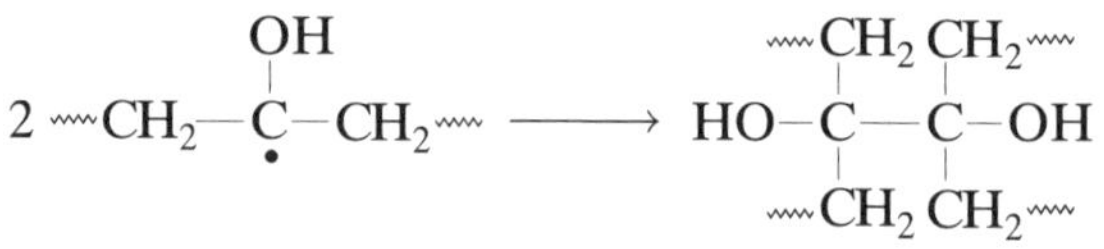

(35)

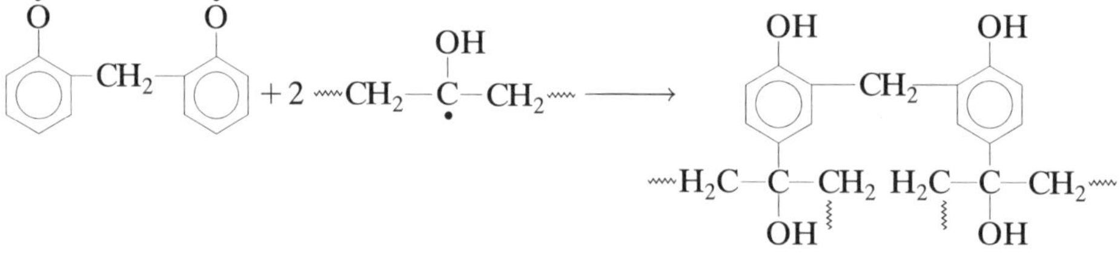

(36)

In all probability the cross-linkage by reactions (35) and (36) does not play the important role because the water insoluble films are easy dissolved at heating in the concentrated hydrogen chloride acid. It is common knowledge[62] that this acid is capable of the phenol ester cleavage on evidence derived from ESR. Besides, the interaction of macroradicals and phenoxy radicals by reactions (35), (36) does not result to the cross linking. Macroradicals $\sim CH_2C(OH)CH_2\sim$ and phenoxy radicals were registered at 77 K by ESR. The formation of these radicals is explained by the transition of primary singlet carbenes to the ground triplet state when they are able the hydrogen atom from C—H bonds to abstract. It should be recorded that no RPs with the average distance between radicals of 0.5–0.6 nm in PVA were detected. No mono and biscyclohexadienone carbenes were likewise registered. These facts testify that the high reactivity BCHC in the hydrogen abstraction and high efficiency of the radical egress from cages exist even at 77 K. The isolated radicals can decay by the PVA warming-up without the cross-linkage. Consequently, one can believe that the macromolecule cross-linkage is a result of the reaction of the singlet BCHC insertion into O—H bonds. The rate of the gel fraction formation is significantly diminished

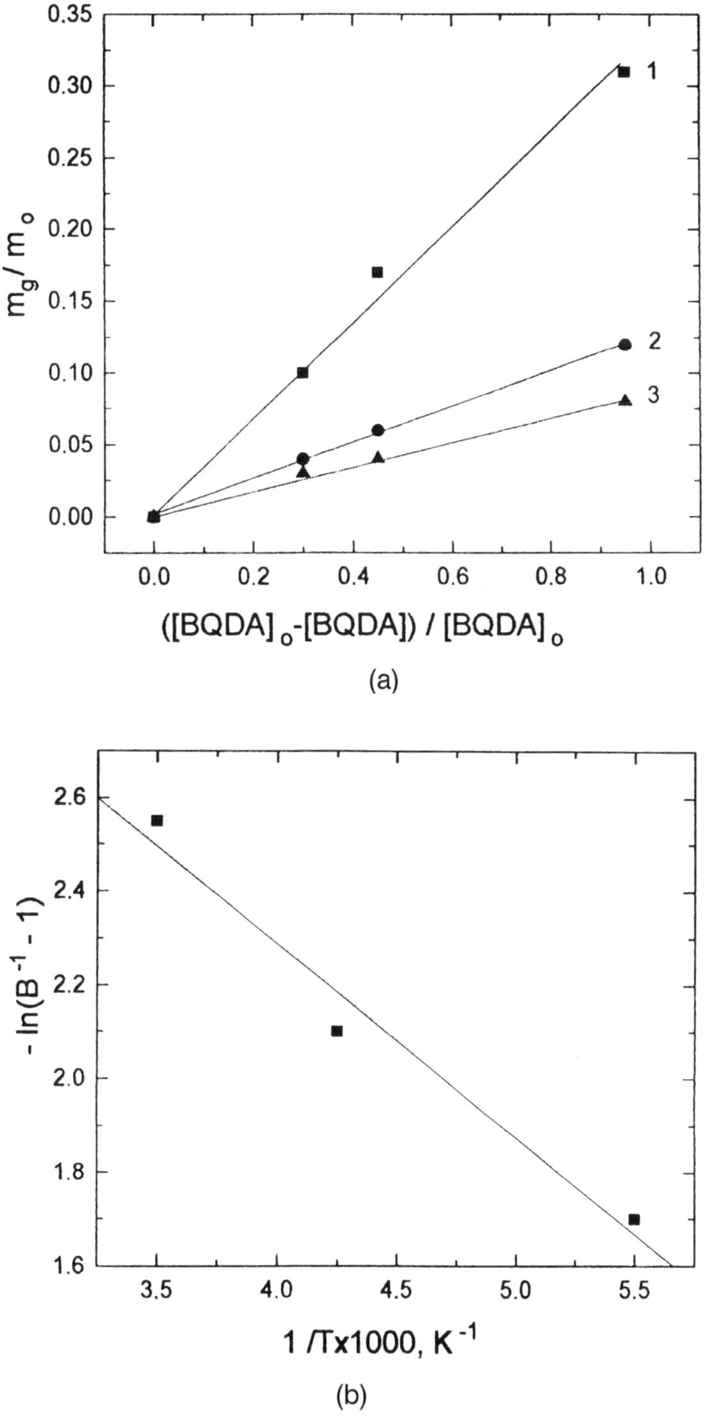

Figure 19 The dependence of gel formation in PVA on BQDA photodecomposition degree at 1—295 K, 2—243 K, 3—183 K (a) and temperature dependence of parameter B (b).

with the temperature decrease. The cross-linkage is observed in samples once the total photolysis of BQDA (10 min). It is evident from plots shown in Figure 19a that during BQDA photodecomposition the cross-linkage is linear related to the degree of the adding conversion. The carbenes likely to be involve in alternative specific reaction. They react in the triplet state by reaction (34) with the formation of radicals that are transformed into some products.

The main carbene reactions in PVA initiated by BQDA photolysis can be represented by the following scheme.

$$\mathrm{BQDA} \longrightarrow {}^{1}\mathrm{BCHC} + \mathrm{RH} \xrightarrow{k_1} \mathrm{S} \tag{37}$$

$$k_{\mathrm{ST}} \Big\Vert k_{\mathrm{TS}}$$

$${}^{3}\mathrm{BCHC} + \mathrm{RH} \xrightarrow{k_2} \mathrm{R} \longrightarrow \text{products} \tag{38}$$

It was found that the optical density of band with $\lambda_{max} = 290\,\mathrm{nm}$ possessed by the cross-linkage groups is changed much as the insoluble fraction proportion m_g that is $m_g/m_0 = \delta[S]$, where S is cross-linkage, m_0 is the film weight. Therefore, if to believe that the carbene concentration is steady-state and carbenes at the relative high temperatures of 183–295 K are kinetic equal then the gel fraction yield would be expressible as

$$\frac{m_0}{m_0} = \frac{[\mathrm{BQDA}]_0 k_1 k_{\mathrm{TS}}}{k_1 k_{\mathrm{TS}} + k_2 k_{\mathrm{ST}}} \left(1 - \frac{[\mathrm{BQDA}]}{[\mathrm{BQDA}]_0}\right) \tag{39}$$

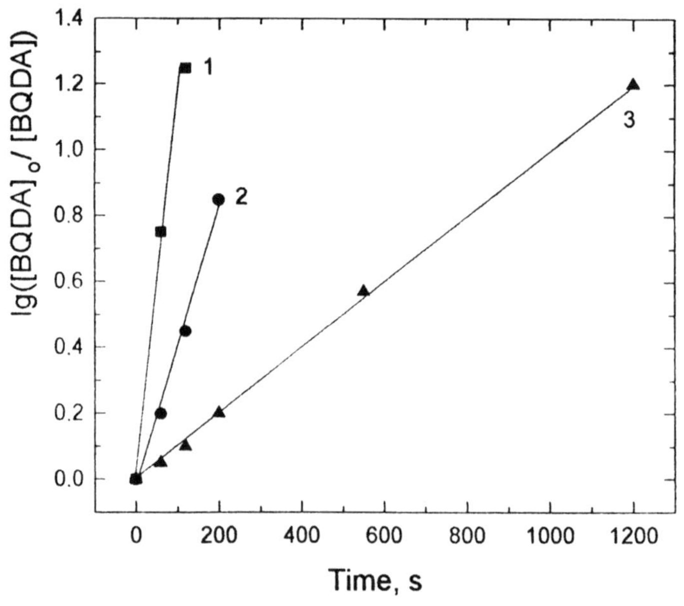

Figure 20 Kinetics of BQDA thermal decomposition in PVA at 1—373 K, 2—343 K and 3—322 K.

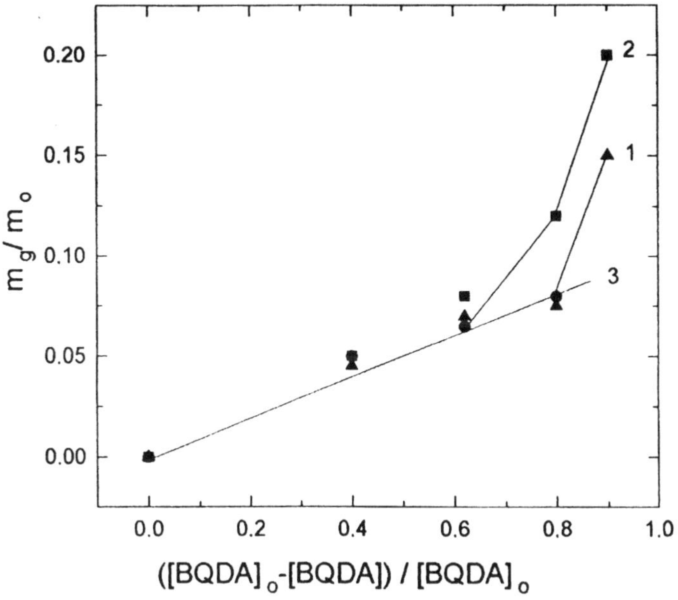

Figure 21 The dependence of gel formation in PVA on BQDA thermal decomposition degree at 1—373 K, 2—343 K and 3—322 K.

From plots of Figure 19a it follows that the efficiency of crosslinking, defined by $B = k_1k_{TS}/(k_1k_{TS} + k_2k_{TS})$, is changed from 0.9 at 295 K to 0.08 at 183 K. The temperature dependence of B can be represented as

$$\ln\left(\frac{1}{B} - 1\right) = A + \frac{\Delta E_{TS} + E_1 - E_2}{RT} \tag{40}$$

where A is constant (Figure 19b).

The retention of this relationship over a fairly wide range of temperatures is evidence of the suggested mechanism of BQDA conversion. The difference of effective activation energies, including ΔE_{TS}, is 2.8 kJ/mol. By this is meant that $E_2 - E_1 < \Delta E_{TS}$. Therefore, the decrease of the efficiency of the cross-linkage by the lowering of the photolysis temperature results because of the increase of the relative population of the ground triplet state similarly the temperature dependence of the product composition in the solid phase reaction of DPC with isobutylene.[8] A build-up of the gel fraction after the BQDA photodecomposition may be attributed to initiation of cross-linkage by products resulting in the carbene reaction (38).

The considerable distinctions of the cross-linkage were observed at the BQDA thermal decomposition. The kinetics of this process is controlled by the first order law at 320–373 K with the rate constant $k = 5 \cdot 10^{10} \exp(-85.6\,\text{kJ/RT}), \text{s}^{-1}$ (Figure 20). In this case insoluble fraction is formed in the wake of the BQDA complete decay similarly to photolysis. As this takes place, the contribution of the BQDA conversion products in cross-linkage is more important at higher temperature. The amount of gel fraction in PVA is proportional to BQDA decomposed up to the high conversion extent (Figure 21). In so doing, the efficiency of cross-linkage is equal at different temperatures and accounts for 0.3. As the yield of products is increased late in the disease of the BQDA decay the abrupt rise of the cross-linkage takes place. Taking the concept of the singlet-triplet equilibrium for carbenes analogously to the BQDA photolysis one can allow their involvement in two competitive reactions. One produces at once the cross-linkage as a result of the singlet BCHC insertion in O—H groups of macromolecules and other reaction of triplet BCHC gives some product. By virtue of the fact that the gel formation efficiency during the BQDA thermal decomposition does not depend on temperature and threefold smaller than during photolysis at 295 K, the mechanism of reaction (38) must be other. The absence of the temperature dependence for the gel yield implies formally $\Delta E_{TS} + E_1 = E_2$ in equation (40), that is triplet carbenes react effectively at high temperatures with larger activation energy than at low temperature conversions. Besides, the reaction product must form itself cross-linkage during heating as evidenced by a drastic gain of the gel formation at high degree of the diazocompound decay (Figure 21).

It is possible that the intramolecular hydrogen atom transfer occurs from methylene group of triplet BQDA.

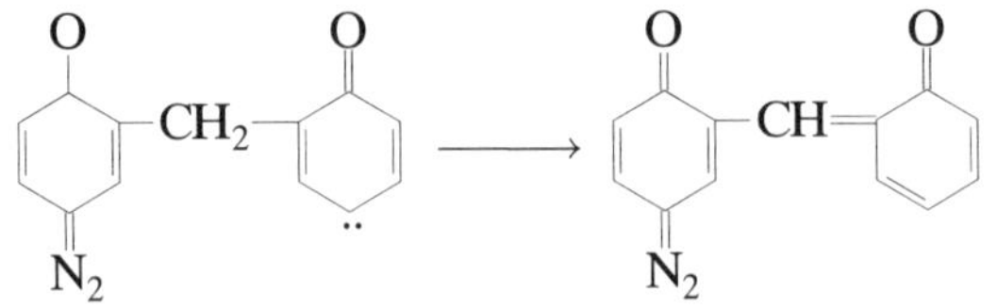

(39)

Such reactions of intramolecular rearrangement with the participation of the hydrogen atom are characteristic of carbenes.[63] By reaction (41) the monodiazocompound containing the methylene quinone group is formed. On further transformation it gives the corresponding product of insertion in O—H bond of PVA.

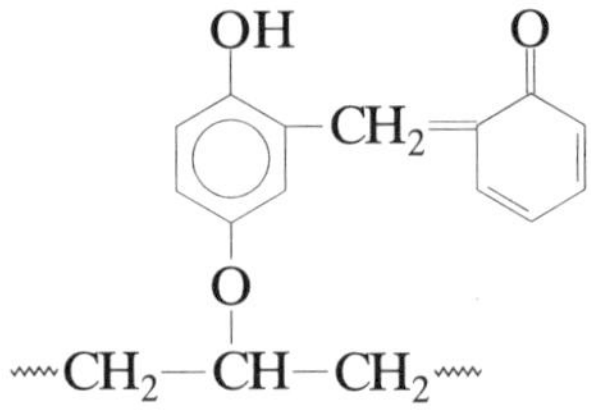

In turn the methylenequinone groups of these products are capable to react with hydroxy groups of macromolecules

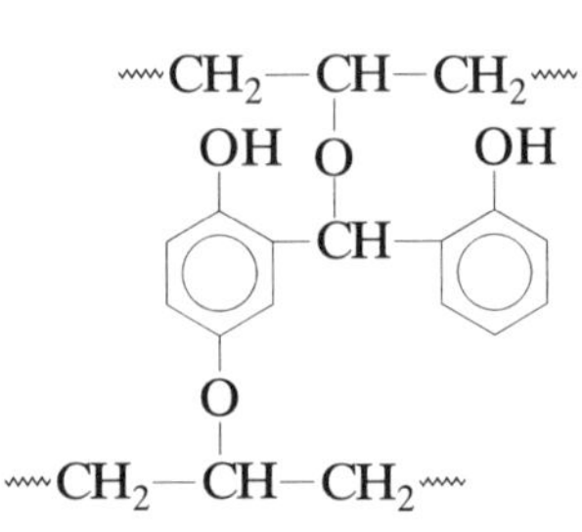

In support of this conclusion one can note that a typical reaction of low molecular alcohols with methylenequinone is the formation of ether $(OH)C_6H_4(CH_2OR)$.[64] The data obtained are primarily important to appreciate the mechanism of influence of the polymer matrix physical condition on the carbene reactivity. PVA shows at the glass transition temperature the high intensity of molecular movements vastly larger than at room and negative temperatures. The different kinds of relaxation processes correspond to these temperature ranges. So the interval of 320–370 K is characteristic of glass transition in randomly packed sites of PVA and the range of 180–279 K corresponds to the relaxation of the hydrogen-unlinked macrochains.[65] The distinctions, observed for the PVA cross-linkage by the BQDA photo and thermal decompositions are analogous to the effect of the low molecular alcohol phase state on products of the carbene reaction.[10] In going from the rigid matrix to $T > T_g$ the change of the triplet carbene conversion mechanism takes place. The bimolecular reaction of the hydrogen atom abstraction is suppressed and the peculiar intramolecular reaction of BQDA is happened. This, it is reasonably safe to suggest that the PVA matrix effect on the carbene reactions is defined by the dependence of their mechanism on molecular relaxation. The change of the product composition of the carbene reactions in polymers may be observed within one phase state in the context of numerous relaxation processes.

d. The kinetics of the carbene reactions in filled polymers

The filling is one of the most commonly encountered way of the polymer modification. The experience thus far gained shows that the filler effect is propagated to the polymer volume non-uniformly[66] that is exhibited by the formation of interfaces. The physical structures of interfaces are distinguished from those in the volume. The influence of filler on the structure of polymers is realised through the interface. The interface thickness evaluated experimentally is effective and reflects the behaviour of the filled systems in reference to the property studied. As a rule, the information on the polymer interfaces can be obtained not by way of their first hand investigation but from the characteristics exhibiting the essential dependence on the filling degree. In the context of the close association between the polymer structural-physical properties and the kinetics of the radical reactions the determination of kinetic plots may be considered as an appropriate technique of the structural characteristic assessment in particular of the interface effective thickness. There is quite voluminous literature devoted to the thermal and thermoxidational degradation of the filled polymers[67] that shows a pronounced role of filler in these processes. But in the high temperature reactions of oxidation, the catalytic properties of filler surface can influence on kinetics besides the structural-physical factors. From this viewpoint the implementation of the low-temperature cage radical reactions, specifically the carbene reactions, has the advantage. These reactions must reflect the molecular organisation features of interfaces practically in pure view. Evidently they are not complicated by the interaction of radicals with the filler surface.

In Figure 22 a, b the kinetic curves of DTBCHC decay at 100 K in PMMA and AC containing up to 65 mass percentage of aerosil are shown. As indicated by figure, the introducing of filler reduces the rate of DTBCHC decay in both polymers. The similar effect was observed throughout the entire temperature range of 100–140 K.

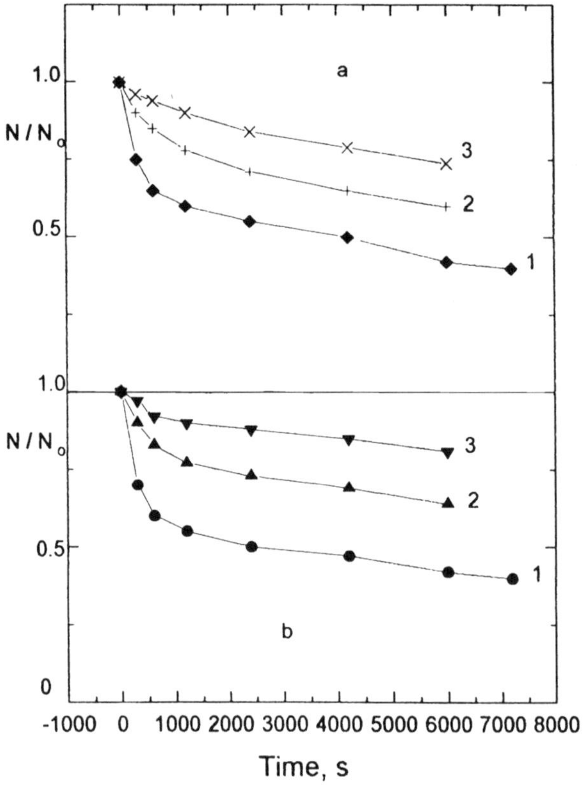

Figure 22 Kinetics of DTBCHC decay at 100 K in PMMA (a) and AC (b) with 1—1, 2—40 and 3—65% of aerosil.

The form of kinetic curves shows the DTBCHC clearly defined non-equivalence. In the studied temperature range, such curves are satisfactorily straightened in coordinates of (10) (Figure 23 a, b).

With the filler content increase, the limiting values of the rate constants k_{max} and k_{min} in PMMA and AC are decreased but the parameter of the distribution width is kept constant. At 100 K lg (k_{max}/k_{min}) are 6.8 and 5.5 respectively in PMMA and AC. The distribution high narrowing is exhibited with increased temperature. The conclusion on uniformity of the distribution width of the DTBCHC decay rate in samples with the different filling is important to understand the nature of the structural-physical modification of polymers. This conclusion has been confirmed by the other method of kinetic analysis involving the approximation by equation put forward in work.[68]

$$\frac{N}{N_0} = (1 + nk_0 t)^{-1/n} \tag{42}$$

where k_0 is the DTBCHC average effective rate constant obtained on the basis of distribution by the decay rate constants $\rho(k_{ef}) : k_0 = \int k_{ef}\rho(k_{ef})dk_{ef}$, n is parameter determining the distribution width. In Figure 24 the straightenings of the carbene

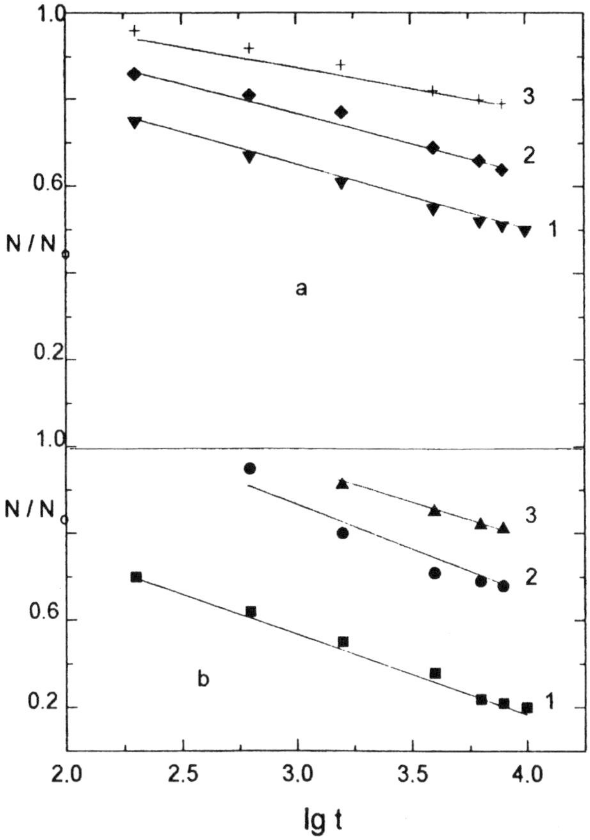

Figure 23 The linear approximations of kinetics of DTBCHC decay in filled PMMA (a) and AC (b) with 1—1, 2—40 and 3—65% of aerosil.

decay kinetics are shown at 100 K in co-ordinates of (42). All curves are approximated by the same anamorphosis regardless of the aerosil content and, therefore, n is constant. The kinetic parameter values obtained are listed in Table 3. Thus the kinetic analysis performed by two methods gives the same result: the distribution by the effective rate constants of the DTBCHC decay in filled polymers does not depend on the filler content.

Figure 25 a, b shows relationships of the average rate constant k_0 and distances between the filler particles. These distances were estimated by equation[66]

$$l = d\left[\left(\frac{0.8}{1-\zeta}\right)^{1/3} - 1\right] \tag{43}$$

where d is the diameter of the aerosil particles ($\approx 20\,\mathrm{nm}$), ζ is the aerosil volume fraction in polymer. As is seen from Figure 23, the k_0 values are moderately decreased with the filler content increase in the range of 1 exceeding 20 nm. If $l < 20\,\mathrm{nm}, k_0$ is decreased more than tenfold.

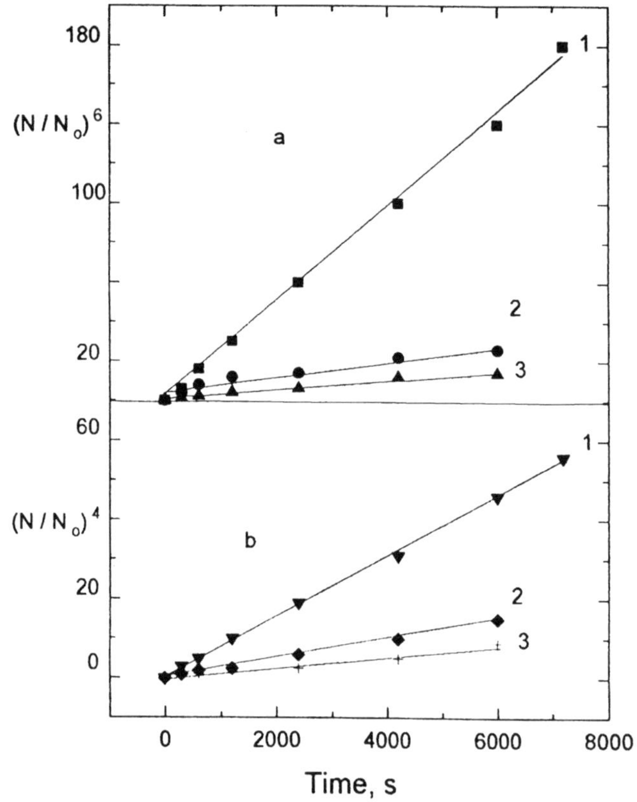

Figure 24 The linear approximations of DTBCHC decay kinetics in filled PMMA (a) and AC (b) in co-ordinates of (42) with 1—1, 2—40 and 3—65% of aerosil.

Along with the physical structure modification of the polymers, the filler effect on the kinetics of the DTBCHC decay can be caused in principle by the change of mechanism on the surface. For instance, one can allow that the fraction of carbenes, decaying on the surface with smaller rate as compared with reaction in the polymer volume, is increased with the filler content. The special experiment was made to elucidate the association of the filler effect with this reason. The sample of the filled polyvinylpyrrolydone was prepared with the DTBCHC precursor tentatively coated on aerosil surface. In this sample, irradiated at 77 K by light with $300\,nm < \lambda < 400\,nm$, the kinetics of the DTBCHC decay was studied at 100–125 K. It turns out that the value of the average rate constant for these samples is two–threefold higher. In so doing, the decay rate increase of carbenes on surface is not due to re-combination because of the average distance between them is 3 nm. By this mean the DTBCHC decay on surface must cause the opposite filler effect. Thus we can conclude that the carbene decay in filled polymers takes place mainly in reaction with macromolecules and essential decrease of this process rate with the increasing of the aerosil content associated with the physical structure changes in polymers accounting for by transformations in the interface state. Its thickness estimated by plots of Figure 25 is 15–20 nm.

TABLE 3
Kinetic parameters of DTBCHC decay in filled PMMA and AC

T, K	aerosil, %	$k_0 10^4, s^{-1}$	n
		PMMA	
100	1	28.0	6
	25	14.5	
	40	4.2	
	65	1.6	
113	1	35.0	4
	25	25.0	
	40	14.7	
	65	1.8	
125	1	38.0	2
	25	25.0	
	40	16.7	
	65	2.1	
		AC	
100	1	13.0	4
	25	11.8	
	40	2.5	
	65	0.7	
125	1	140.0	3
	25	–	
	40	87.0	
	65	6.9	
135	1	1000	2
	25	580	
	40	200	
	65	12	

On the basis of kinetic data obtained the following conclusions can be reached about the nature of the matrix structure changes by filling. As the width of distribution by the DTBCHC reactivity is not changed with the conversion of polymer into the interface state the structural-physical modification does not influence the distribution by the rate constants of primary reaction of the hydrogen atom transfer from C—H bonds of macromolecules to carbenes (18) which is the limiting step of their decay. This step determines precisely the kinetic non-equivalence of carbenes in reaction with macromolecules through the dispersion of distances between the carbene centre and C—H bonds of matrix. In this connection one can believe that the structural changes by filling effect on efficiency of the intermediate RP recombination defined by $[(k_{-1}P_T/k_2P_S)+1]$ in (19). It was found that as the filled polymer is prepared from solution the formation of more friable packing of macromolecules is possible in interfaces.[66] Such structural realignment can change the relation between the recombination rate of singlet RP and back hydrogen atom transfer together with the relative population P_T/P_S as a result of the RP configuration changes. So, for example, more departure from complimentary perpendicular orientation of the non-pair electron axis the more the change energy value and the more the triplet level population of RP.[39]

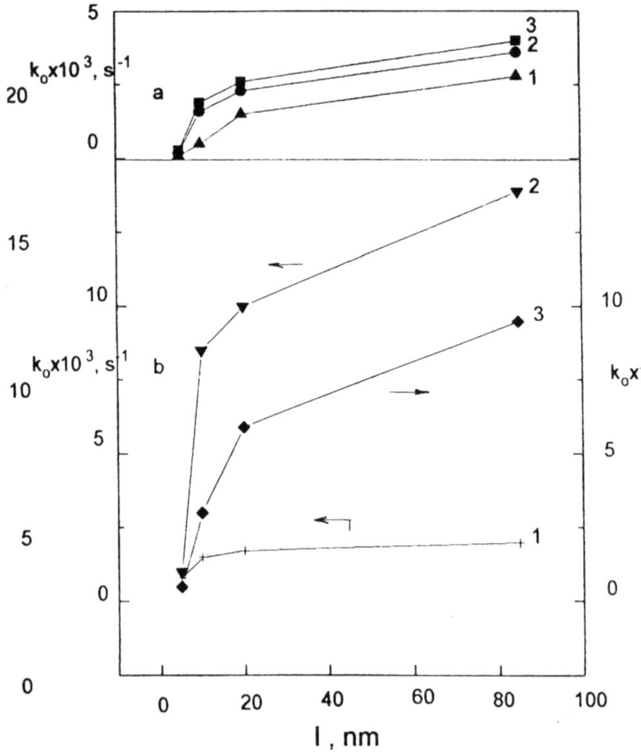

Figure 25 Relationships of average rate constant on distances between aerosil particles in PMMA at 1—100 K, 2—113 K, 3—125 K (a) and AC at 1—100 K, 2—125 K, 3—135 K (b).

The Thermostabilisation of Polyisoprene by Phenol Grafting in the Carbene Synthesis

A convenient method for stabiliser fixation in polymers is the reaction of suitable carbenes with macromolecules. This method enables physical losses of stabilisers to be avoided owing to volatilisation and washing-off by water and other organic solvents. The grafted antioxidants can be effective under service conditions of polymeric materials at high temperatures and also during reprocessing. There are examples of effective use of carbenes to stabilise polyolefines by 2,6-di-*t*-butylphenol (DTBP). The fixed phenol shows better protective properties at 300–500 K than non-grafted phenols.[70]

To fix DTBP on polyisoprene (PI) films with DTBQDA additives ($6 \cdot 10^{-3}$–$4 \cdot 10^{-2}$ M) were heated for one hour at 343 K.[71] In this case the appearance of the 280 nm phenol band in the UV spectrum is observed. The reprecipitation of PI samples does not lead to the band disappearance. The estimation shows that the phenol concentration is about 90% of that of DTBQDA inserted in PI. The oxidation of PI with grafted DTBP at 353 K and 363 K was performed on 50μ films placed on CaF_2 plates. The thermoxidation kinetics was determined by the accumulation of the carbonyl (1720 cm^{-1}) and hydroxyl (3200–3600 cm^{-1}) absorptions in IR spectrum and by the oxygen sorption. The oxidation of PI stabilised by 2,6-di-*t*-butyl-4-methylpropionatephenol (DTBMP) was studied by the same technique to compare at both antioxidants from the point of view of their stabilising capabilities.

The formation of phenol derivatives in carbene synthesis is possible in PI by reactions of triplet carbenes with C—H allyl bands and as a result of spirodienone conversion.[72]

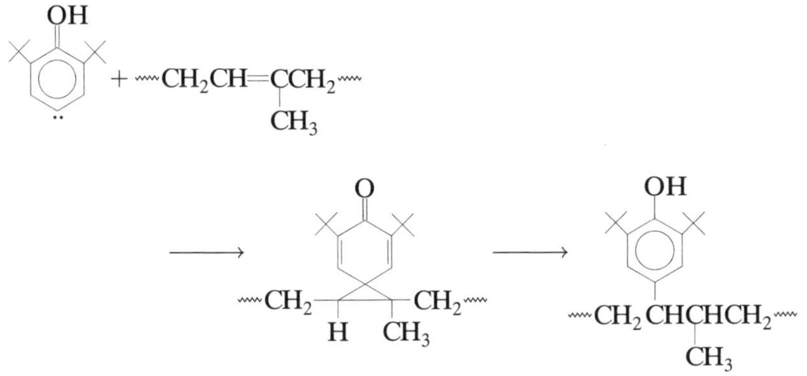

(44)

The kinetic curves of carbonyl group accumulation in PI with DTBP are shown in Figure 26. The same type of curves were obtained for hydroxyl production and oxygen sorption.

The dependence of induction periods of oxidation on grafted antioxidant concentrations is shown in Figure 27. The analogous relationships are presented for low-molecular phenol. Clearly, the concentration dependence observed has essential differences. The induction period is increased linearly for grafted antioxidant with concentration. The evident departure from linearity was observed for DTBMP in the concentration range up to $3.8 \cdot 10^{-2}$ M. The induction period values are similar for both antioxidants at low concentrations. The difference of τ rises largely with the antioxidant concentration increase. This result suggests that the deviation from linearity of the concentration dependence of τ for DTBMP does not result from the sweating-out that is typical of low-molecular antioxidants.

It is known that the dependence of τ on the inhibitor concentration of therm-oxidation is defined by the kinetics of antioxidant consumption. Thus, PhOH consumption with constant rate corresponds to the linear concentration dependence of τ.[73,74] The kinetics of phenol consumption does not fall from the zero order until the end of the induction period when the phenol concentration approaches a critical value. Yet neither the proportionality of the induction period values and phenol concentration nor the zero order of its consumption kinetics are accomplished commonly in practice.

The origin of this effect consists in unexpected side reactions with assistance of phenoxy radicals, resulting at the termination of oxidation chains,[75] as well as direct interaction of phenols with oxygen in the course of inhibited oxidation.[76] One can consider possible reasons for the resulting decrease of DTBMP antioxidational

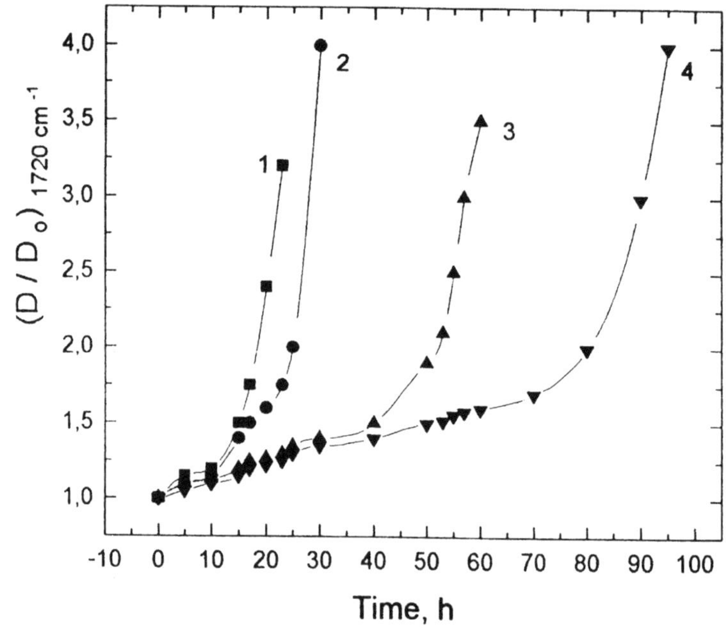

Figure 26 Kinetics of C=O formation at 353 K in PI with grafted DTBP: 1—$6.36 \cdot 10^{-3}$ M, 2—$1.27 \cdot 10^{-2}$ M, 3—$2.12 \cdot 10^{-2}$ M, 4—$4.24 \cdot 10^{-2}$ M.

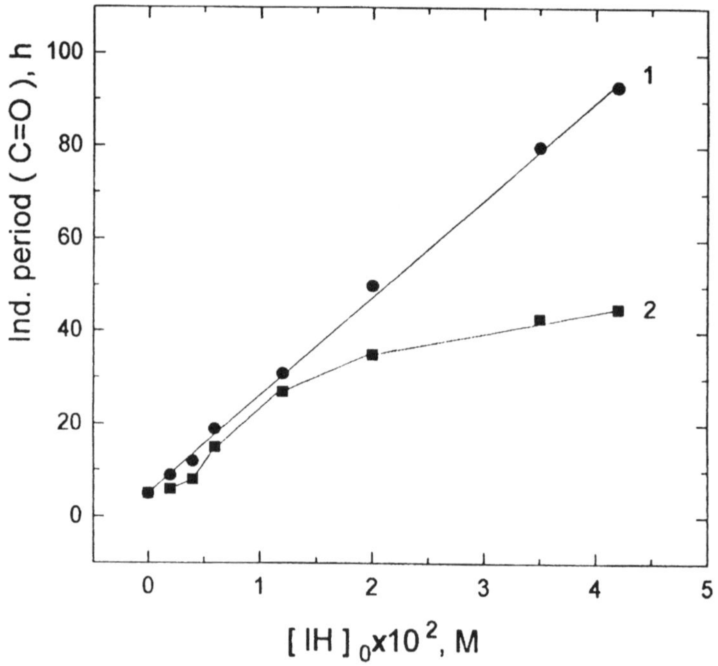

Figure 27 The dependence of τ of C=O formation at 353 K in PI on antioxidant concentrations: 1—grafted DTBP, 2—DTBMP.

activity in PI as compared with grafted DTBP. The direct oxidation of low-molecular weight phenol does not take place, apparently for lack of this process for its grafted analogue. The possibility of β-dissociation of phenoxy radicals with substitutes in the p-position can be assumed with the result that slightly active inhibitor radicals are coverted to active substitute radicals. Similar reactions are typical of *p*-alkoxyderivatives of phenols.[77] Then the PhOH consumption is accelaerted greatly in a range of the phenol high concentrations. This reaction can be ignored for phenoxy radicals containing alkyl substitutes in *p*-position.[77] Thus, grafted DTBP is not affected by undesirable β-dissociation decreasing its efficiency.

The comparison of activity of traditional and grafted antioxidants shows that the last has qualitative advantages in addition to non-volatility. The grafted DTBP is an "ideal" antioxidant in the overall studied concentration range, the upper limit of which corresponds to concentrations used in real working conditions. Its consumption within the induction period occurs as a result of linear termination of oxidation chains and is evidently not attended by side reactions. These advantages permit making use of hindered phenols grafted by carbene synthesis on macromolecules to stabilise PI and other elastomers.

CONCLUSIONS

One can note a series of the common features of the carbene reactions in solid polymers. The physical structure of medium results in the non-equivalence of carbene reactivity and non-uniformity of distribution of the carbene precursors. The main reason of kinetic non-equivalence is the space-orientation variety of the carbene centre arrangement with relation to the C—H bonds of matrix. This variation defines the dispersion of the rate constants of the hydrogen atom transfer at low temperature. The reaction is described in the framework of one model of the hydrogen atom tunneling through the potential barrier oscillating in response to intermolecular vibrations.

Some fraction (up to 20%) of carbenes are clustered in two, three or more particles both in polymers and frozen organic glasses. The dimerisation, trimerisation and so on with the BR formation takes place in such clusters. But the mechanism of the carbene transformation in polymers has essential dissimilarity determined by molecular organisation. The stepwise kinetics of the low temperature carbene decay in polymers is often governed by a "degree of conversion—logarithm of time" law. The dispersion of $3–5 \cdot 10^{-2}$ nm in equilibrium distances between carbene and the C—H bonds of macromolecule accords to the difference in 5–6 orders for the carbene decay rate constants.

The established strong structure effect on the carbene reactivity allows to use their reactions as a sensitive technique of the structural-physical characteristic estimation. One can determine in part the interface thickness of filled polymers by the kinetic data of the triplet carbene decay. The reaction of the BR formation in clusters of arylcarbenes allows investigation of the molecular dynamics at cryogenic temperatures. The kinetics of this process reflects a very wide spectrum of the orientational movement with frequencies from 10^5 to $10^{-6}\,s^{-1}$.

In parallel with investigation of the cage environment influence on kinetics of elementary reactions in solid polymers, carbenes can be used for solving practical problems of the rubbers stabilisation by grafting, for instance, of hindered phenols.

REFERENCES

1. S. Siddiqui and R.E. Cais, *Macromolecules*, 1986, **19**(3), pp. 595–603.
2. J.H. Bradbury and M.C.S. Perera, *British. Polym. J.*, 1986, **18**(2), pp. 127–134.
3. M. Aglietto, R. Alterio, R. Bertani, F. Galleschi and G. Ruggeri, *Polymer*, 1989, **30**(6), pp. 1133–1136.
4. N.M. Emanuel and A.L. Buchachenko, *Chemical physics of molecular degradation and stabilization of polymers*, 1988, Moscow, Nauka, p. 133.
5. A.L. Kovarsky and V.N. Saprygin, *Vysokomolek. soed.*, 1984, **A29**(9), pp. 1949–1956.
6. P.S. Skell, *Tetrahedron*, 1985, **42**(8), pp. 1427–1428.
7. O.R. Hoffman, *J. Amer. Chem. Soc.*, 1969, **90**(6), pp. 1475–1485.
8. B.B. Wright, *Tetrahedron*, 1985, **42**(8), pp. 1517–1523.
9. R.A. Moss and U.H. Dolling, *J. Amer. Chem. Soc.*, 1971, **93**(4), pp. 954–960.
10. H. Tomioka, T. Inagaki, S. Nakamura and Y. Izawa, *J. Chem. Soc. Perkin I*, 1979, 1, pp. 130–134.
11. H. Tomioka, G.W. Griffin and K. Nishigama, *J. Amer. Chem. Soc.*, 1979, **101**(20), pp. 6009–6012.
12. E.C. Palik and M.S. Platz, *J. Org. Chem.*, 1983, **48**(7), pp. 963–969.
13. S.G. Boxer, C.E.D Chidsey and M.G. Roelofs, *J. Amer. Chem. Soc.*, 1982, **104**(9), pp. 2674–2675.
14. V.A. Schevelev, *Vysokomolek. soed.*, 1971, **A13**(10), pp. 2316–2323.
15. M.S. Platz, V.P. Senthilnathan, B.B. Wright and C.W. McCurdy, *J. Amer. Chem. Soc.*, 1982, **104**(24), pp. 6494–6501.
16. M.S. Platz, *Acc. Chem. Res.*, 1989, **21**(6), pp. 236–242.
17. M. Iwasaki and K. Toriyama, *J. Chem. Phys.*, 1967, **46**(7), pp. 2852–2853.
18. M. Iwasaki, T. Ichikawa and T. Ohmori, *J. Chem. Phys.*, 1969, **50**(5), pp. 1984–1990.
19. V.S. Pudov, L.L. Yasina and A.L. Buchahenko, *Kinetika i kataliz*, 1974, **15**(5), pp. 1110–1114.
20. B.B. Wright and M.S. Platz, *J. Amer. Chem. Soc.*, 1984, **106**(15), pp. 4175–4180.
21. B.B. Wright, K. Kanakarajan and M.S. Platz, *J. Phys. Chem.*, 1985, **89**(16), pp. 3574–3577.
22. A.P. Vorotnikov, E.Ya. Davydov and D.Ya. Toptygin, *Vysokomolek. soed.*, 1984, **B26**(9), pp. 664–669.
23. W. Siebrand and A.T. Wildman, *Acc. Chem. Res.*, 1986, **17**(1), pp. 238–243.
24. A.P. Vorotnikov, E.Ya. Davydov, G.B. Pariyskii and D.Ya. Toptygin, *Khimicheskaya Fizika*, 1983, **2**(6), pp. 818–822.
25. V.V. Korshak, A.P. Vorotnikov, E.Ya. Davydov, N.M. Kozyreva, A.I. Kirillin, S.B. Skubina and D.Ya. Toptygin, *Dokl. Akad. Nauk SSSR*, 1986, **291**(2), pp. 376–381.
26. Ya.S. Lebedev, *Kinetika I kataliz*, 1978, **19**(6), pp. 1367–1376.
27. A.P. Vorotnikov, E.Ya. Davydov and D.Ya. Toptygin, *Izv. Akad. Nauk SSSR, ser. khimich.*, 1985, 6, pp. 1275–1281.
28. A.P. Vorotnikov, E.Ya. Davydov and D.Ya. Toptygin, *Izv. Akad. Nauk SSSR, ser. khimich.*, 1983, 7, pp. 1499–1505.
29. R.J. Le Roy, *J. Phys. Chem.*, 1980, **84**(26), pp. 3508–3521.
30. L.I. Trakhtenberg, V.L. Klochikhin and S.Ya. Pshezhetsky, *Chem. Phys.*, 1981, **59**(1), pp. 191–198.
31. E.R. Lippincott and R. Schroeder, *J. Chem. Phys.*, 1955, **23**(8), pp. 1131–1141.
32. G. Brunton, D. Griller, K.R. Barclay and K.U. Ingold, *J. Amer. Chem. Soc.*, 1976, **98**(22), pp. 6803–6807.
33. V.L. Klochikhin and L.I. Trakhtenberg, *Khimicheskaya Fizika*, 1983, **2**(6), pp. 810–817.
34. A.P. Vorotnikov, E.Ya. Davydov and D.Ya. Toptygin, *Khimicheskaya Fizika*, 1987, **6**(5), pp. 639–644.
35. E.Ya. Davydov, A.P. Vorotnikov and D.Ya. Toptygin, *Int. J. Polym. Mat.*, 1990, **13**(1), pp. 191–194.
36. U.E. Steiner and T. Ulrich, *Chem. Rev.*, 1989, **89**(1), pp. 51–147.
37. F.J.J. De Kanter and R. Kaptein, *J. Amer. Chem. Soc.*, 1982, **104**(17), pp. 4759–4766.
38. R. Kaptein, *J. Amer. Chem. Soc.*, 1972, **94**(18), pp. 6269–6280.
39. R.N. Musin and P.V. Schastnev, *Jurn. Struct. Khimii*, 1976, **17**(3), pp. 419–425.
40. A.M. Trozzolo, *Acc. Chem. Res.*, 1968, **1**(1), pp. 329–335.
41. W.A. Gibbons and A.M. Trozzolo, *J. Amer. Chem. Soc.*, 1966, **88**(1), pp. 172–173.

42. R.L. Barcus, B.B. Wright, E. Leyva and M.S. Platz, *J. Phys. Chem.*, 1987, **91**(24), pp. 6677–6683.
43. B.B. Wright and M.S. Platz, *J. Amer. Chem. Soc.*, 1983, **105**(3), pp. 628–630.
44. E. Wasserman and R.W. Murray, *J. Amer. Chem. Soc.*, 1964, **86**(19), pp. 4203–4204.
45. J.L. Roebber, *J. Chem. Phys.*, 1962, **37**(9), pp. 1974–1981.
46. E.Ya. Davydov, G.B. Pariyskii and D.Ya. Toptygin, *Vysokomolek. soed.*, 1977, **A19**(5), pp. 977–983.
47. E.Ya. Davydov, G.B. Pariyskii and D.Ya. Toptygin, *Vysokomolek. soed.*, 1975, **A17**(7), pp. 1504–1509.
48. E.Ya. Davydov, L.A. Dobrovinskii, G.B. Pariyskii and D.Ya. Toptygin, *Lakokrasochnye materialy*, 1982, **3**, pp. 15–17.
49. A.M. Trozzolo, R.W. Murray, E. Wasserman and W.A. Yager, *J. Amer. Chem. Soc.*, 1962, **84**(16), pp. 3213–3214.
50. A.M. Trozzolo and W.A. Gibbons, *J. Amer. Chem. Soc.*, 1967, **89**(2), pp. 239–243.
51. A.P. Vorotnikov and E.Ya. Davydov, *Khimicheskaya Fizika*, 1991, **10**(11), pp. 1475–1479.
52. E.Ya. Davydov, A.P. Vorotnikov and V.P. Pustoshnyi, *Oxidation Communications*, 1995, **18**(3), pp. 230–241.
53. A.P. Mar'in and Yu.A. Shlapnikov, *Dokl. Akad. Nauk SSSR*, 1974, **215**, pp. 1160–1163.
54. S.N. Kuzina and A.I. Mihailov, *Dokl. Akad. Nauk SSSR*, 1976, **231**(6), pp. 1395–1398.
55. A.L. Kovarskii and J. Placek, F. Szocs, *Polymer*, 1978, **19**(9), pp. 1137–1141.
56. A.M. Vaserman and A.L. Kovarskii, *Spin labels and probes*, 1986, Nauka, Moscow, pp. 132–146.
57. F.P. Grigor'eva and Yu.Ya. Gotlib, *Vysokomolek. Soed.*, 1968, **A10**(2), pp. 339–348.
58. K.B. Eisental, N.J. Turro, E.V. Sitzmann, I.R. Gould, G. Hefferon, J. Langen and Y. Cha, *Tetrahedron*, 1985, **41**(8), pp. 1543–1554.
59. G.A. Nikifirov and V.V. Ershov, *Mendeleev's JVHO*, 1979, 5, pp. 523–528.
60. R. Baird and S. Winstein, *J. Amer. Chem. Soc.*, 1963, **85**(5), pp. 567–578.
61. A.P. Vorotnikov, E.Ya. Davydov and D.Ya. Toptygin, *Vysokomolek. soed.*, 1986, **A28**(9), pp. 510–516.
62. J.D. Roberts and M.C. Caserio, *Basic Principles of Organic Chemistry*, 1964, Benjamin, New-York, p. 235.
63. H. Tomioka, H. Ueda, S. Kondo and Y. Izawa, *J. Amer. Chem. Soc.*, 1980, **102**(26), pp. 7817–7918.
64. P.I. Kudinova, A.A. Volod'kin and V.V. Ershov, *Izv. Akad. Nauk SSSR, ser. khimich*, 1978, 7, pp. 1661–1663.
65. P.D. Garrett and D. Grubb, *J. Polymer Sci.*, 1988, **26**(12), pp. 2507–2523.
66. Yu.S. Lipatov, *Fizicheskaya khimiya napolnennyh polimerov*, 1977, Moscow, Khimiya, p. 304.
67. M.T. Bryk, *Destructsiya napolnennyh polimerov*, 1989, Moscow, Khimiya, p. 191.
68. I.R. Mardaleyshvili, V.A. Kutyrkin, O.N. Karpuhin and V.M. Anisimov, *Vysokomolek. Soed.*, 1979, **B21**(10) pp. 834–836.
69. D. Barnard and P. Lewis, *Natural Rubber Science and Technology*, ed. A.D. Roberts, 1988, Oxford university Press, Oxford, 1988, p. 130.
70. M.L. Kaplan, P.G. Kelleher, G.H. Bebbeington and R. Hartless, *J. Polymer Sci.*, Polymer Lett. Ed., 1973, **11**(6), pp. 357–361.
71. E.Ya. Davydov, V.P. Pustoshnyi and A.P. Vorotnikov, *Polymers and Polymer Composites*, 1994, **2**(6), pp. 387–390.
72. V.V. Ershov, G.A. Nikiforov and A.A. Volod'kin, *Space-hindered Phenols*, 1972, Khimiya, Moscow, p. 204.
73. E.C. Horswil and K.U. Ingold, *Canad. J. Chem.*, 1966, **44**(3), pp. 263–268.
74. V.A. Roginskii, *Kinetika I Kataliz*, 1982, **24**(9), pp. 1808–1827.
75. J.A. Howard and K.U. Ingold, *Canad. J. Chem.*, 1965, **43**(10), p. 2724.
76. E.L. Shanina, V.A. Roginskii and G.E. Zaikov, *Vysokomolek. Soed.*, 1986, **A28**(9), pp. 1971–1976.
77. V.A. Roginskii, V.Z. Dubinskii and V.B. Miller, *Izv. Akad. Nauk SSSR, ser. Khimich.*, 1985, 6, pp. 2808–2812.

Properties of Constitutive Equations for Undiluted Linear Polymers Based on the Molecular Theory

V.N. POKROVSKII and YU. G. YANOVSKY

Institute of Applied Mechanics of Russian Academy of Sciences, Moscow, Russia, 117334

YU. A. ALTUKHOV and G.V. PYSHNOGRAI

Altai State Technical University, Barnaul, Russia, 656099

1 INTRODUCTION

There is a long history of molecular approaches to the dynamic properties of a polymer system.

Dilute polymer solutions were considered by 1960 by Kirkwood and Riseman (1948), Rouse (1953), Bueche (1954), Cerf (1958), and others. One of the main models known as the Rouse model can be conceived as a set of Brownian particles in a viscous liquid linearly connected to one another by elastic forces due mainly to entropy forces. It is well known that the Rouse model with properly defined hydrodynamic interaction, excluded volume effects, and internal viscosity is consistent with experimental data.

The theory of dilute polymer solutions is the starting point of the theory of the dynamical properties of non-dilute solutions and polymer melts that can be considered as a system of weakly-coupled macromolecules. The viscoelastic behavior of such a system was the object of investigation of many groups in recent decades.

The strong elasticity of polymer solutions and melts was attributed initially to the network formed owing to temporary knots and/or entanglements. The network theory for the system was elaborated by Green and Tobolsky (1947), Lodge (1956), and Yamamoto (1956–1958).

Later the network concept was found to be wrong, nevertheless the concept of the intermediate length as the length between adjacent entanglements was retained in the reptation/tube theory advanced by de Gennes (1971) and Doi and Edwards (1978, 1979). The reptation concept was developed further in detail by many authors, but it appears to be inadequate to explain all the phenomena in polymer dynamics. A comprehensive discussion of the problem was given by Lodge *et al.* (1990). Despite the popularity of the theory of Doi and Edwards among rheologists, its predictions concerning several phenomena of pivotal significance such as the viscoelasticity of blends and the optical anisotropy of slowly changing motions of macromolecules differ drastically from available data.

Below we discuss the theoretical concepts of the viscoelasticity mechanism of a system of weakly coupled macromolecules developed by Russian scientists beginning from the 1970s. The description of the dynamics of a macromolecule in the system is the corner stone of our theory. We do not assume that a macromolecule moves in a tube as it was done by de Gennes (1971) and Doi and Edwards (1986), nevertheless a scale of localization or an internal length appears in our theory. This localization scale can be interpreted as the radius of a "tube" containing a wriggling macromolecule. But calculations show that its possible reptations above the first order approximations do not contribute substantially to relaxation processes underlying the main features of the viscoelastic behavior of a polymer liquid; the reptations must be considered when dealing with effects of "higher orders". Our theory is indeed a first approximation.

Below we shall consider the initial tenets and prerequisites of the molecular theory of the viscoelastic behavior of concentrated polymer solutions and melts, the basic nonlinear constitutive equations of the theory, and its corollaries for various cases of flow.

2 MACROMOLECULAR FOUNDATION OF CONSTITUTIVE EQUATION

2.1 Dynamics of a Macromolecule in a Concentrated System

To understand the mechanical behavior of an individual macromolecule in its motion among its kindred, it is sufficient to limit oneself to large-scale or slowly changing motions thereof. This makes it possible to model a macromolecule as a system of subchains. Such an approach was employed widely by many investigators when modeling the viscoelasticity and flow of polymers (Ferry, 1980 and Graessley, 1974). Each macromolecule is represented in the form of a chain of linearly bonded Brownian particles numbered from 0 to N and with the coordinates r^0, $r^1, \ldots, r^N$. The ν-th particle experiences the elastic force

$$K_i^\nu = -2\mu T A_{\nu\gamma}\, r_i^\gamma, \tag{2.1}$$

where $\mu = 3N/2\langle R^2\rangle_0$, $\langle R\rangle_0$ is the mean-square end-to-end distance, T is the temperature in energy units, while matrix $A_{\nu\gamma}$ is a Rouse matrix and determines the bond of $N+1$ particles into a linear chain.

In the flow of a system, every Brownian particle moves in the flow with the velocity gradient

$$\nu_{ij} = \partial v_i / \partial x_j.$$

Using the symbols for a symmetrized and antisymmetrized tensor of the velocity gradients, we can write

$$\gamma_{ij} = \frac{1}{2}(\nu_{ij} + \nu_{ji}); \quad \omega_{ij} = \frac{1}{2}(\nu_{ij} - \nu_{ji}).$$

We can thus say that every Brownian particle experiences the effect of the additional forces of hydrodynamic drag F_i^α and internal friction G_i^α. The equation of motion of each of the particles can be written in the form of the Langevin equation:

$$m(\mathrm{d}^2 r_i^\alpha/\mathrm{d}t^2) = -\zeta r_i^\alpha + F_i^\alpha + G_i^\alpha + K_i^\alpha + \Phi_i^\alpha, \tag{2.2}$$

where $\Phi_i^\alpha(t)$ is a random process whose characteristics are defined from a fluctuating-dissipative expression (Pokrovskii and Pyshnograi, 1990).

Such an expression holds both for the motion of a macromolecule in a viscous liquid (in a very simple case $F = G = 0$) and for its motion among its kindred. In the latter case, the after effect must be considered in the expressions for the forces of external F_i^α and internal friction G_i^α respectively:

$$\begin{aligned} F_i^\alpha &= -\int_0^\infty \beta(s)(r_i^\alpha - \nu_{ij} r_j^\alpha)_{t-s}\,\mathrm{d}s \\ G_i^\alpha &= -\int_0^\infty \varphi(s)(r_i^\alpha - \omega_{kj} r_i^\alpha)_{t-s}\,\mathrm{d}s \end{aligned} \tag{2.3}$$

the expressions in parentheses in the integrand were calculated for the $(t - s)$ moment of time.

One can readily see that the equation of dynamics (2.2) with the expressions for the forces (2.1) and (2.3) is the general form of the equation of the dynamics of a macromolecule in a flow to a linear approximation with respect to the coordinates and velocities of the particles. However, if the general form of the equation of dynamics (2.2) and (2.3) is written unambiguously in this case (a linear approximation), the memory functions in (2.3) cannot be established from general considerations. The involving of quite simple model considerations allowed Astarita and Marrucci (1974) to write the memory functions in the form

$$\begin{aligned} \beta(s) &= (\zeta/\tau)Be^{-s/\tau} \\ \varphi(s) &= (\zeta/\tau)Ee^{-s/\tau} \end{aligned} \tag{2.4}$$

As in Equation (2.2), in (2.4) ζ is the coefficient of friction of a Brownian particle in a "monomer" viscous liquid, and τ is a relaxation time of the surroundings that coincides with the calculated main time of mechanical relaxation (Pokrovskii and Volkov, 1978). In other words, the theory is self-consistent. The parameters B and E reflect the influence of the surroundings on the single molecule being considered. With a view to the nonlocal nature of the friction forces, one can estimate the change in these parameters depending on the length of the surrounding macromolecules M. For instance, Pokrovsky (1992) found that

$$B \approx M^\delta, \quad \delta > 2. \tag{2.5}$$

Let us introduce the dimensionless parameters

$$\chi = \tau/2B\tau^* \quad \text{and} \quad \psi = E/B, \tag{2.6}$$

where $\tau^* = \zeta N^2/2T\mu\pi^2$ has the meaning of the characteristic time. From the physical viewpoint, τ^* is the maximum relaxation time of a macromolecule in a "monomeric" viscous liquid.

The theory being considered is featured by the absence of the usually postulated intermediate length that is like the chain length between entanglements of the macromolecules M_e, or tube diameter. It was understood lately that the localization of a macromolecule in "a tube" postulated by de Gennes follows from a formal approach based on equations (2.2)–(2.4). An intermediate length appears that can be identified by the tube radius. Here

$$\chi = (2\zeta)^2/\langle R^2\rangle_0 \approx (M_e/M) \tag{2.7}$$

The last addend in the equation of dynamics (2.2) reflects the presence of a random heat force whose statistical properties, as usually (Chandraskhar, 1943), are determined in such a way that in an equilibrium situation the quantities being calculated would coincide with known ones. With this definition of the random force, Equation 2.2 can be considered as a first approximation (linearity in coordinates, velocities, and velocity gradients) when describing nonequilibrium phenomena in undiluted polymers. With this approach, the effects associated with nonlinear addends, e.g. reptations (De Gennes, 1971) are eliminated. The latter appear with a different mobility of a particle along and across a chain and can be described by using addends higher than the first order.

2.2 Normal Modes and Markov Form of Equation of Dynamics

For convenience of further calculations, we shall use transformed coordinates. They will be introduced with the aid of the orthogonal and normalized matrix Q

$$\begin{aligned} Q^T A Q &= \lambda_\alpha E \\ \lambda_\alpha &= (\pi\alpha/N^2); \quad \alpha = 0, 1, 2, \ldots < N. \end{aligned} \tag{2.8}$$

By introducing the quantities transformed in this way and designated as

$$\rho_i^\alpha = Q^T\, r_i^\alpha; \quad \psi_i^\alpha = Q^T\, \dot{r}_i^\alpha; \quad \Gamma_i^\alpha = Q^T\, F_i^\alpha; \quad T_i^\alpha = Q^T\, G_i^\alpha; \quad f_i^\alpha = Q^T \Phi_i^\alpha; \tag{2.9}$$

into the equation of dynamics (2.2), we obtain a system of differential equations (Pokrovskii and Pyshnograi, 1990).

$$\begin{aligned} \mathrm{d}\rho_i^\alpha/\mathrm{d}t &= \psi_i^\alpha; \\ m(\mathrm{d}\psi_i^\alpha/\mathrm{d}t) &= -\zeta(\psi_i^\alpha - \nu_{ij}\rho_j^\alpha) + \Gamma_i^\alpha + T_i^\alpha - 2T\mu\lambda_\alpha\rho_i^\alpha + f_i^\alpha; \\ (\mathrm{d}\Gamma_i^\alpha/\mathrm{d}t) - \nu_{il}\Gamma_l^\alpha &= (1/\tau)\Gamma_i^\alpha - (\zeta/\tau)B_{ij}(\psi_j^\alpha - \nu_{jl}\rho_l^\alpha); \\ (\mathrm{d}T_i^\alpha/\mathrm{d}t) - \omega_{il}T_i^\alpha &= (1/\tau)T_i^\alpha - (\zeta/\tau)E_{ij}(\psi_j^\alpha - \omega_{jl}\rho_l^\alpha); \end{aligned} \tag{2.10}$$

To achieve generality of the equation of dynamics of a macromolecule in both linear and nonlinear cases, in Equations (2.10) the scalars B_{ij} and E_{ij} were replaced by the tensor B and E, respectively. With a view to the monomolecular approximation, the medium in which a Brownian particle moves is assumed to be anisotropic (on an average), and the anisotropy is determined only by the extended macromolecular coils, i.e. by the tensor (Pyshnograi and Pokrovskii, 1988).

$$a_{ik} = \sum \langle \rho_i^\alpha \rho_k^\alpha \rangle / \langle \rho_j^\alpha \rho_j^\alpha \rangle_0 - \frac{1}{3}\delta_{ik},$$

where $\langle \rho_i^\alpha \rho_k^\alpha \rangle_0$ is the equilibrium value of the correlation moment $\langle \rho_i^\alpha \rho_k^\alpha \rangle$. The averaging is performed over the assembly of realizations of the random process f_i^α.

Hence, B_{ik} and E_{ik} are functions of the indicated tensor. In a linear approximation, the general form of the functions is as follows:

$$\begin{aligned} B_{ik} &= B\left[\delta_{ik} - 3\beta\left(a_{ik} - \frac{1}{3}a_{ll}\,\delta_{ik}\right) - \kappa a_{ll}\,\delta_{ik}\right] \\ E_{ik} &= E\left[\delta_{ik} - 3\varepsilon\left(a_{ik} - \frac{1}{3}a_{ll}\,\delta_{ik}\right) - \nu a_{ll}\,\delta_{ik}\right]. \end{aligned} \tag{2.11}$$

The addends with constant β and ε determine the change in the coefficient of friction of a particle when the shape of the surrounding coils changes and the addends with constant κ and ν when the volume of the coils changes (expansion).

Since at large velocity gradients the deformation of a coil cannot be considered small, linear approximation (2.11) is inadequate. For the more general case considered by Pokrovskii and Pyshnograi (1990), we can employ the convenient approximations

$$\begin{aligned} B_{ik} &= B\left(\delta_{ik} - 3\beta\left(a_{ik} - \frac{1}{3}a_{ll}\,\delta_{ik}\right) - \kappa a_{ll}\,\delta_{ik}\right)^{-1} \\ E_{ik} &= E\left(\delta_{ik} + 3\varepsilon\left(a_{ik} - \frac{1}{3}a_{ll}\,\delta_{ik}\right) + \nu a_{ll}\,\delta_{ik}\right)^{-1}. \end{aligned} \tag{2.12}$$

At low changes of the size of a macromolecular coil, with an accuracy up to first-order terms with respect to the components of the anisotropy tensor, expressions (2.11) and (2.12) coincide.

2.3 Stresses in Deformation

A concentrated polymer solution or melt is a system of entangled chains. When modeling such a system in a monomolecular approximation, we consider that it can be represented in the form of a set of noninteracting macromolecules whose behavior is considered with a view to their neighbors. Each macromolecule is schematized by a chain with $N+1$ Brownian particles so that the system as a whole can be considered as a suspension of Brownian particles in a viscoelastic liquid. The set of Brownian particles can be characterized by the mean density

$$\rho(x,t) = \sum_\alpha m\langle \delta(x - r^\alpha)\rangle = m(N+1)\,n(x,t) \tag{2.13}$$

and the mean pulse density

$$\rho(x,t)\, v(x,t) = \sum_{\alpha} m\langle \dot{r}^{\alpha}\delta(x - r^{\alpha})\rangle \tag{2.14}$$

The angular brackets signify averaging over the ensemble of realizations of the random forces in the equations of motion of the particles. Summation in (2.13) and (2.14) is performed over all the Brownian particles.

When formulating the equations of motion, which consists in deriving an expression for the stress tensor, one must consider the presence of two interacting continuums inserted into each other. They are formed by a carrying viscoelastic liquid and interacting Brownian particles which macromolecules are modeled by. However, the contribution of the carrying medium when dealing with a concentrated solution is insignificant and is no longer considered.

To find the stress tensor, we proceed from the determination of the pulse density (2.14) holding for an arbitrary set of Brownian particles.

By differentiating expression (14) with respect to time and employing quite simple transformations of Equation (2.2) (Pyshnograi and Pokrovskii, 1988), we obtain a standard form of the equation of motion of a continuum:

$$\rho(\mathrm{d}v_i/\mathrm{d}t) = (\partial\sigma_{ij}/\partial x_j)$$

where the stress tensor has the form

$$\sigma_{ij} = -nT\delta_{ij} + n\sum(2\mu\lambda_{\alpha}T\langle\rho_i^{\alpha}\rho_j^{\alpha}\rangle - m\langle\dot{\rho}_i^{\alpha}\dot{\rho}_j^{\alpha}\rangle - \langle\rho_j^{\alpha}T_i^{\alpha}\rangle) \tag{2.15}$$

T_i^{α} is the transformed force of "internal" friction of a macromolecule determined according to (2.9).

Assuming a locally equilibrium distribution by velocities, we can write the stress tensor in the form:

$$\sigma_{ij} = -p\delta_{ij} + 3nT\sum_{\alpha}\left(x_{ij}^{\alpha} - \frac{1}{3}\delta_{ij} - u_{ij}^{\alpha}\right) \tag{2.16}$$

The pressure p includes both the partial pressure of the gas of Brownian particles and $n(N+1)T$, and the pressure of a "monomer" liquid whose viscosity in our opinion could be ignored.

By the monomolecular approach, the stress tensor of a system is determined by the sum of the contributions of all the macromolecules, i.e. by simple multiplication by the number of macromolecules n.

$$x_{ij}^{\alpha} = \frac{2}{3}\mu\lambda_{\alpha}\langle\rho_i^{\alpha}\rho_j^{\alpha}\rangle, \quad u_{ij}^{\alpha} = \frac{1}{3T}\langle\rho_j^{\alpha}T_j^{\alpha}\rangle \tag{2.17}$$

that must be calculated.

The first group of variables in Equation (2.17) characterizes the size and shape of a macromolecular coil and is determined so that in equilibrium $x_{ij}^{\alpha} = \frac{1}{3}\delta_{ij}^{\alpha}$.

The second group of variables is associated with the "internal" stresses appearing because each macromolecule is intertwined with its neighbors.

2.4 Relaxation Equations

To obtain determining equations, we must establish relaxation equations for the internal macroscopic parameters (2.17). To do this, we shall revert to the equation of the dynamics of a macromolecule in form (2.10) with account taken of approximation (2.12). After transformations, we obtain a system of relaxation equations for the internal moments (Pokrovskii and Pyshnograi, 1991)

$$\begin{aligned}(D/Dt)x_{ik}^{\alpha} - (B\tau_{\alpha}^{R}/\tau_{\alpha})(x_{ij}^{\alpha}\gamma_{jl}c_{lk}^{\alpha} + x_{kj}^{\alpha}\gamma_{jl}c_{lk}^{\alpha}) \\ = \frac{1}{2}\tau_{\alpha}\left(x_{ij}^{\alpha} - \frac{1}{3}\delta_{ij}\right)b_{jk}^{\alpha} + \left(x_{kj}^{\alpha} - \frac{1}{3}\delta_{kj}\right)b_{ji}^{\alpha};\end{aligned} \tag{2.18}$$

$$\begin{aligned}(D/Dt)u_{ik}^{\alpha} - (B\tau_{\alpha}^{R}/\tau_{\alpha})e_{ij}^{\alpha}\gamma_{jl}u_{lk}^{\alpha} = -\left(\frac{1}{\tau}\delta_{ij} + \frac{1}{2}\tau_{\alpha}b_{ij}^{\alpha}\right)u_{jk}^{\alpha} \\ + \psi(B\tau_{\alpha}^{R}/\tau\tau_{\alpha})\left(\left(x_{ij}^{\alpha} - \frac{1}{3}\delta_{ij}\right)d_{jk}^{\alpha} - 2B\tau_{\alpha}^{R}x_{il}^{\alpha}\gamma_{lj}f_{jk}^{\alpha}\right).\end{aligned}$$

The auxiliary quantities b_{ik}^{α}, c_{ik}^{α}, d_{ik}^{α}, e_{ik}^{α} and f_{ik}^{α} are determined in terms of the previously introduced parameters characterizing the dynamics of an individual macromolecule in a system

$$b_{ik}^{\alpha} = \left(\delta_{ik} - (B\tau_{\alpha}^{R}/\tau_{\alpha})(\beta_{ik} + \psi\varepsilon_{ik})\right)^{-1};$$

$$c_{ik}^{\alpha} = (\delta_{ij} - \beta_{ij})b_{jk}^{\alpha}; \quad e_{ik}^{\alpha} = b_{ij}^{\alpha}(\delta_{ji} - \beta_{jk});$$

$$d_{ik}^{\alpha} = \mathrm{b}_{ij}^{\alpha}(\delta_{kj} - \varepsilon_{kj}); \quad f_{ik}^{\alpha} = c_{ij}^{\alpha}(\delta_{kj} - \varepsilon_{kj});$$

$$\beta_{ik} = 3\left(\frac{1}{3}\kappa a_{ll}\,\delta_{ij} + \beta\left(a_{ij} - \frac{1}{3}a_{ll}\,\delta_{ij}\right)\right)\left(\delta_{jk} + \left(\kappa a_{ll}\,\delta_{jk} + 3\beta\left(a_{jk} - \frac{1}{3}a_{ll}\,\delta_{jk}\right)\right)\right)^{-1};$$

$$\varepsilon_{ik} = 3\left(\frac{1}{3}\nu a_{ll}\,\delta_{ij} + \varepsilon\left(a_{ij} - \frac{1}{3}a_{ll}\,\delta_{ij}\right)\right)\left(\delta_{jk} + \left(\nu a_{ll}\,\delta_{jk} + 3\varepsilon\left(a_{jk} - \frac{1}{3}a_{ll}\,\delta_{jk}\right)\right)\right)^{-1}.$$

The system of relaxation equations includes the relaxation times

$$\tau; \quad \tau_{\alpha} = \tau/2 + B\tau_{\alpha}^{R}(1+\psi), \quad \tau_{\alpha}^{R} = \tau^{*}/\alpha^{2} \tag{2.19}$$

The relaxation processes by (2.18) are featured, in particular, by anisotropy of relaxation, *viz.* in a deformed system different components of the tensors x_{ik}^{α} and u_{ik}^{α} relax at a different rate.

We shall consider below the conclusions of the theory and its applications for various cases of deformation.

2.5 Discussion of the Approach

Initially our concept was based on some rather formal approaches of macromolecule dynamics and some suggestions of a general kind (Pokrovskii and Volkov, 1978).

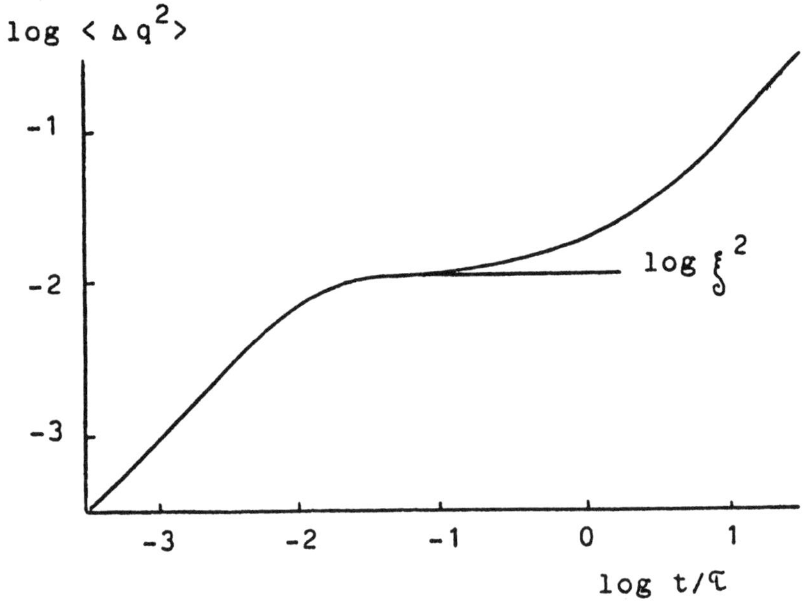

Figure 1 The displacement of the center of mass of a macromolecule depends on the intermediate length ξ-scale. The displacement is measured in units of $(\tau\langle R^2\rangle/\pi^2\tau^*)^{\frac{1}{2}}$.

Later the picture of thermal motion of macromolecules in non-dilute system was clarified step by step (Pokrovskii and Kokorin, 1985, 1987). The thermal motion is featured by localization of a macromolecule near its initial position. Figure 1 shows the displacement of a macromolecule and the intermediate length ξ that is similar to the length ξ between adjacent entanglements. The motion of macromolecule is so constrained by the surrounding chains that its motion is essentially equivalent to the motion of the macromolecule in an effective tube. But this does not mean that there is reptation inside the tube.

We can discuss this in more detail as answers to the questions posed by Lodge *et al.* (1990, pp. 16–17).

1. Do linear polymer chains execute primarily reptation over a nonvanishing region of parameter space?

No. Reptation is a very weak effect that can be manifest in special cases noted by Lodge *et al.* (1990, p. 117) as strict reptation: "sufficiently long tracer chains surrounded by a matrix of much longer chains, and unattached chains in a regular network". It is incorrect to consider reptation as a first approximation of the theory of relaxation of macromolecules.

- What is fundamentally incorrect in the reptation model?

The postulation of reptation as the main form of thermal motion of macromolecules is incorrect.

- What is the strongest evidence against reptation?

The strongest evidence against reptation is the discrepancies of the results for the viscoelasticity of a dilute blend of a linear polymer (Yanovsky *et al.* 1980, Vinogradov *et al.* 1982, Pokrovskii and Kokorin 1985, Yanovsky 1993).

- What is the most promising alternative approach?

We most likely set out the best monomacromolecular approach that includes all the features of behavior of linear polymers.

The Schweizer's (1989a, 1989b, 1991) monomacromolecular approach is naturally better, but it is not completed yet.

- Why does the reptation picture seem to agree with so many observations?

Some effects are consequences not of reptation, but of constraints of motion with an internal length postulated in the reptation theory that appears in our theory as a localization effect. Besides, the reptation theory has its region of validity as pointed out by Lodge *et al.* (1990, p. 117).

2. What further experiments, if any, are required to answer question 1 without any reasonable doubt?

A comparison of dynamic birefringence and the dynamic modulus. Investigation of birefringence and viscoelasticity of a dilute blend of polymers. The predictions of the reptation theory and our theory are quite different (Pokrovskii and Kokorin, 1985, 1987).

3. In what direction should future theoretical efforts be aimed?

The main direction of future theoretical efforts should be investigation of multi-macromolecular approaches.

These are replies to the questions of Lodge *et al.* (1990, pp. 16–17).

Despite the continuing research into the problem there is no evidence of any conflict between the large volume of experimental data that has now accumulated and the discussed theory.

3 UNIFORM MOTION WITH LOW VELOCITY GRADIENTS

System of equations (2.16) and (2.18) determines the stresses in a polymer liquid as functions of velocity gradients, in other words system of equations (2.16) and (2.18) is a constitutive equation of a polymer liquid that was formulated by proceeding from principles based on the dynamics of individual macromolecules. To compare the theoretical predictions with experimental results, let us first consider low velocity gradients.

3.1 Dynamic Modulus

The viscoelastic behavior of a polymer system is manifest in the typical way in uniform oscillating motion:

$$\nu_{12} \sim e^{-i\omega t}$$

The expressions for the stresses and moments in a linear case also determine the expression for the dynamic modulus, which in the general case has the form (Yanovsky *et al.* 1988, Pokrovskii 1992, Yanovsky 1993)

$$G^*(\omega) = nTf(\tau^*\omega, B, \chi, \psi). \tag{3.1}$$

The frequency dependence of the dynamic modulus is shown in Figure 2 and in the approximation considered here (at low frequencies) is determined by relaxation processes with two sets of relaxation times whose values are determined by equations (2.18)

$$\tau_\alpha = B\tau^*[\chi + \alpha^{-2}(1+\psi)], \quad \tau_\alpha^0 = 2\tau\tau_\alpha/(\tau + 2\tau_\alpha). \tag{3.2}$$

It should be noted that the indicated curve has two relaxation branches. The one with slower relaxation processes due to the change in the average size of a macromolecule is hardly manifest on the frequency dependence of the dynamic modulus, though the reptation relaxation processes ought to be identified exactly with this branch.

The intermediate plateau in the modulus is associated with the intermediate length

$$G_e = \frac{\pi^2}{12} nT\chi^{-1}. \tag{3.3}$$

It is clear from the picture that the main relaxation branch is the one numbered 2. Its set of relaxation times (3.2) is not wide and can be approximated with a single relaxation time τ that coincides with the introduced relaxation time τ. Hence at $\psi \to \infty$ we have self-consistency without any extra requirement. The requirement of the equality of relaxation times of macro- and microviscoelasticity gives a first order a relation with respect to ψ^{-1}

$$\psi = \frac{4}{\pi^2}\chi^{-1} \tag{3.4}$$

Recently Leonov (1994) attempted to improve the theory by focusing on the formulation of the true self-consistency condition for the model, that is the requirement of equality of the micro- and macroviscoelasticities.

However, simple reasoning shows that "the true self-consistency condition" cannot be reached. Indeed, a macromolecule in a viscous fluid gives one set of relaxation times, in a fluid with one relaxation time gives a several sets of relaxation times, and so on. That is why in our papers we stopped using the "true self-consistency condition" and discussed the correlation between the relaxation times of micro- and macroviscoelasticity. A self-consistency condition of this kind was discussed by Pokrovskii (1992).

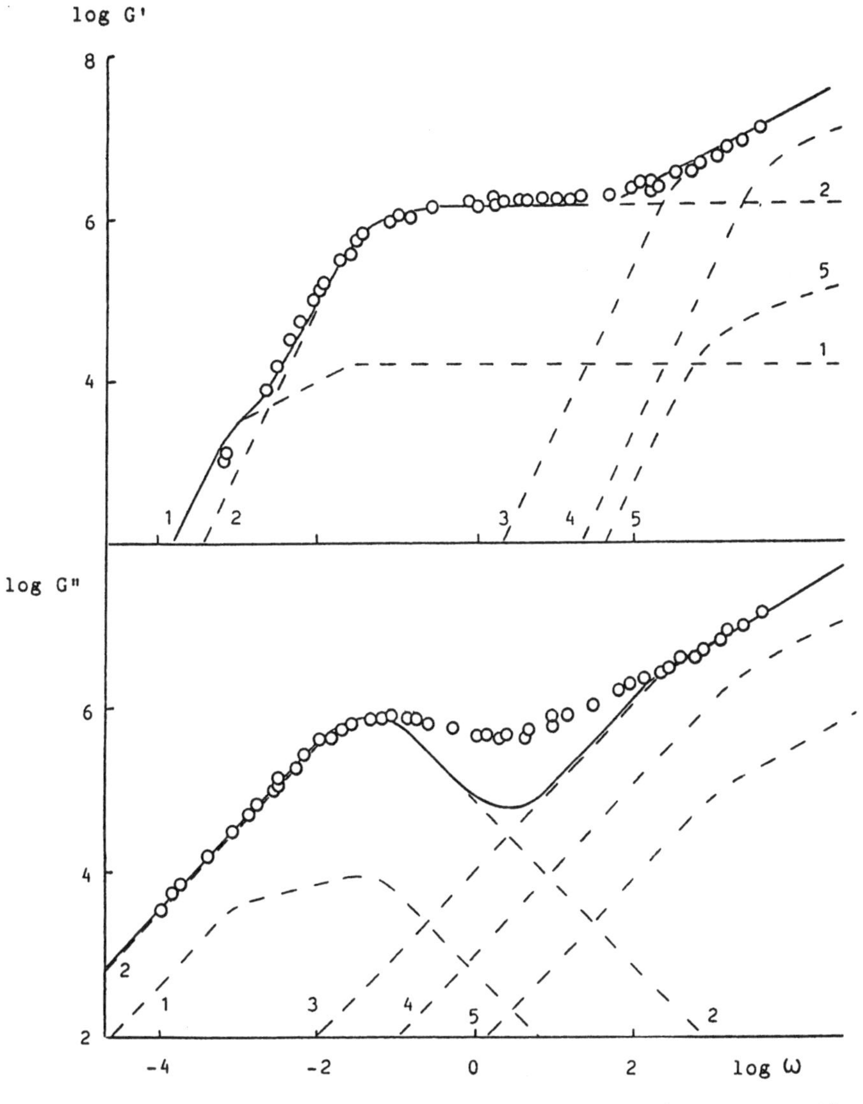

Figure 2 Experimental and theoretical frequency dependences of the real G' and imaginary G'' components of the dynamic shear modulus. The points were reproduced from S. Onogi, *et al.* (1970) for polystyrene with a molecular weight of 215000 at 160°C. The theoretical values indicated by the dashed lines were calculated for values of $B = 3 \times 10^6$; $E = 2 \times 10^4$; $\chi = 0.08$; τ^*; $\tau^* = 5 \times 10^{-5}$ s and $nT = 1.7 \times 10^5$ dyn.cm^{-2}.

3.2 Steady Simple Shear

In steady shear, to a first approximation according to the velocity gradient, only the shear stress differs from zero:

$$\sigma_{12}^0 = \eta_0 \nu_{12}; \quad \eta_0 = \frac{\pi}{6} nTB\tau^*. \tag{3.5}$$

Approximations of a higher order reveal that normal stresses are also needed to realize shear strain. For low values of the parameters χ, ψ and β (here $\beta = \kappa, \varepsilon = \nu$), it was found that (Pokrovskii and Kokorin, 1985)

$$\sigma_{12} = \eta\nu_{12}$$

$$\eta = \eta_0\left[1 - \left(\frac{\sigma_{12}^0}{nT}\right)^2\left(\frac{72}{315}\psi + \frac{72}{15}\pi^2\chi\right)\right]$$

$$\sigma_{11} + p = nT\left(\frac{\pi^4}{45} + \frac{\pi^2}{6}\chi - \frac{\pi^4}{90}\beta\right)(B\tau^*\nu_{12})^2 \tag{3.6}$$

$$\sigma_{22} + p = nT\left(\frac{\pi^2}{6}\chi + \frac{\pi^4}{90}\beta\right)(B\tau^*\nu_{12})^2$$

$$\sigma_{33} + p = 0$$

In summarizing the results obtained in (3.4), we must note three factors causing the appearance of nonlinear effects in shear, namely, (i) the effective nonlinear rigidity of a macromolecule (ψ), (ii) the after effect of the surroundings (χ), and (iii) the effects connected with a change in the size and shape of the macromolecular coils (β).

We can obtain relations for shear strain from expressions (3.4):

$$\sigma_{11} - \sigma_{33} = \frac{1}{nT}\left(\frac{4}{5} + \frac{6}{\pi^2}\chi - \frac{4}{10}\beta\right)\sigma_{12}^2$$

$$\frac{\sigma_{22} - \sigma_{33}}{\sigma_{11} - \sigma_{33}} = -\frac{15}{2\pi^2} - \frac{1}{2}\beta \tag{3.7}$$

They can be verified experimentally by data typical for concentrated polymer systems (Graessley, 1974), the first difference of the normal stresses $\sigma_{11} - \sigma_{33}$ is proportional to the square of the shear stresses in the region of low velocity gradients. The second difference of the normal stresses $\sigma_{22} - \sigma_{33}$ is low in comparison with the first one, which conforms with the previous statement on the smallness of the parameters β and χ.

3.3 Extentional Flow

Steady uniaxial extentional flow is studied on the basis of equations (2.16) and (2.18).

Stickfort (1986) showed that the steady extentional viscosity could be represented vs. the shear stress σ as follows:

$$\lambda(\sigma) = \frac{3}{2\gamma(\sigma)} \cdot \frac{1}{1 - \frac{1}{3}\alpha(\sigma)\sigma}$$

where $\gamma(\sigma)$ and $\alpha(\sigma)$ are phenomenological functions, the slip and anisotropy of the flow coefficients, respectively. On the basis of the constitutive equations (2.16) and (2.18), Pyshnograi (1994) calculated the first terms in the series of $\gamma(\sigma)$ and $\alpha(\sigma)$ by degrees of tensile stresses. With precision of the second order with respect to σ, we have

$$\gamma(\bar{\sigma}) = \gamma_0\left(1 - \frac{16}{525}\left(\frac{4}{3} - 11\beta\right)\bar{\sigma}^2\right)$$
$$\alpha(\bar{\sigma}) = \frac{2\pi^2}{15}\cdot\frac{\gamma_0^2}{\gamma(\bar{\sigma})}\left(1 - 3\beta - \frac{4}{3}\left(\frac{8}{105} + 7\beta\right)\bar{\sigma}^2\right) \tag{3.8}$$

where $\gamma_0 = 3/\pi^2 nTB\tau^*$ and $\bar{\sigma} = \sigma/nT$.

This relations correspond to the information given by Stickforth (1986) on the functions $\gamma(\sigma)$ and $\alpha(\sigma)$, which was obtained from experimental data. The last relation in (3.8) determines the relation between the phenomenological (macro) anisotropy and micro anisotropy coefficient β.

4 CONSTITUTIVE EQUATION FOR FLOWABLE SYSTEM

It can be seen from the preceding section that the system of constitutive equations (2.16) and (2.18), not with standing the simplifying assumptions, is quite cumbersome. To facilitate further calculations, it is expedient to employ additional assumptions, in particular, low values of some parameters of the theory. (It must be stressed, however, that in principle the investigation of a quite general case is also possible.)

4.1 Condition of Flowability

The irreversible flow of a system becomes appreciable for observation times longer than the relaxation times of a macromolecule, the longest of which is, according to (3.2)

$$\tau_1 = \tau(1 + \chi + \psi)/2\chi \tag{4.1}$$

In analyzing the system of equations, we can note that the parameter χ by the meaning of the problem posed [see expression (2.7)] changes within the range of values from 0.01 to 0.1 We can consider it to be small with adequate grounds. At the same time, the parameter ψ may have either large or small values, which corresponds to two different cases of behavior of the system. At large values of ψ and low velocity gradients, the relaxation times [see Equation 3.2] of the first set of variables considerably exceed the relaxation times of the second set, for which $\tau_\alpha^0 = \tau$ holds in this case. Actually, these relaxation times are manifest as a single main one—the most noticeable relaxation time determining the viscoelastic behavior of a system as a whole. Since the relaxation processes with the first set of relaxation times contribute only slightly to the stresses, i.e. are actually not noticeable, the durations of flow are compared with the relaxation time τ and the system is perceived as a non flowing one.

In the other limiting case when $\psi \ll 1$, the systems are perceived as flowing ones. This case is the most interesting for applications connected, in particular, with the theory of polymer article molding.

Since for cases of flow, the system of equations (2.16) and (2.18) can be simplified because of the low values of the parameters χ and ψ, we shall discuss below the results obtained exactly in the approximation to first-order terms with respect to χ and ψ.

4.2 Zero-Order Approximation

We shall now discuss the possible simplification of the indicated expressions with respect to χ and ψ holding for any arbitrary velocity gradients. In this case from equations (2.16) and (2.18) in the zero approximation in parameters χ and ψ we obtain a system of constitutive relations.

Then we retain the only internal variable characterizing the highest relaxation times and obtain relations for the stress tensor and an equation for the internal variable

$$\begin{aligned}
\sigma_{ij} &= -p\delta_{ij} + 3\frac{h_0}{\tau_0}\left(\xi_{ij} - \frac{1}{3}\delta_{ij}\right) \\
\frac{d\xi_{ij}}{dt} - \nu_{il}\,\xi_{lj} - \nu_{jl}\,\xi_{li} &= -\frac{1}{\tau_0}(1 + (\kappa - \beta)\xi_{ss})\left(\xi_{ij} - \frac{1}{3}\delta_{ij}\right) \\
&\quad - 3\frac{\beta}{\tau_0}\left(\xi_{il} - \frac{1}{3}\delta_{il}\right)\left(\xi_{lj} - \frac{1}{3}\delta_{lj}\right)
\end{aligned} \tag{4.2}$$

The system includes the characteristics of the material: η_0 is the initial shear viscosity, τ_0 is the initial relaxation time, κ and β determine the effect of changing of the volume (κ) and form (β) of a molecular coil on the macromolecule dynamics.

One of the properties of constitutive equations (4.2) is the anisotropy of relaxation: different components of the tensor ξ_{il} approach equilibrium at a different rate. When anisotropy is disregarded ($\beta = 0$), system of equations (4.2) takes on a simpler form

$$\begin{aligned}
\sigma_{ij} &= -p\delta_{ij} + 3\frac{\eta}{\tau}\left(\xi_{ij} - \frac{1}{3}\delta_{ij}\right) \\
\frac{D\xi_{ij}}{Dt} - \gamma_{il}\xi_{lj} - \gamma_{jl}\xi_{li} &= -\frac{1}{\tau D}\left(\xi_{ij} - \frac{1}{3}\delta_{ij}\right) \\
\tau D &= \frac{\tau_0}{1 + \kappa D/3}; \qquad a_{ss} = \xi_{ss} - 1.
\end{aligned} \tag{4.3}$$

The quantity η in system (4.3) has the meaning of the shear viscosity coefficient and depends on the invariance of the tensor a_{ij} in the same way as the relaxation time

$$\frac{\eta}{\eta_0} = \frac{\tau}{\tau_0} = \left(1 + \frac{1}{3}\kappa D\right)^{-1} = \varphi(D) \tag{4.4}$$

The subscript "0" signifies the initial (independent of the argument) values of the relevant quantities.

The argument of the shear viscosity coefficient and relaxation time in the approximation being considered has the meaning of the first invariant of the tensor of additional stresses

$$D = 3a_{ss} = 3(\xi_{ss} - 1) = \frac{\tau_0}{\eta_0}(\sigma_{ss} + 3p) \tag{4.5}$$

Consequently, in a very simple variant, the system of determining equations (4.3)–(4.5) contains two rheological parameters: the initial shear viscosity η_0 and the initial relaxation time τ_0, as well as the dimensionless function $\varphi(D)$.

4.3 Steady Simple Shear

In practice, the properties of a polymer liquid were mainly studied by uniform shear, that is, only one component of the gradient rate tensor differs from 0, namely, $\nu_{12} \neq 0$. However, in analyzing the shear deformation of viscoelastic media, we have to take into account not only the tangential stresses σ_{12}, as for linear viscoelastic liquids, but also the normal stresses. The latter can be set as the difference of the normal stresses $\sigma_{11} - \sigma_{22}$ and $\sigma_{22} - \sigma_{33}$. The stresses under consideration are defined as

$$\sigma_{12} = \eta\nu_{12}; \quad \sigma_{11} - \sigma_{22} = \psi_1\nu_{12}^2; \quad \sigma_{22} - \sigma_{33} = \psi_2\nu_{12}^2 \tag{4.6}$$

In a theoretical interpretation of the coefficients of shear viscosity η and normal stresses ψ_1 and ψ_2, in general, one can assume $\beta \neq 0$. In this case the system of equations (2.2) defines the above coefficients as functions of the gradient rates.

Figures 3, 4 shows the steady shear viscosity η versus the dimensionless shear rate $\tau_0\nu_{12}$ for various values of the parameters κ and β. The curves in Figure 3 show that as β increases, the deviation of η from η_0 also increases. It should be noted that variation of the parameter κ has a small affect on the values of the viscosimetric functions. Figure 5 shows the shear stress versus the dimensionless shear rate for various values of the parameters β. If $\beta < \kappa$, the value of the shear stress is an increasing function of the shear rate that is consistent with experimental data.

In Figure 6, the first normal stress coefficient ψ_1 is plotted versus the shear rate and diminishes when the latter grows.

The dependence of the ratio of the second normal stress difference to the first one ψ_2/ψ_1 is given in Figure 7. This ratio is negative and decreases depending on the magnitude of a function of the dimensionless shear rate. This also agrees with experimental data.

If the gradient rates are small, the parameters η, ψ_1 and ψ_2 with a second order approximation can be written as follows:

$$\eta = \eta_0\left[1 - \frac{1}{3}(2\kappa + 7\beta)\right]; \quad \psi_1 = 2\eta_0\tau_0; \quad \psi_2 = -\beta\eta_0\tau_0 \tag{4.7}$$

Comparison of the theoretical calculated data (Figures 3–7) and the experimental results shows that the above theory gives sufficiently reliable relations, observed experimentally. Particularly, the second difference of normal stresses is negative and small in comparison with the first one (Graessley, 1974). It shows the anisotropy coefficient to be a small quantity.

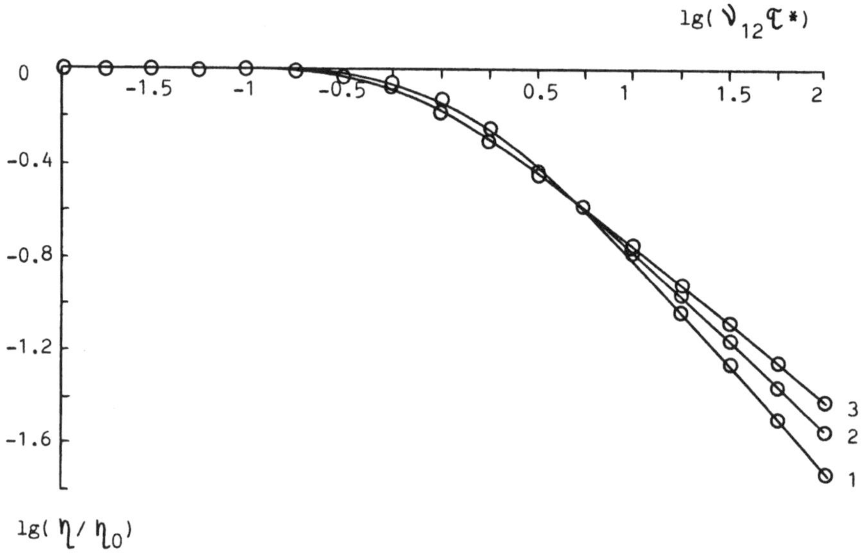

Figure 3 Viscosity vs. shear rate for different values of the parameter κ: 1—0.2; 2—0.3; 3—1.0. $\beta = 0.2$.

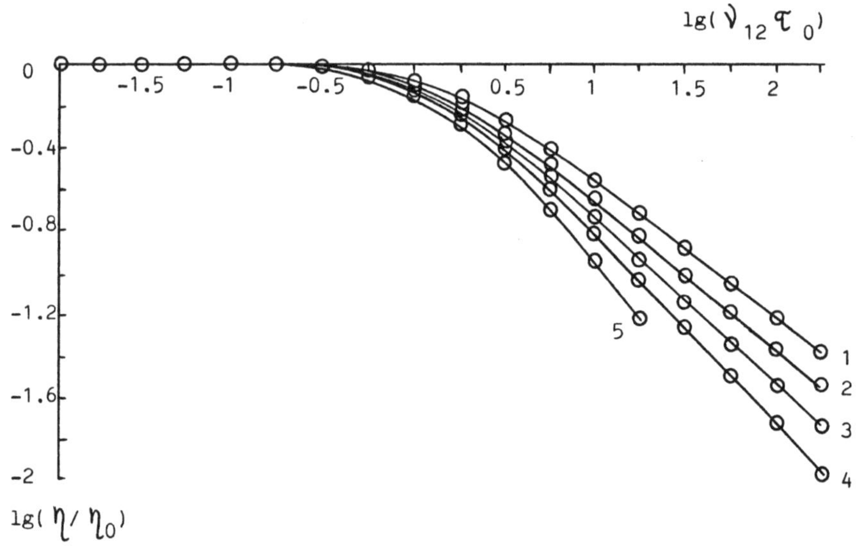

Figure 4 Viscosity vs. shear rate for different values of the parameter β: 1—0.05; 2—0.1; 3—0.15; 4—0.2; 5—0.3. $\kappa = 0.2$.

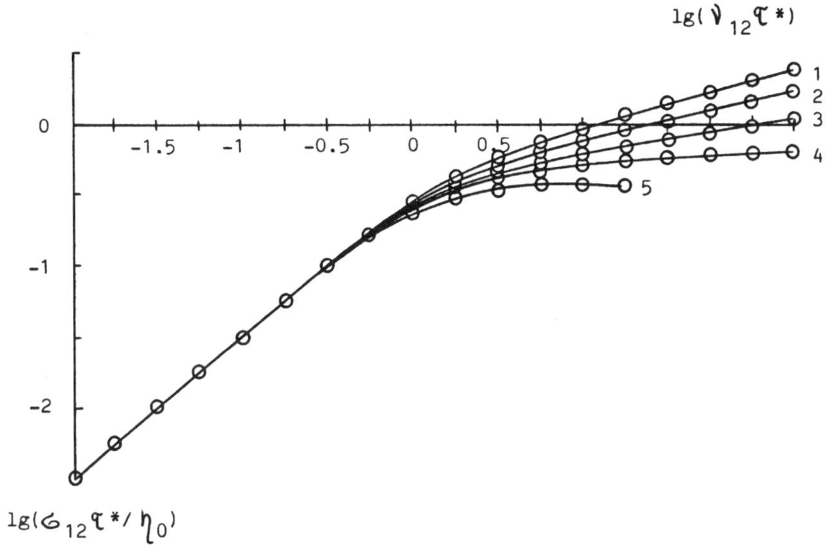

Figure 5 Shear stress vs. shear rate for different values of the parameter β (see Figure 4 for the curves). $\kappa = 0.2$.

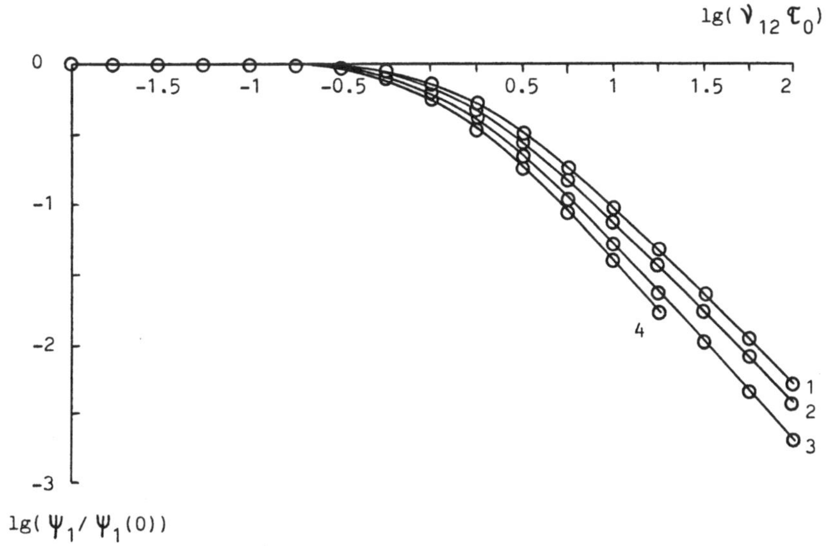

Figure 6 First normal stress coefficient vs. the shear rate for different values of the parameter β: 1—0.05; 2—0.1; 3—0.2; 4 —0.3. $\kappa = 0.2\beta$: 1—0.05; 2—0.1; 3—0.2; 4— 0.3. $\kappa = 0.2$.

At small magnitudes of the gradient rates, the ratio of the normal stress difference depends only on the anisotropy coefficient:

$$\frac{\sigma_{22} - \sigma_{33}}{\sigma_{11} - \sigma_{33}} = -\frac{1}{2}\beta \tag{4.8}$$

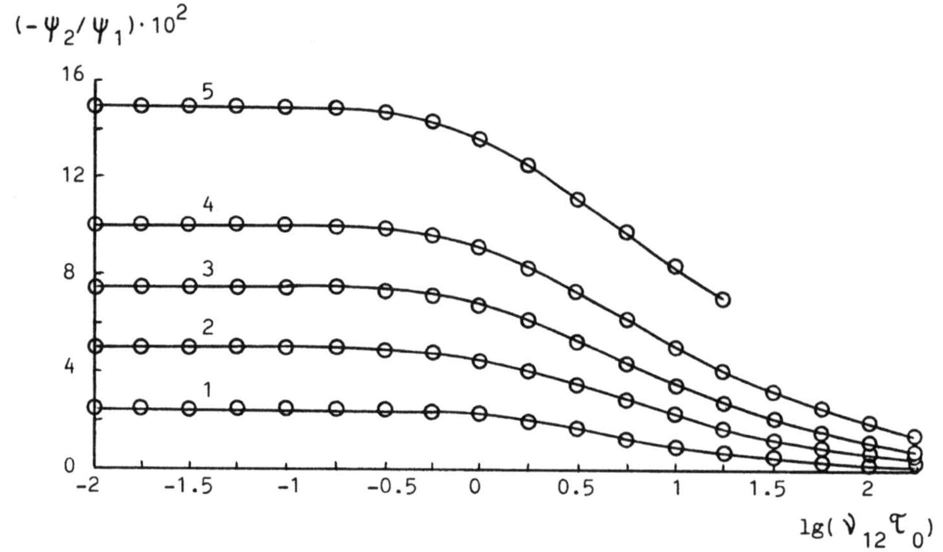

Figure 7 Ratio of the second normal stress difference to the first one vs. the shear rate for different values of the parameter β (see Figure 4 for the curves). $\kappa = 0.2$.

Figure 7 shows such a ratio for an arbitrary value of the gradient rate.

In the zero approximation of a viscoelastic flow, the ratio of the normal stress difference should not depend on the macromolecule length.

For experimental verification of the above inference, one must obtain the value of this ratio for samples characterized well by the molecular parameters. Unfortunately, in view of the problems connected with difficulties of measuring the second normal stress difference investigations of this kind still remain incomplete.

One can notice that when $\beta = 0$ for simple shear, the following expressions can be obtained from systems (4.3)

$$\eta = \eta_0 \Big/ \left(1 + \frac{1}{3}\kappa D\right); \quad \tau = \tau_0 \Big/ \left(1 + \frac{1}{3}\kappa D\right); \quad \psi_1 = 2\eta\tau; \quad \psi_2 = 0; \qquad (4.9)$$

where $D = \tau_0/\eta_0(\sigma_{ss} + 3p)$ is the first dimensionless invariant of the additional stress tensor. Expressions (4.9) are more approximate in comparison with (4.6) and (4.7).

4.4 Relation Between Shear and Extentional Viscosity Coefficients

Consider the case of employing system (4.3) to describe the uniaxial tension of a polymer liquid with an extentional viscosity coefficient λ(λ is determined by the ratio of the tensile stress σ to the velocity gradient ν_{11}). We shall calculate the ratio between the coefficients of extentional λ and shear viscosity η, namely, the quantity λ/η by using system of equations (4.2). For uniform uniaxial tension of a polymer liquid along axis 1, the tensor of the velocity gradients (the values of ν_{11} do not depend on the coordinates) with a view to the conditions of incompressibility can be written in the form

$$\nu_{ik} = \begin{Vmatrix} \nu_{11} & 0 & 0 \\ 0 & -\frac{1}{2}\nu_{11} & 0 \\ 0 & 0 & -\frac{1}{2}\nu_{11} \end{Vmatrix}$$

Excluding the pressure from the relations for the stresses [see system of equations (4.3)] because we are considering uniaxial tension, we obtain an expression for the tensile stress

$$\sigma = 3\frac{\eta}{\tau}(\xi_{11} - \xi_{22}) = 3\eta(2\xi_{11} + \xi_{22})\nu_{11} \tag{4.10}$$

where

$$\xi_{ii} = \frac{1}{3} + \frac{2\tau\nu_{ii}}{1 - 2\nu_{ii}\tau} \tag{4.11}$$

The tensile stress in the steady case characterizes the apparent extentional viscosity

$$\lambda = 3\frac{\eta}{1 - \tau\nu_{11} - 2(\tau\nu_{11})^2} \tag{4.12}$$

Figure 8 shows the steady extentional viscosity λ versus the dimensionless elongational rate $\nu_{11}\tau_0$ for different values of the parameters $\kappa = \beta$. Here the extentional viscosity increases with the extentional rate.

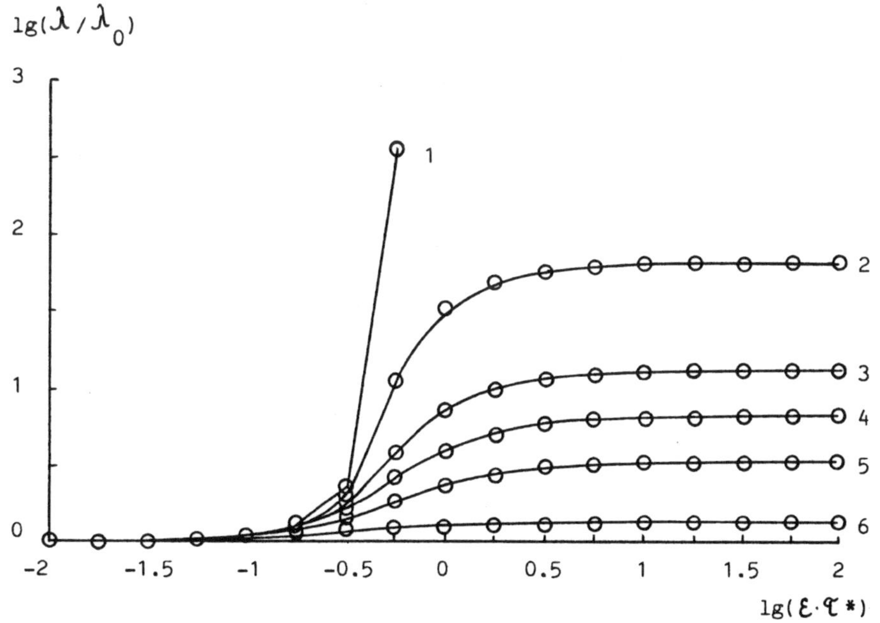

Figure 8 Elongational viscosity vs. elongational rate for different values of the parameter $\beta = \kappa$: 1—0.0; 2—0.01; 3—0.05; 4—0.1; 5—0.2; 6—0.5.

The viscosity coefficients η and λ are functions of the first invariant of the tensor of stresses

$$D = \frac{\tau_0}{\eta_0}(\sigma_{ii} + 3p)$$

which with the aid of expressions (4.7) and (4.8) is written in terms of the velocity gradient

$$D = \frac{\lambda}{\eta} 2(\tau\nu_{11})^2 \tag{4.13}$$

Analysis of expressions (4.9) and (4.10) enables us to obtain an expression for the ratio of the coefficients of extentional and shear viscosity

$$\frac{\lambda}{\eta} = 3 + \frac{5}{4}D + \sqrt{\left(\frac{3}{2}D + \frac{9}{16}D^2\right)} \tag{4.14}$$

For shear strain, the invariant D has the form:

$$D = 2\left(\frac{\tau_0}{\eta_0}\sigma_{12}\right)^2 \tag{4.15}$$

and for uniaxial tension

$$D = \frac{1}{2}\left[-3 - \frac{\tau_0}{\eta_0}\sigma + \left(9 + 6\frac{\tau_0}{\eta_0}\sigma + 9\left(\frac{\tau_0}{\eta_0}\sigma\right)^2\right)^{\frac{1}{2}}\right] \tag{4.16}$$

It should be noted that when deriving expression (4.14) we used the assumption that η and λ are functions of D, but we did not give the specific form of this function.

Expression (4.14) makes it possible to see whether the system of equations (2.3) discussed above can be employed to describe flows of polymer liquids differing in their nature.

Figure 9 presents experimental values of λ/η depending on D for numerous polymer systems in comparison with theoretical calculations by formula (4.16). The experimental results can be seen to have a definite scatter relative to the theoretical curve, which can be ascribed to both natural experimental errors and the necessity of introducing theoretical corrections associated with the parameters χ and ψ. However, the observed consistence of the experimental and theoretical appraisals can be considered satisfactory. This points to the possibility of employing the proposed theoretical relations for describing the properties of various types of polymer systems.

We draw attention to the fact that expression (4.12) equals infinity when $\nu_{11} = \frac{1}{2}\tau$. This feature has no real physical meaning, but is connected with the fact that expression (4.12) holds for small tensions and, consequently, for low velocity gradients, when the following condition is observed for the velocity gradient:

$$2\tau\nu_{11} \ll 1$$

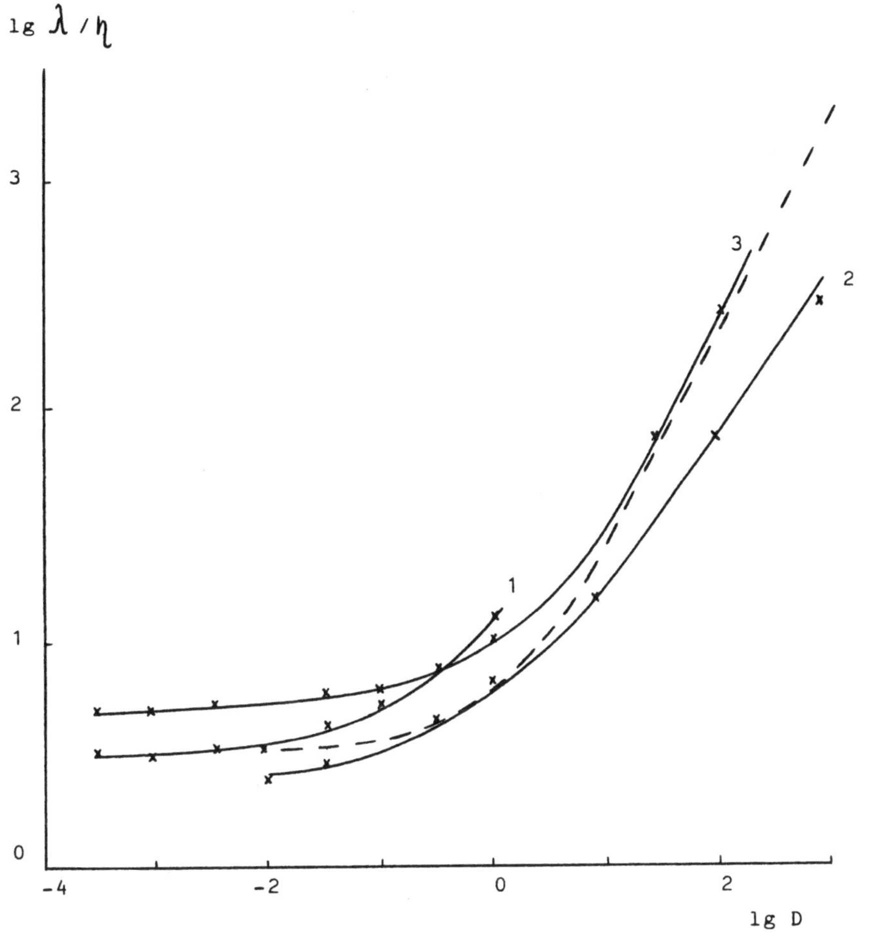

Figure 9 Theoretical (dashed line) and experimental (solid lines) dependences of the ratio of the longitudinal and shear viscosity coefficients on the invariant tensor of additional stresses for the systems listed in the table.

or an equivalent condition is observed for the applied stress

$$\frac{\tau_0}{\eta_0}\sigma \ll \frac{1}{2}\frac{\lambda}{\eta}$$

The values of λ/η calculated by formulas (4.14) for large stress values approach the boundary of the applicability region asymptotically. Hence, theory does not lead to infinite stresses that may exceed the actually observed ones. The use of Equation 4.14 with large stress values also has restrictions because of an initial prerequisite introduced into the theory, namely, on the unlimited stretching of a macromolecule. This condition is naturally not observed in a real situation because a macromolecule can stretch only to a certain limit.

4.5 Nonsteady Simple Shear

To consider the problem, let us compile constitutive equations for small velocity gradients. In this case, we consider a quite simple case when the nonlinear effects are associated only with a change in the volume of the macromolecular coils. In expressions (2.18), the values of $\beta = \varepsilon = 0$ correspond to this condition. We can see here that the effects connected with anisotropy of relaxation are eliminated, and the system of relaxation equations acquires the form:

$$\tau_\alpha\left(Dx_{ik}^\alpha/Dt\right) - \left[B\tau_\alpha^R/(1+\kappa a_{ss})\right]\left(\gamma_{il}x_{ik}^\alpha + \gamma_{kl}x_{li}^\alpha\right) = -\left(x_{ik}^\alpha - \frac{1}{3}\delta_{ik}\right) \tag{4.17}$$

$$\begin{aligned} &\tau_\alpha^0\left(Du_{ik}^\alpha/Dt\right) - \left(B\tau_\alpha^R/(1+\kappa a_{ss})\right)\left(\tau_\alpha^0/\tau_\alpha\right)\gamma_{il}u_{lk}^\alpha \\ &\quad = u_{ik}^\alpha - \left(B\tau_\alpha^R/(1+\kappa a_{ss})\right)\left(E\tau_\alpha^R/(1+\nu a_{ss})\right)\left(2\tau_\alpha^0/\tau\tau_\alpha\right)\gamma_{il}x_{lk}^\alpha \\ &\quad + \left(E\tau_\alpha^R/(1+\nu a_{ss})\right)\left(\tau_\alpha^0/\tau\tau_\alpha\right)\left(x_{ik}^\alpha - \frac{1}{3}\delta_{ik}\right) \end{aligned} \tag{4.18}$$

where the following values are used for the relaxation times:

$$\begin{aligned} \tau_\alpha &= \tau/2 + \tau_\alpha^R(B/(1+\kappa a_{ss}) + E/(1+\nu a_{ss}) \\ \tau_\alpha^0 &= (2\tau\tau_\alpha)/(\tau + 2\tau_\alpha); \quad \tau_\alpha^R = \tau^*/\alpha^2; \end{aligned}$$

Equations (2.16), (4.17) and (4.18) form a system of constitutive equations of a linear polymer with two sets of internal relaxation variables.

According to the structure of Equation (4.19), the quantities u_{ik}^α are proportional to E, hence in the indicated equation we can assume that

$$\tau_\alpha = (B\tau_\alpha^R)/(1+\kappa a_{ss}); \quad \tau_\alpha^0 = \tau \tag{4.19}$$

This enables us to write the following expression instead of (4.18)

$$\begin{aligned} \tau(Du_{ik}^\alpha/Dt) - \tau\gamma_{il}u_{lk}^\alpha &= -u_{ik}^\alpha + \psi[(1+\kappa a_{ss})/(1+\nu a_{ss})]\left(x_{ik}^\alpha - \frac{1}{3}\delta_{ik}\right) \\ &\quad - 2\psi[(1+\kappa a_{ss})/(1+\nu a_{ss})](\tau_\alpha\gamma_{il}x_{lk}^\alpha); \end{aligned} \tag{4.20}$$

and hence the system of equations (2.16), (4.17) and (4.20) with an accuracy within first-order terms with respect to χ and ψ is exactly a system of constitutive equations for flowing polymer systems.

As an example confirming the possibilities of employing the above expressions for practical estimates, we shall compare the results of theoretical calculations with experimental ones. This is shown in Figure 10 in the form of a plot of the shear stresses vs. the shear strain. (It should be noted that the normal stresses evaluated for this case also vary nonmonotonically (Grebnev and Pokrovskii, 1987).) The comparison of the experimental and theoretical relations (Figure 10) can be considered as satisfactory only for comparatively low velocity gradients. This is not surprising, by the way, because considerable velocity gradients should lead to considerable anisotropy, which in the given example was not considered.

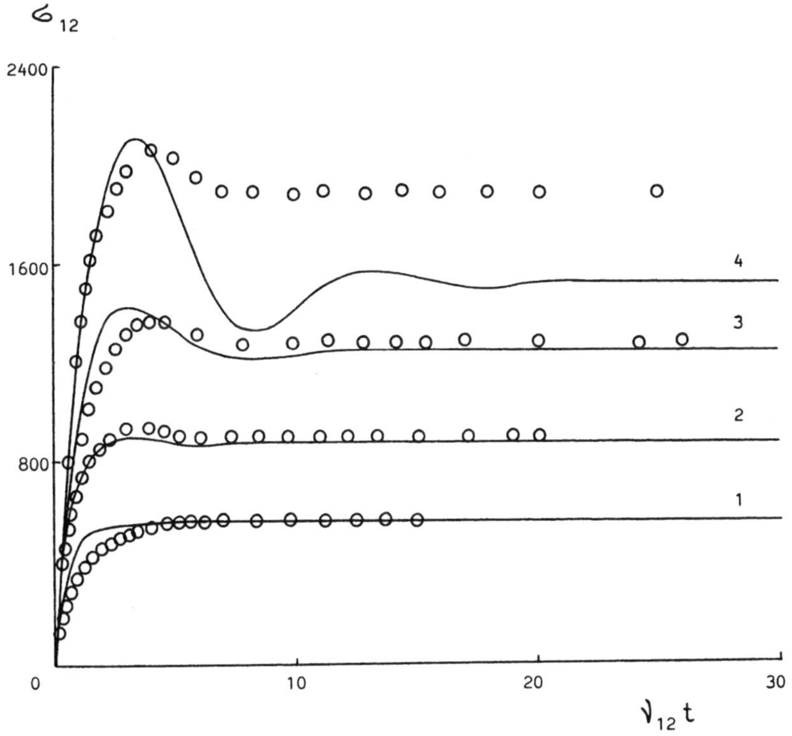

Figure 10 Experimental values (dots, according to Trapeznikov A. and Korotina T., 1971) and theoretical plot of the shear stress vs. the shear strain (solid lines) for velocity gradients of: 1—0.0182; 2—0.0313; 3—0.0627; 4—0.125 s^{-1}. The theoretical curves were plotted for values of $nT = 1270\,\text{dyn.cm}^{-2}$; $\eta_0 = 27.5$ s; $\chi = 0.11$; $\psi = 12$.

It can be seen from (4.6) that the time dependences of the shear and normal stresses with a steady shear flow (a constant velocity gradient) with a view to the adopted simplifications are monotonic. (Compare with the results in Figure 5).

5 PULSATING AND OSCILLATING FLOWS IN TUBES

In giving above examples of reducing the determining equations to simpler forms, the authors understood that any simplification is associated with the exclusion of the possibility of analyzing a number of quite fine effects. However, when these effects are secondary or unimportant with respect to the main process, such simplifications are quite justified.

In many specific practical cases, in particular with nonuniform movements of a flowing polymer system in channels having an intricate configuration, it becomes necessary to employ a quite simple system of equations approximating the flow process in the region of arbitrary velocity gradients. We have already given a system of constitutive equations (4.2) or (4.3) obtained for the flow of a polymer liquid. When investigating a complex nonuniform flow, it is also convenient to employ system (4.2) or (4.3), setting definite simplifications beforehand. We shall indicate as an example the results of studying the influence of pressure oscillations when a polymer liquid flows in a tube. For this purpose, consider the polymer liquid to flow in a long tube of radius R under the effect of an oscillating pressure difference:

$$p = p_0(1 + A \sin \omega t).$$

5.1 Motion Equations

The basic motion and relaxation equations describing the oscillating and pulsating flows of a viscoelastic fluid (undilute polymer solution) in annular ducts with sinusoidal variations of the pressure gradient in time, as follows from (4.3), are:

$$\begin{aligned} Re_f \frac{\partial u}{\partial t} &= \frac{dp}{dz} + \frac{3}{4} We^{-1} \frac{\partial}{r\partial r}(r\xi_{rz}) \\ De \frac{\partial \xi_{rz}}{\partial t} &= \frac{1}{3} We \frac{\partial u}{\partial r} - \frac{\xi_{rz}}{f(D)} \\ De \frac{\partial \xi_{zz}}{\partial t} &= 2We\xi_{rz} \frac{\partial u}{\partial r} - \frac{\xi_{zz} - 1/3}{f(D)} \\ f(D) &= (1 + kD)^{-n} \end{aligned} \tag{5.1}$$

where $dp/dz = (dp/dz)_0(1 + A \sin \omega t)$ and $(dp/dz)_0$ is the steady pressure gradient.

The physical meaning of the criteria is as follows: $Re_f = \rho R^2 \omega/(8\pi\eta_0)$ is the pulsational Reynolds number; $De = \omega\tau_0/(2\pi)$ is the Deborah number; $We = -(dp/dz)_0 R\tau_0/(4\eta_0)$ is the Weissenberg number. When analyzing pulsating flows, the dimensionless elasticity number El equal to the ratio between the Deborah number and pulsational Reynolds number $El = De/Re_f = \eta_0\tau_0/(\rho R^2)$, is frequently used. The set of values of these criteria defines the deviation of the velocity profiles and volumetric flow rates at different phases of the pulsation period from their equilibrium values.

The flow rate characteristics of a pulsating flow of viscoelastic fluids over a wide range of Weissenberg and Deborah numbers and pulsational Reynolds number ($Re_f = 10^{-4} - 0.2$; $We = 0.4 - 5$; $De = 0.01 - 5$) were studied theoretically (Astarita and Marrucci, 1974 and Doi and Edwards, 1986).

We compared calculated results with data for an aqueous polyacrylamide solution. Its rheological properties (the parameter $\kappa = 0.06$, $n = 0.55$, the value of zero-shear-rate viscosity $\eta_0 = 0.323\, Pa.s$ and the value of $\tau_0 = 1.35$s in the equation (5.1)) were determined by conventional methods of stationary rotational viscosimetry (Astarita and Marrucci, 1974 and Doi and Edwards, 1986).

5.2 Velocity Fields

The frequency of oscillations in the experiments (Altukhov *et al.*, 1986) with the polyacrylamide solution changed in the range of 0.15–0.5 Hz. In this case, the Deborah numbers varied in the range of 0.04–0.13. The pulsating Reynolds number remained small ($Re_f < 10^{-3}$). The oscillating flow of the polyacrylamide solutions is characterized by a pronounced phase shift between the velocity and pressure gradient. The phase shift increased with the frequency and amounted to $\varphi \sim 35-45°$ under the experimental conditions. In glycerin (Newtonian fluid) flow, the pressure gradient changed by a sinusoidal law, but in a polyacrylamide solution the pressure gradient increased more sharply than it decreased.

A pulsating flow is more complicated than an oscillating one, as the extent of the pressure pulsation effect depends on the value of the steady pressure gradient in the flow (Weissenberg number We), which defines the variation rheological properties of the fluid.

In the experiments conducted under inertia less conditions at a constant value of the mean pressure drop (We = const), the frequency f and amplitude A of the pressure gradient variations were changed. In this case, the values of Deborah number were in the same ranges as in oscillating flow, while the amplitude of the oscillations was higher (A = 0.65–0.8).

The values of the axial velocity and changes in velocity over a tube section obtained in experiments were compared with calculations by equations (5). The results of the calculations for relative velocity values are shown in Figure 11 and Figure 12 by solid lines (the experimental values are shown by dots). One can see from the figures that the calculations describe satisfactorily both the experimentally observed features of the axial velocity changes in different phases of the pulsation period and the velocity profile flatness over the tube section.

5.3 Flow Enhancement

Similar to velocity profiles, the flow rate characteristics of the pulsating flow of a nonlinear viscoelastic fluid depend on their rheological properties and the flow conditions. Measurements were performed with both the sinusoidal and stepwise pressure gradient variation. The change in the flow rate of a pulsating flow in comparison with that of a steady-state one is usually determined by the flow enhancement $I = (Q_p/Q_0) - 1$, where Q_p and Q_0 are the mean flow rates of the pulsating and steady-state flows, respectively. According to the available results of theoretical and experimental studies, the effect of the above criteria on the value of I appeared to be different not only qualitatively, but also quantitatively. The system of determining equations (3)–(4) was used to study this theoretically.

It had previously been shown theoretically and confirmed experimentally up to values $A \leq 0.45$ that $I \sim A^2$. Our experiments showed that this dependence is valid at substantially higher values of the relative amplitude of the pressure-gradient pulsation. Therefore, in the following, the experimental results will be represented as the basic flow enhancement I/A^2.

By using aqueous polyacrylamide solutions of different concentrations and changing the pulsation frequency and mean values of the steady pressure gradient, we were able to combine some dimensionless criteria in the experiments.

If $Re_f \gg 1$, the pulsating component of the shear wave does not propagate over the entire tube section during the pulsation period and the pulsation effect on the fluid flow rate will be small.

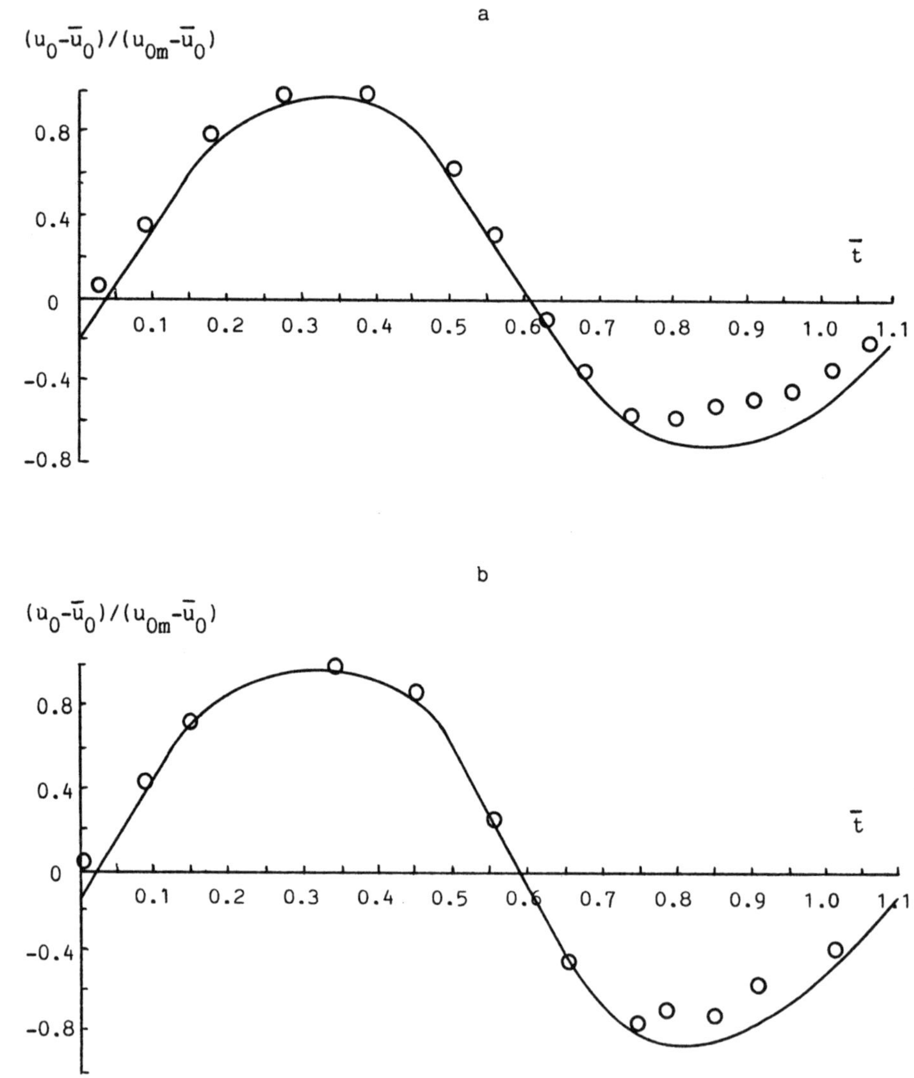

Figure 11 Comparison of experimental values (dots) of axial velocity pulsations and calculated ones (solid line). The frequencies of oscillations are: a—0.15 Hz; b—0.5 Hz.

At *De* $\ll 1$ one can speak of the equilibrium nature of the flow, when the relaxation properties of the fluid are not practically exhibited. In this case, the pulsation effect will be defined solely by the nonlinear viscous properties of the fluid. This case was considered earlier by a number of authors. One should also not expect a substantial effect of nonlinear viscoelastic properties of fluid at small values of reversible deformations, i.e. at small values of the Weissenberg number.

Case $Re_f \ll 1$; $De < 1$. Figure 13 shows the experimental and theoretical values of I/A^2 as a function of *We* for a fixed *De*. This range of data corresponds to the curve for the theoretically-predicted dependence of I/A^2 on *We*.

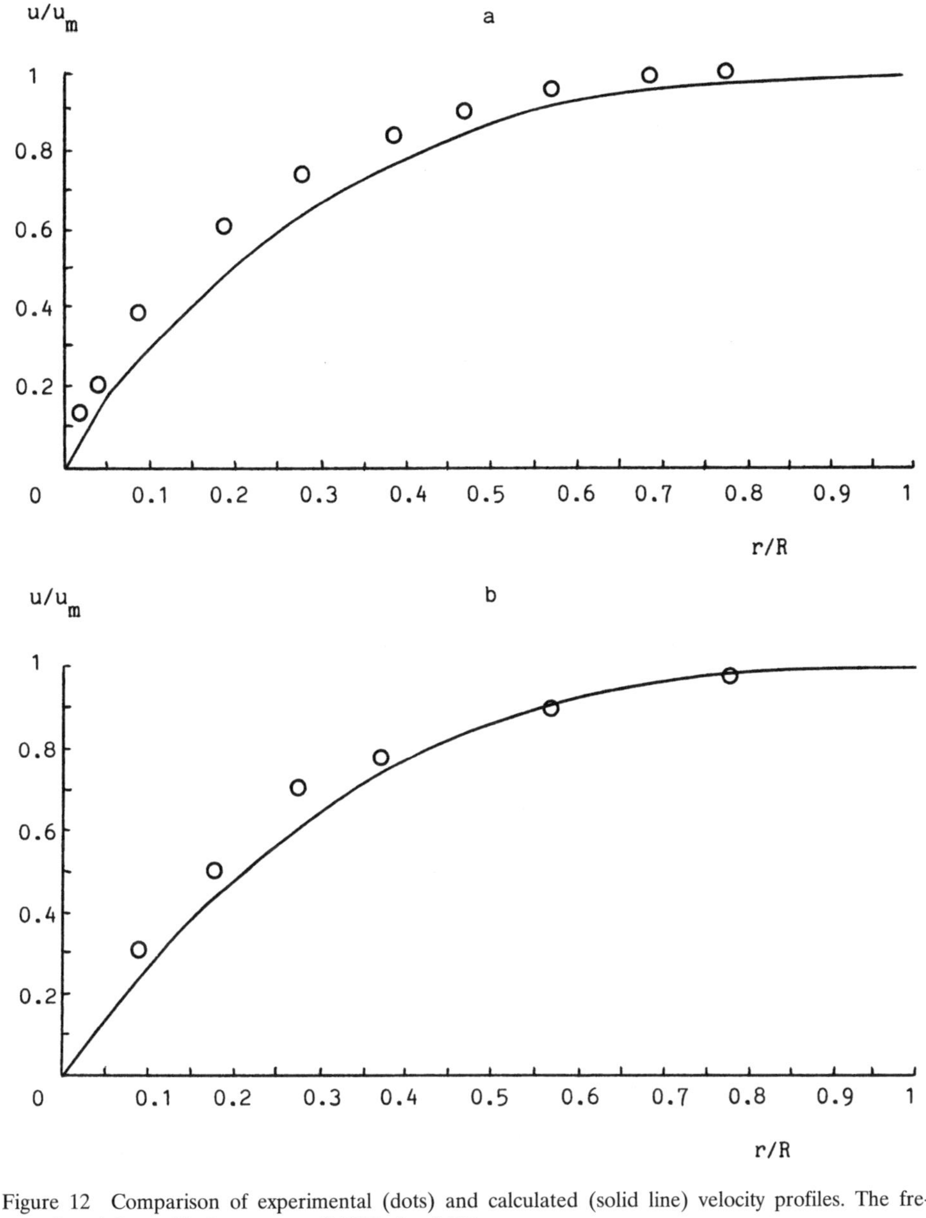

Figure 12 Comparison of experimental (dots) and calculated (solid line) velocity profiles. The frequencies of the oscillations are: a—0.15 Hz; b—0.5 Hz.

Case $Re_f \ll 1$; $We \approx 4$; $0 < De < 1.2$. Figure 14 presents the values of basic flow enhancement I/A^2 as a function of the Deborah number, obtained for two different values of the Weissenberg number. With an increase in *De*, the value of I/A^2 decreases at $We = 3.7$, but that of I/A^2 increases weakly at $We = 5.2$.

It was shown theoretically earlier (Altukhov *et al.*, 1986) that the flow enhancement curve *I* as a function of the dimensionless pulsation frequency had both

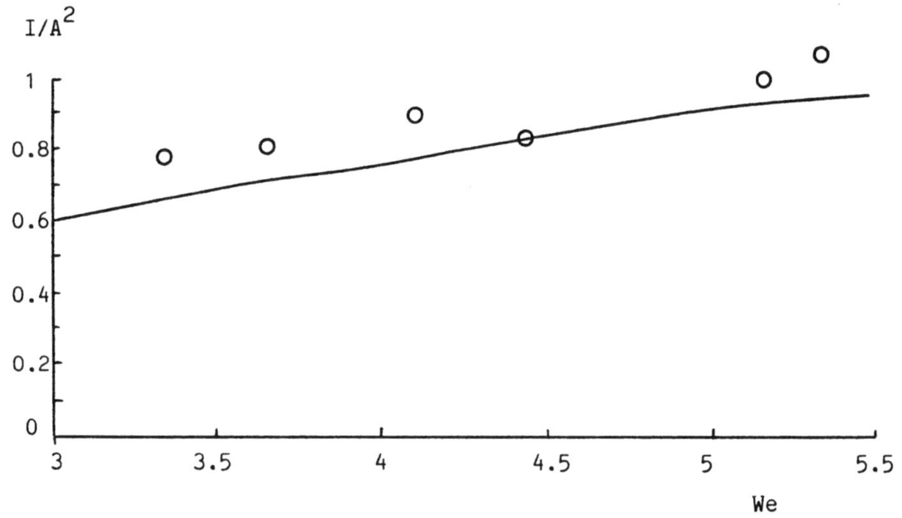

Figure 13 Basic low enhancement I/A^2 vs. *We* for the stepwise law of pressure gradient variation ($De = 0.3$). The dots are experimental values, the solid line—theoretical ones.

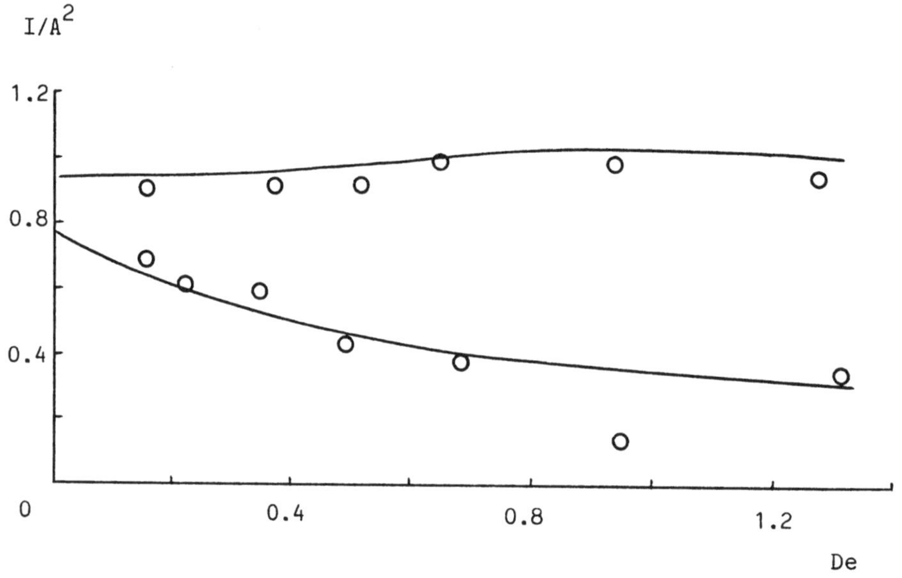

Figure 14 Basic flow enhancement I/A^2 vs. *De* for the stepwise law of pressure gradient variation (*We*: 1—5.2; 2—3.7).

descending and ascending branches. Previously, experiments could obtain only one branch of the flow enhancement curve *I*(*De*), generally, a curve dropping with a growing frequency. In our experiments, for the first time, both branches of the curve of flow enhancement vs. Deborah number were obtained in one experimental setup. The calculations performed for equations (3)–(5) confirm this result (Figure 15).

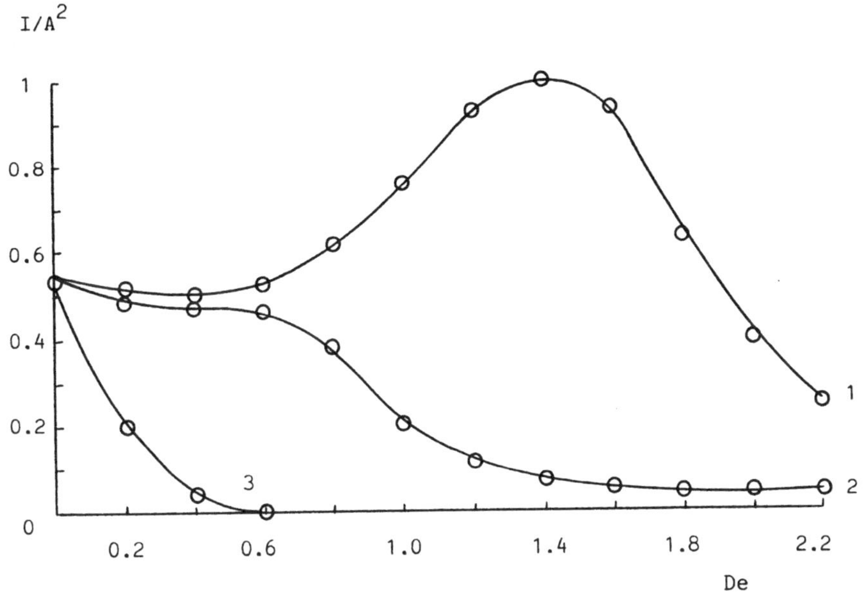

Figure 15 Basic flow enhancement I/A^2 vs. *De*. (We = 0.28).

Both the regions of decreasing and of increasing flow rates with an increasing Deborah number were found.

One can see from the experiments and calculations that at certain combinations of the viscoelastic fluid properties and parameters of pressure gradient pulsations, a considerable increase in the fluid flow rate can be attained as compared with steady flow with the same mean values of the pressure gradient. However, according to calculation (Astarita and Marrucci, 1974 and Edwards, 1982), this can be achieved only by increasing the power necessary for viscoelastic fluid pumping.

5.4 Nonisothermal Flows

The heat transfer in oscillating flows of viscoelastic fluids with sinusoidal variations of the pressure gradient in time are studied theoretically. The system (4), (5) together with energy equation

$$
\begin{gathered}
Fo^{-1}\frac{\partial T}{\partial t} + Peu\frac{\partial T}{\partial z} = \frac{\partial^2 T}{\partial r^2} + \frac{\partial^2 T}{\partial z^2} \\
r = 0,\ \partial u/\partial r = \partial T/\partial r = 0;\ r = 1,\ u = 0,\ T = 1; \\
x = 0,\ T = 0,\ x \to \pm\infty,\ \partial T/\partial x = 0
\end{gathered}
\tag{6}
$$

where T is a dimensionless temperature; Fo is the Fourier number and Pe is the Pecle number, was used as the basic system to study unsteady-state heat transfer in a round tube (Popov and Altukhov, 1992).

The chief results of the calculations are shown in Figures 16–17. As can be seen from the calculations, a resonance regime of heat transfer may exist in oscillating flows.

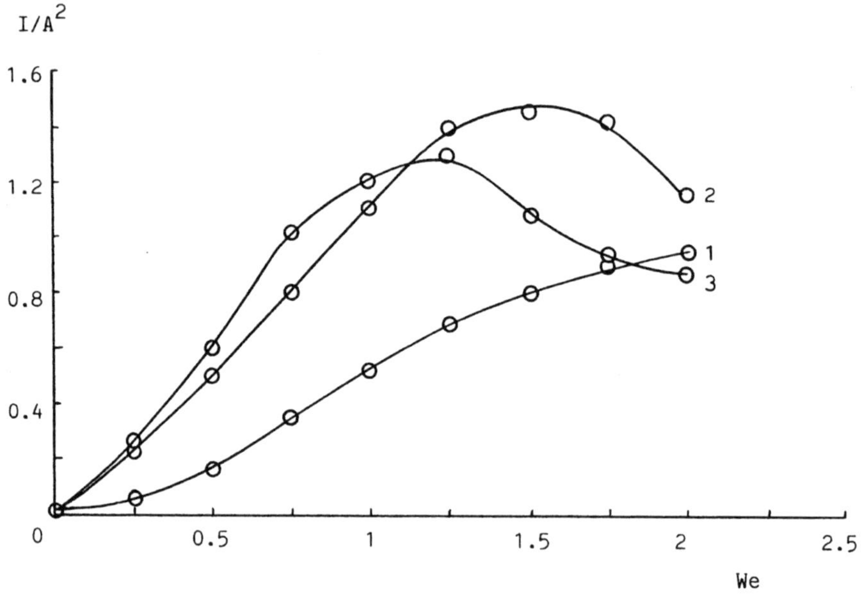

Figure 16 Basic flow enhancement I/A^2 vs. *We*. (El = 50).

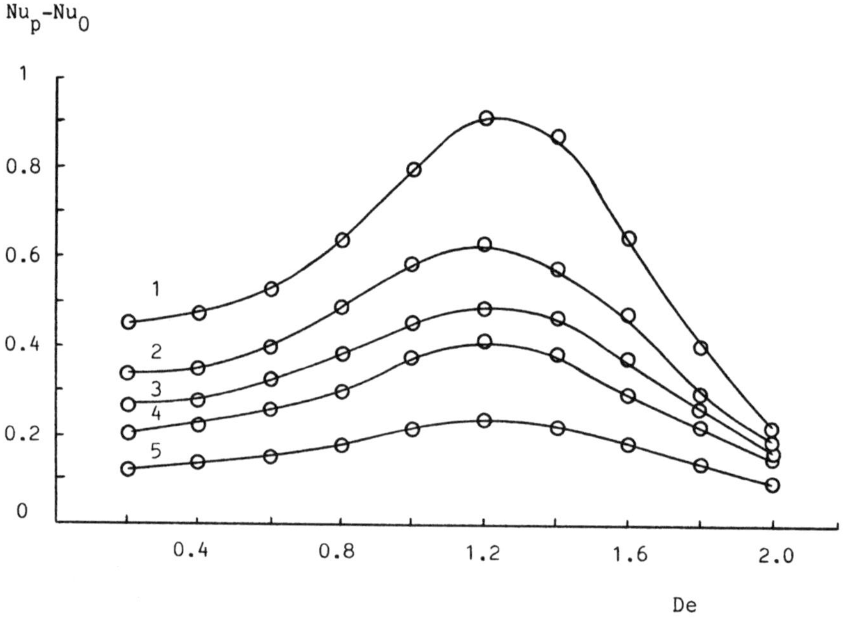

Figure 17 The difference of unsteady Nusselt number and steady one vs. *De*. Curves 1–5 are the values of $Pe^{-1}\ x/d$: 1—0.128; 2—0.266; 3—0.5; 4—0.675; 5—1.9, respectively.

Let us note in conclusion that a numerical and experimental studies of the secondary flows that occur in the laminar pressure-driven motion of polymer solutions in ducts of noncircular cross-section were performed. A numerical and experimentally study of the secondary flows that occur in the laminar pressure-driven motion of dilute polymer solutions in ducts of a rectangular cross-section is presented. The full nonlinear two-dimensional equations of motion for a viscoelastic fluid with shear thinning are solved by an explicit finite-difference technique. The results are presented that indicate the existence of the previously observed vortex secondary flow in ducts of a noncircular cross-section. It was demonstrated experimentally and theoretically that the laminar pressure driven flow of a viscoelastic fluid in noncircular ducts is not unidirectional like its Newtonian counterpart. A weak secondary flow occurs in the transverse planes of the ducts that causes fluid particles to undergo a spiraling motion down the duct in contrast to the rectilinear particle paths in a Newtonian fluid.

6. CONCLUSION

The use of the methods of statistical mechanics to derive rheological equations of state made significant progress in recent years and made possible a unified approach (based on an ideal model) that gives a satisfactory description of the experimental date on the viscoelasticity of polymers in connection with their molecular structure. At any rate the results are useful in understanding the approaches used in the phenomenological theories of polymer dynamics.

We considered the constitutive equations of the theory obtained on the basis of the hypothesis of the dynamics of a macromolecule presuming its motion in an aftereffect medium. Subsequently, the hypothesis was discussed in detail in works of Russian investigators. A number of experimental appraisals of the theory undertaken by the authors (Vinogradov *et al.* 1972, Pokrovskii and Yanovsky 1973, Yanovsky *et al.* 1988, Yanovsky 1993, Pyshnograi *et al.* 1994), and also other estimates showed that the considered nature of the thermal motion of a macromolecule is close to the real one. The conclusions of the theory and its results were also extended to nonlinear phenomena. In their corollaries, the conclusions of the theory correspond to the observed experimental results. The determining equations can be formulated in various approximations.

It should be noted that the proposed dynamics of a macromolecule in an undilute system can be used to study behavior of the surface layers. Unlike the previous case, we must add the forces attracting a macromolecule to the surface-nonlinear terms.

We should use computer simulation methods to analyze the behavior of a macromolecule on the basis of non-linear macromolecular dynamics. These methods allow us to follow the trajectory of a macromolecule and calculate the averaged values under different surface forces.

The investigation of macromolecules gives the mean length of a surface layer. The investigation of the time correlation function gives the set of relaxation times of the macromolecule near the surface.

Consequently, the length of the surface layer and its relaxation times can be calculated from the dynamics of a single macromolecule.

TABLE 1
Characteristics of presented systems.

System	$T°$, C	c, %	η_0/τ_0	η_0, Pa.s	τ_0, s	N
High Density Polyethylene [Park H.J. *et al.*, 1992]	180	100	2.5×10^4	2.8×10^4	1.12×10^0	1
Low Density Polyethylene [Luo X.L. and Mitsoulis E., 1990]	160	100	1.45×10^3	5.65×10^4	3.89×10^1	2
Aqueous solution of Polyacrilamide (0.05% w.) [Deiber J.A. and Schowalter W.R., 1981]	22	—	9.45×10^0	1.37×10^0	1.45×10^{-1}	3

REFERENCES

1. Yu.A. Altukhov, A.N. Kekalov, V.N. Pokrovskii, V.I. Popov and E.M. Khabakhpasheva, Description of pulsating flow of elastic polymer solutions in Structure of Hydrodynamic Flows (Forces Flow, Thermal Convection). 1986, Coll. Institute of Thermophysics, Novosibirsk, pp. 5–12. (in Russian).
2. G. Astarita and G. Marrucci, Principles of Non-Newtonian Fluid Mechanics. (New York, McGraw-Hill, 1974).
3. F. Bueche, The viscoelastic properties of plastics, *J. Chem. Phys.*, 1954, **22**, pp. 603–609.
4. R. Cerf, Statistical mechanics of chain macromolecules in a velocity field, *J. de Phys. et-Radium*, 1958, **19**, pp. 122–134.
5. S. Chandrasekhar, Stochastic Problems in Physics and Astronomie, *S. Rev. Mod. Phys.*, 1943, **25**, pp. 1–35.
6. P.G. De Gennes, Reptation of a polymer chain in the presence of fixed obstacles, *J. Chemical Physics*, 1971, **55**, pp. 572–579.
7. J.A. Deiber and W.R. Schowalter, Modeling the flow of viscoelastic fluids through porous media, *AIChE J.*, 1981, **27**, pp. 912–920.
8. M. Doi and S.F. Edwards, Dynamics of concentrated polymer systems, *J. Chem. Soc. Faraday Trans.*, 1978, **74**, pp. 1789–1801, 1802–1817, 1818–1832.
9. M. Doi and S.F. Edwards, The Theory of Polymer Dynamics. (Oxford Univ. Press, Oxford, 1986).
10. S.F. Edwards, Dynamics of entangled polymers. Proceedings of the Royal Society A., 1982, **385**, pp. 267–288.
11. J.D. Ferry, Viscoelastic Properties of Polymers, 3rd edn. (New York, Wiley, 1980).
12. W.W. Graessley, The entanglement concept in polymer rheology, *Advances Polymer Sci.*, 1974, **16**(1), pp. 1–179.
13. V.L. Grebnev and V.N. Pokrovskii, Viscoelasticity of linear polymer: the second order effects, *Vysokomolek. Soed.*, 1987, **29**(9), pp. 704–710 (Russian).
14. M.S. Green and A.V. Tobolsky, A new approach to the theory of relaxing polymeric media, *J. Chem. Phys.*, 1947, **14**, p. 80.
15. J.G. Kirkwood and J. Rieseman, The intrinsic viscosities and diffusion constants of flexible macromolecules in solution, *J. Chem. Phys.*, 1948, **16**, pp. 565–573.
16. R.G. Larson, Constitutive Equations for Polymer Melts and Solutions. (Butterworth, Boston, 1988).
17. A.I. Leonov, On a self-consistent molecular modeling of linear relaxation phenomena in polymer melts and concentrated solutions, *J. Rheol. Acta.*, 1994, **38**, pp. 1–11.
18. A.S. Lodge, A network theory of flow birefringence and stress in concentrated polymer solutions. Trans. Faraday Soc., 1956, **52**, pp. 120–130.
19. T.P. Lodge, N.A. Rotstein and S. Prager, Dynamics of entangled polymer liquids. Do linear chains reptate, *Adv. Chem. Phys.*, 1990, **79**, pp. 1–132.
20. X.L. Luo and E. A Mitsoulis, numerical study of the effect of elongational viscosity on vortex growth in contraction flows of polyethylene melts, *J. Rheology*, 1990, **34**(3), pp. 309–342.

21. S. Onogi, T. Masuda and K. Kitagawa, Rheological properties of anionic polystyrenes. I. Dynamic viscoelasticity of narrow-distribution polystyrenes, *Macromolecules*, 1970, **3**(2), pp. 109–116.
22. H.J. Park, D.G. Kiriakidis and E. Mitsoulis, Birefringence studies in die flows of an HDPE melt, *Journal of Rheology*, 1992, **36**(8), pp. 1563–1589.
23. V.N. Pokrovskii and Yu.G. Yanovsky, A new molecular model for description of viscoelastic behavior of linear polymers and their concentrate solutions, *Rheol. Acta.*, 1973, **12**(4), pp. 280–292.
24. V.N. Pokrovskii and V.S. Volkov, The calculation of relaxation time and dynamical modulus of linear polymers on one-molecular approximation with self-consistency. (A new approach to the theory of viscoelasticity of linear polymers), *Polymer Science USSR*, 1978, **20**, pp. 3029–3037.
25. V.N. Pokrovskii and Yu.K. Kokorin, Theory of viscoelasticity of dilute blends of linear polymers. *Vysokomolek. Soed.*, 1985, B, **26**, pp. 573–577 (Russian).
26. V.N. Pokrovskii and Yu.K. Kokorin, The theory of oscillating birefringence of solutions of linear polymers. Dilute and concentrated systems, *Polymer science USSR*, 1987, **29**, pp. 2385–2393.
27. V.N. Pokrovskii and G.V. Pyshnogray, Non-linear effects in the dynamics of concentrated polymer solutions and melts, *Fluid Dynamics*, 1990, **25**, pp. 568–576.
28. V.N. Pokrovskii and G.V. Pyshnogray, The simple forms of constitutive equation of polymer concentrated solution and melts as consequence of molecular theory of viscoelasticity, *Fluid Dynamics*, 1991, **26**, pp. 58–64.
29. V.N. Pokrovskii, Dynamics of weakly-coupled linear macromolecules, *Add. Phys. Sci.*, 1992, **162**, pp. 87–121 (Russian).
30. V.N. Pokrovskii, Low frequency dynamics of dilute solutions of linear polymers, *Adv. Phys. Sci.*, 1994, **164**, pp. 157–176 (Russian).
31. V.I. Popov, Yu.A. Altukhov, On the resonance regime of flow and heat transfer of non-linear viscoelastic liquid in the duct, *Sibirskii fizikotekhnicheskii journal*, 1992, 4, pp. 22–26 (Russian).
32. G.V. Pyshnogray and V.N. Pokrovskii, Dependence of stationary shear viscosity of linear polymers on stress in the theory of the molecular field, *Polymer Science USSR*, 1988, **30**, pp. 2624–2629.
33. G.V. Pyshnogray, Influence of macromolecular coils anisotropy on nonlinear properties of polymer fluids by uniaxial tension, *J. Applied Mechanics and Theoretical Physics*, 1994, 4, pp. 525–532 (Russian).
34. G.V. Pyshnogray, V.N. Pokrovskii, Yu.G. Yanovsky, Yu.N. Karnet and I.F. Obraztsov, Constitutive Equation on nonlinear viscoelastic (polymer) media in nought approximation by parameter of molecular theory and conclusions for shear and extension. The Russian Academy of Sciences Reports, 1994, **335**(8), pp. 1235–1241 (Russian).
35. P.E. Rouse, A theory of the linear viscoelastic properties of dilute solutions of coiling polymers, *J. Chem. Phys.*, 1953, **21**, pp. 1272–1280.
36. K.S. Schweizer, Microscopic theory of the dynamics of polymeric liquids: General formulation of a mode-mode coupling approach, *J. Chem. Phys.*, 1989a, **91**, pp. 5802–5821.
37. K.S. Schweizer, Mode-coupling theory of the dynamics of polymer liquids: Qualitative predictions for flexible chain and ring melts, *J. Chem. Phys.*, 1989b, **91**, pp. 5822–5839.
38. K.S. Schweizer, Mode-coupling theory of the dynamics of polymer liquids, *J. Non-Cryst. Solids*, 1991, **131–133**, pp. 643–649.
39. J. Stickforth, The rational mechanics and thermodynamics of polymeric fluids based upon the concept of a variable relaxed state, *Rheol. Acta*, 1986, **25**(5), pp. 420–433.
40. A.A. Trapeznikov and T.V. Korotkova, Normal, tangential stresses vs. recovery deformation in prestationary stage of deformation for concentrated polymer solutions by high range of deformation rate, The USSR Academy of Sciences Reports, 1971, **201**(6), pp. 1402–1405.
41. G.V. Vinogradov, V.N. Pokrovskii and Yu.G. Yanovsky, Theory of viscoelastic behavior of concentrated polymer solutions and melts in one-molecular approximation and their experimental verification, *Rheol. Acta*, 1972, **VII**, pp. 258–274.
42. G.V. Vinogradov, Yu.G. Yanovsky L.I. Ivanova, Viscoelasticity of solutions and blends of narrow molecular mass distribution polymers, *Int. J. Polym. Mater.*, 1982, **9**, pp. 257–277.
43. M. Yamamoto, The viscoelasticity properties of network structure, *J. Phys. Soc. Jpn.*, 1956, **11**, pp. 413–421; 1957, **12**, pp. 1148–1158, 1958; **13**, pp. 1200–1211.
44. Yu.G. Yanovsky, G.V. Vinogradov, V.S. Volkov and L.I. Ivanova, Microviscoelasticity and viscoelastic properties of blends of linear flexiblechain polymers. Proceedings of VIII-th International Congress on Rheology. (Plenum Press, New York, 1980, pp. 483–486).

45. Yu.G. Yanovsky, V.N. Pokrovskii, Yu.K. Kokorin, Yu.N. Karnet and Titkova, Superslow, relaxation processes in amorphous linear polymers and their interpretation, *Polymer Science USSR*, 1988, **30**, pp. 1037–1046.
46. Yu.G. Yanovsky Polymer, Rheology: Theory and Practice (Chapman and Hall, London, 1993).

Investigation of Organosiloxane Equilibrium Reactions

V.M. KOPYLOV and V.A. KOVJAZIN

Russian Federation State Scientific Research Institute of Chemistry and Technology of Organoelement Compounds. 38 Entuziastov chausse, Moscow, Russia

1 INTRODUCTION

We extensively studied the regularities of the equilibrium rearrangement reactions of monomeric and oligomeric organosilicon compounds with ≡Si—O—Si≡, ≡Si—Cl, ≡Si—O— bonds participation. The reactions were carried out in the presence of nucleophilic and electrophilic catalysts. The results of these studies are presented in publications.[1–10]

These reactions are widely used in laboratory and industrial practices for directed synthesis of a variety of organosilicon compounds. However, in spite the widespread use of these reactions their regularities at quantitative levels have not been adequately investigated. There are not available summarized articles wherein a correlation of the regularities of equilibrium rearrangement reactions and participation of the most broadly used reactive bonds at silicon ≡Si—O—Si≡, ≡Si—Cl, ≡Si—O— is carried out. In the present article we analyse the principal results of our published and nonpublished investigations are considered. Analysis of this data allowed to summarize the features common for all reactions under consideration.

2 FUNDAMENTALS

2.1 Investigations of Equilibrium Reactions at Catalytic Rearrangements of Organodisiloxanes

Asymmetrical organodisiloxanes are obtained by the cohydrolysis,[11] co-condensation[12] and catalytic redistribution reactions in the presence of nucleophilic or electrophilic catalysts.[13] The last reaction allows one to obtain these compounds quantitatively due to the reuse of unreacted reagents.

The effect of substituent nature on the process of asymmetrical organodisiloxanes formation through reaction of symmetrical organodisiloxanes, catalized by heterogenous electrophilic catalysts—sulphocationite "KU-23" (sulphonated copolymer styrene with divinylbenzene with sulpho group containing of 3.8 mg-eq/l and 7% mass.water) has been studied. The reactions of pentamethyldisiloxane (I) formation through 1,1,3,3-tetramethyldisiloxane interaction with hexamethyldisiloxane (system A); 1-chloromethyl-1,1,3,3-tetramethyldisiloxane (II) at 1,1,3,3-tetramethyldisiloxane interaction with 1,3-bis-(chloromethyl)tetramethyldisiloxane (system B); pentamethyl(chloromethyl)disiloxane (III) at hexamethyldisiloxane interaction with 1,3-bis(chloromethyl)tetramethyldisiloxane (system C) and pentamethyl-(chloroformiatomethyl)disiloxane (IV) at hexamethyldisiloxane interaction with 1,3-bis (chloroformiatomethyl)tetramethyldisiloxane (system D) have been studied. The reaction may be shown as follows:

$$\underset{\mathrm{M}}{\mathrm{X\,SiMe_2OSiMe_2X}} + \underset{\mathrm{L}}{\mathrm{Y\,SiMe_2OSiMe_2\,Y}} \xrightleftharpoons{\text{Cat.}} \underset{\mathrm{Q}}{\mathrm{2X\,SiMe_2OSiMe_2Y}} \tag{1.1}$$

The reaction is conducted without solvent at temperatures over 10–40°C in the presence of 5 mass% of "KU-23" sulphocationite. The reaction proceeding is controlled by GLC method against the changes in the contents of initial symmetrical and formed asymmetrical organodisiloxanes. Time of reaction systems arriving to the equilibrium is diminished in a series:

$$\underset{\text{“A”}}{(\mathrm{Me_3Si})_2\mathrm{O} + (\mathrm{HMe_2Si})_2\mathrm{O}} > \underset{\text{“C”}}{(\mathrm{HMe_2Si})_2\mathrm{O} + (\mathrm{ClCH_2SiMe_2})_2\mathrm{O}} >$$

$$\underset{\text{“B”}}{(\mathrm{Me_3Si})_2\mathrm{O} + [\mathrm{ClC(O)OCH_2\,SiMe_2}]_2\mathrm{O}} > \underset{\text{“D”}}{(\mathrm{Me_3Si})_2\mathrm{O} + (\mathrm{ClCH_2SiMe_2})_2\mathrm{O}}$$

Due to electrophilic nature of the catalysts reactivity for the organodisiloxane pair under consideration should be diminished with diminishing of electronodonor properties of oxygen atom in siloxanes and should be the lowest for the system $(HMe_2Si)_2O$—$(ClCH_2SiMe_2)_2O$ (B) since the initial siloxanes have more electronoacceptor substituents X and Y (H and $ClCH_2$, respectively) at silicon. Characteristically, however, high reactivity is observed for this pair. The lowest reactivity is observed for pair $(Me_3Si)_2O$—$(ClCH_2SiMe_2)_2O$. Observed order of the change in reactivity allows to suggest that the reaction rate is considerably determined by substituent sizes (X and Y) at silicon. Equilibrium content of compound (II) for B system is near to the calculated for the statistical composition. Value of the equilibrium constant is equal to 4.7 ± 0.7 and is near to the constant value at statistical composition (4.0). For A, C and D systems equilibrium content of asymmetrical organodisiloxanes is higher than calculated. Values of the constants are higher than at the statistical composition and amounted to 5.4 ± 1.0; 6.5 ± 1.0 and 5.5 ± 1.0 respectively. The kinetic parameters of this reaction have been investigated. According to the scheme (1.1) the process under consideration is a reversible reaction of the second order and is described in [14] by equation (1.2):

$$\frac{\mathrm{d}x}{\mathrm{d}t} = k(\mathrm{M}_0 - x)(L_0 - x) - k'x^2 \tag{1.2}$$

Integral form of equaltion (1.2) has the following form:

$$\ln\left(\frac{|\bar{x}|}{|x'|} \cdot \frac{|\bar{x}' - x|}{|\bar{x} - x|}\right) \cdot \left(\frac{1}{\bar{x}' - x}\right) = a.t \quad \text{or} \quad F(x) = a.t \tag{1.3}$$

where

$$x = M_0 - M = L_0 - L = 0.5Q \tag{1.4}$$

$$x = M_0 - M_e = L_0 - L_p = 0.5Q_e \tag{1.5}$$

$$\bar{x}' = \frac{4K(M_0 + L_0)}{K - 4} - \bar{x} \tag{1.6}$$

$$K = k/k' = Q_e^2/(M_e L_e) \tag{1.7}$$

$$a = k - 4k', \quad k' = a/(K - 4), \quad k = a - 4k' \tag{1.8}$$

M_0, L_0—initial; M, L, Q—running; M_e, L_e, Q_e—equilibrium concentrations of organodisiloxanes in reaction mixture (equation 1.1); k, k'—rate constants of direct and reverse reaction; K—equilibrium constant; t—time.

Experimental data show that in accordance with reaction scheme the process with high correlation coefficient (r) is described by the equation (1.3). Values of rate constants of direct and reverse reaction estimated by equation (1.4–1.8) are presented in Table 1. From Table 1 it follows that obtained rate constants of reactions depend on initial ratios of starting reagents.

Correlation of rate constants of reverse reactions (on equation 1.1) showed that the reactivity of asymmetrical organodisiloxanes is changed in a series:

$$\text{(I)} > \text{(II)} > \text{(IV)} > \text{(III)}$$

Study of the B system at different temperatures showed that equilibrium constant values are essentially unaffected by temperature. Thus, a conclusion is made that the process is determined by enthropy factor since reaction enthalpy is near the zero. The same values of activation energy of direct (ΔE) and reverse ($\Delta E'$) reactions (44.8 kJ/mol) point out to the zero value of the reaction enthalpy. Observed dependence of reaction rate constants on the type of substituents (X and Y) at silicon and on initial concentrations of starting symmetrical organodisiloxanes may be provided by reaction mechanism features.

At the interaction of organodisiloxanes with reaction centers of the catalysts two types of the intermediate centers are formed including fragments of any either of siloxanes:

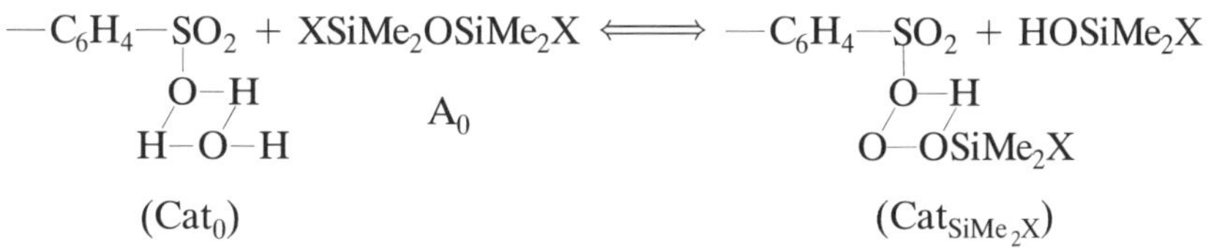

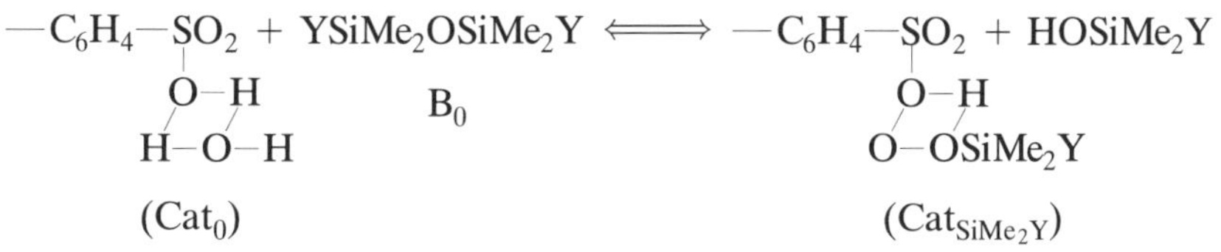

TABLE 1
Rate constants of direct (k) and reverse (k') reactions and equilibrium (K) of reactions of redistribution of symmetrical organodisiloxanes.

Initial concentration of organodisiloxanes l/mol.sec A_0, mol/l	B_0, mol/l	t, °C	r	k l/mol.sec	k' l/mol.sec	K
System A: $HMe_2SiOSiMe_2H + Me_3SiOSiMe_3$						
4.39	0.99	12	0.999	$14.3 \cdot 10^{-4}$	$2.6 \cdot 10^{-4}$	5.4±1.0
2.91	2.12	12	0.979	$12.7 \cdot 10^{-4}$	$2.4 \cdot 10^{-4}$	
1.01	3.81	12	0.984	$9.5 \cdot 10^{-4}$	$1.8 \cdot 10^{-4}$	
System B: $HMe_2SiOSiMe_2H + ClCH_2Me_2SiOSiMe_2CH_2Cl$						
4.39	1.02	22	0.999	$14.0 \cdot 10^{-5}$	$3.0 \cdot 10^{-5}$	4.7±0.7
3.86	1.75	22	0.993	$16.0 \cdot 10^{-5}$	$3.4 \cdot 10^{-5}$	
2.42	2.50	22	0.999	$25.0 \cdot 10^{-5}$	$5.3 \cdot 10^{-5}$	
1.67	3.17	22	0.982	$34.5 \cdot 10^{-5}$	$7.3 \cdot 10^{-5}$	
0.99	3.68	22	0.996	$67.0 \cdot 10^{-5}$	$14.2 \cdot 10^{-5}$	
2.63	2.46	33	0.997	$52.8 \cdot 10^{-5}$	$11.2 \cdot 10^{-5}$	4.4
2.68	2.42	39	0.998	$81.7 \cdot 10^{-5}$	$17.4 \cdot 10^{-5}$	4.4
System C: $Me_3SiOSiMe_3 + ClCH_2Me_2SiOSiMe_2CH_2Cl$						
3.80	0.95	22	0.999	$5.0 \cdot 10^{-7}$	$7.7 \cdot 10^{-8}$	6.5±1.0
3.01	1.69	22	0.992	$6.2 \cdot 10^{-7}$	$9.5 \cdot 10^{-8}$	
2.33	2.50	22	0.997	$6.9 \cdot 10^{-7}$	$10.5 \cdot 10^{-8}$	
1.65	3.03	22	0.970	$21.9 \cdot 10^{-7}$	$33.4 \cdot 10^{-8}$	
0.87	3.72	22	0.981	$73.3 \cdot 10^{-7}$	$112 \cdot 10^{-8}$	
System D: $Me_3SiOSiMe_3 + ClC(O)OCH_2Me_2SiOSiMe_2CH_2O(O)CCl$						
2.45	2.05	17	0.996	$5.5 \cdot 10^{-5}$	$1.01 \cdot 10^{-5}$	5.5

Since dehydrated "KU-23" sulphocationate is unsuited as catalyst redistribution reaction water participation in the formation of active centers is indispensable and it is consistent with previously obtained data upon water activation effects in the case of acidic catalysis.[15] Amount of active reaction centers of both forms is constant, it is determined by initial concentration of starting components—M_0, L_0, Cat_0. Formation of asymetrical organodisiloxanes doesn't change content of the reaction centers because they interact with catalyst resulting information of the same centers. The reaction centers may interect with component of reaction mixture according to equations (1.11) and (1.12):

$$\text{Cat-SiMe}_2\text{X} + \text{YSiMe}_2\text{OSiMe}_2\text{Y} \Longleftrightarrow \text{Cat-SiMe}_2\text{Y} + \text{YSiMe}_2\text{OSiMe}_2\text{X} \quad (1.11)$$

$$\text{Cat-SiMe}_2\text{Y} + \text{XSiMe}_2\text{OSiMe}_2\text{X} \Longleftrightarrow \text{Cat-SiMe}_2\text{X} + \text{YSiMe}_2\text{OSiMe}_2\text{X} \quad (1.12)$$

Taking into account the availability of two types of the reaction centers and two types of reagents it is belived that observed decreasing of the rate constant values at reagent ratio changes is depended by that the interaction of less active substance with reaction center as a principal stage.

2.2 Investigation of Disproportionation process of Oligoethoxysiloxanes

A great number of works[16–29] are devoted to the investigations on reaction of hydrolytic polycondensation of tetraethoxysilane (TES) in the presence of acidic and alkaline catalysts. In the case of alkaline hydrolysis NaOH, KF, NH_3 are used as catalysts, at acidic hydrolysis—inorganic acids: HCl, HNO_3, H_3PO_4.[20,22–27] It is supposed that hydrolysis process of TES, catalyzed by acids consists in a series of successive and parallel stages involving the hydrolysis reactions as well as inter-and intramolecular homofunctional condensation of ≡Si—OH and ≡Si—O—Et groups. As a result of reaction at partial hydrolysis linear and cyclic ethoxysiloxanes are formed and at complete hydrolysis—silicon dioxide.[20] However description of the process in above mentioned works has mainly quantitative character. In work [26] the dependence of TES, hexaethoxydisiloxane (L_2) and octaethoxytrisiloxane (L_3) contents at change of H_2O:TES molar ratio from 0 up to 1 is described. Under examination of these results it follows that composition of the products is considerably different from statistic one that could be obtained at polycondensation of tetrafunctional compounds.[30] The present investigation evaluation on disproportionation of model individual oligoethoxysiloxanes L_2 and L_3 has been carried out, they correspond to reactions:

$$2(\mathrm{EtO})_4\mathrm{Si} + \mathrm{H_2O} \longrightarrow \mathrm{Et[OSi(OEt)_2]_2OEt} + 2\mathrm{EtOH} \tag{2.1}$$

$$3(\mathrm{EtO})_4\mathrm{Si} + 2\mathrm{H_2O} \longrightarrow \mathrm{Et[OSi(OEt)_2]_3OEt} + 4\mathrm{EtOH} \tag{2.2}$$

The investigation was conducted by GLC method through determination of ethoxysiloxane contents with number of silicon atoms over 1 to 5. The disproportionation of ethoxysiloxanes may be presented by equation:

$$\begin{aligned} q_n\mathrm{Et[OSi(OEt)_2]}_n\mathrm{OEt} \Longleftrightarrow\ & (\mathrm{EtO})_4\mathrm{Si} + q_{n-1}\mathrm{Et[OSi(OEt)_2]}_{n-1}\mathrm{OEt} + \\ & + q_{n+1}\mathrm{Et[OSi(OEt)_2]}_{n+1}\mathrm{OEt} + q_i\mathrm{Et[OSi(OEt)_2]}_i\mathrm{OEt} \end{aligned} \tag{2.3}$$

where $q_1 \ldots q_i$—molar ethoxysiloxane concentrations with siliconatom number from 1 to 5.

The composition of ethoxysiloxanes disproportionation could be given by statistic Flory equation indicating the product contents with various molecular mass at polyfunctional monomers polycondensation.[30]

$$q_i = \frac{(f_i - i)!f}{(i-1)!(f_i - 2i + 2)!i} \cdot P^{(i-1)} \cdot (1-P)^{(fi-2i+2)} q_{no} \tag{2.4}$$

where i—a number of silicon atoms in molecule; $f = 4$; $p = 0.25$ for L_2 and 0.33 for L_3; q_n—number of starting reagent moles.

The disproportionation reaction was carried out with use of nucleophilic catalysts: L_2—in the presence of KF, Me_4 NOH, Me_4NF, L_3—in the presence of Me_4NOH and KF. To determine equilibrium composition and disproportionation process rate—reaction temperature dependence in the presence of Me_3SiONa and Me_4NOH. The disproportionation reaction rate depends on catalyst nature and reaction temperature. Thus, L_2 disproportionation in the presence of KF proceeded with remarkable rate at temperature over 150°C, that is why the reaction was studied at 160°C. As a result of disproportionation reaction formation of TES, L_3, decaethoxytetrasiloxane (L_4) and decreasing of L_3 concentration (Table 2) were observed. System reaches the equilibrium within 9.5 hr. Time of the equilibrium to be reached was determined versus time the equilibrium is reaching by TES, because with TES the constant concentration is reached much slower. Disproportionation in the presence of Me_4NOH proceeds even at 19°C. In the presence of this catalyst even at 19°C the reaction rate is well above than in the case of KF. The equilibrium is reached within 3 hrs with obtaining of similar products. Time of equilibrium reaching is reduced and at 100°C accounts for 2 min. In the presence of Me_3SiONa the disproportionation begins at 35°C and at 108°C the rate increases by five times and time of equilibrium achieving accounts to 35 min.

Effect of Me_4NF in contrast to above catalysts is characterized by given prolonged induction period. In the process of heating at 100°C the reaction begins within 1.5 hr and then is accompanied by rather sharp increasing of the rate, and the equilibrium is reached within 5.5 hr including induction period. The disproportionation reaction of L_3 in the presence of KF at 160°C proceeds much slower than in the case of L_2 and the equilibrium is reached in about 11 hr. In the equilibrium state a system already contains even five components: TES, L_2, L_3, L_4 and dodecaethoxypentasiloxane (L_5); the latter appears within 5 hrs after the reaction begins. The process of L_3 disproportionation in the presence of Me_4NOH undergoes conversions similarly to L_2 even at 19°C but much slower than for L_2. For L_3 the equilibrium is reached in 3.5 hr and the system contains the same five components. As in the case of L_2 the process rate in the presence of Me_4NOH is higher than in the presence of KF.

TABLE 2

Equilibrium composition of disproportionation reaction products of oligoethoxysiloxanes $[L_2]_0 = 2.3$ mol/l (at use of KF, Me_4NOH, Me_4NF) and 1.68 mol/l (Me_3SiONa); $[L_3]_0 = 1.25$ (KF) and 1.36 mol/l (Me_4NOH).

Components	Components contents in reaction mixture, mol/l — Disproportionation $Et[OSi(OEt)_2]_2OET$										
	KF	ME_4NOH				ME_4N	Estimated	Me_3SiONA			Estimated
	160°	19°	40°	60°	100°	100°		35°	70°	108°	
$Si(OEt)_4$	1.41	1.46	1.43	1.48	1.50	1.52	1.52	1.06	1.06	1.06	1.07
$ET[OSi(OEt)_2]_2OEt$	0.42	0.43	0.42	0.42	0.41	0.42	0.41	0.30	0.32	032	031
$ET[OSi(OEt)_2]_3OEt$	0.20	0.20	0.21	0.20	0.19	0.18	0.18	0.13	0.13	0.13	0.13
$ET[OSi(OEt)_2]_4OEt$	0.09	0.09	0.10	0.09	0.08	0.09	0.09	0.06	0.07	0.07	0.07
$ET[OSi(OEt)_2]_5OEt$	—	—	—	—	—	—	—	—	—	—	—

	Disproportion $Et[OSi(OEt)_2)]_3OEt$			
	KF	Estimated	Me_4NOH	Estimated
	160°	—	19°	—
$Si(OEt)_4$	0.71	0.74	0.81	0.81
$ET[OSi(OEt)_2]_2OEt$	0.31	0.22	0.24	0.24
$ET[OSi(OEt)_2]_3OEt$	0.10	0.10	0.10	0.11
$ET[OSi(OEt)_2]_4OEt$	0.09	0.05	0.06	0.06
$ET[OSi(OEt)_2]_5OEt$	0.032	0.033	0.034	0.035

The equilibrium concentrations found experimentally are in agreement with estimated from the formula (2.4) (Table 2) within the range of experiment error. The activity of used catalysts in the disproportionation reaction is diminished in a series $Me_4NOH > Me_3SiONa > Me_4NF > KF$. In the presence of Me_4NOH and Me_3SiONa disproportionation reaction proceeds as follows:

$$\equiv SiOEt + MX \Longleftrightarrow \equiv Si{-}O{-}M + EtX \tag{2.5}$$

$$\begin{aligned} \equiv Si{-}O{-}M + Et[OSi(OEt)_2]_m OEt \Longleftrightarrow & \equiv OSi{-}O{-}Et + \\ & MO[Si(OEt)_2O]_m Et \end{aligned} \tag{2.6}$$

$$\begin{aligned} Et[OSi(OEt)_2]_m OM + EtO[Si(OEt)_2O]_m Et \Longleftrightarrow & \; EtO[Si(OEt)_2O]_{m+q} Et \\ & + Et[OSi(OEt)_2]_{m-q} OM \end{aligned} \tag{2.7}$$

where $M = Me_4N$, Na; $X = OH$, $OSiMe_3$.

In the presence of Me_4NF and KF the following scheme by analogy with other reactions catalyzed by fluorides[31] may be suggested:

$$Et[OSi(OEt)_2]_{m-1}OSi(OEt) + 2MF \Longleftrightarrow$$

$$\begin{array}{l} \quad EtO \;\; FM \\ EtOSi{-}[OSi(OEt)_2]_{m-1}OEt \Longleftrightarrow Et[OSi(OEt)_2]_{m-1}OM + FSi(OEt)_3 + MF \\ \quad EtO \;\; FM \end{array} \tag{2.8}$$

$$\begin{aligned} Et[OSi(OEt)_2]_{m-1}OM + Et[OSi(OEt)_2]_m OEt & \Longleftrightarrow \\ Et[OSi(OEt)_2]_{m+q} OEt + Et[OSi(OEt)_2]_{m-q} OM & \end{aligned} \tag{2.9}$$

where $M = Me_4N$, K.

The disproportionation reaction proceeds at the expense of ethoxysiloxanes redistribution at interaction with nucleophilic catalysts upon $\equiv Si{-}O$ bond in the fragments $\equiv Si{-}O{-}Si \equiv$ and $\equiv Si{-}O{-}Et$. For compounds under study the disproportionation reactions running up to the equilibrium reaching may be described in general manner with use of the system of reversible reactions. Thus, at L_2 disproportionation the formation of all products in accordance with equilibrium composition may be presented by three principal equations:

$$\underset{A}{2\,Et[OSi(OEt)_2]_2OEt} \overset{K_1}{\Longleftrightarrow} \underset{B}{(EtO)_4\,Si} + \underset{C}{Et[OSi(OEt)_2]_3\,OEt} \tag{2.10}$$

$$A + C \overset{K_2}{\Longleftrightarrow} B + \underset{D}{Et[OSi(OEt)_2]_4\,OEt} \tag{2.11}$$

$$A + D \overset{K_4}{\Longleftrightarrow} 2C \tag{2.12}$$

These equations comply with equilibrium constants K_1, K_2, K_4 that may be estimated from formulas:

$$K_1 = \frac{[C][B]}{[A]^2} \quad (2.13); \qquad K_2 = \frac{[B][D]}{[A][C]} \quad (2.14); \qquad K_4 = \frac{[C]^2}{[A][D]} \quad (2.15)$$

In the case of L_3 disproportionation to foregoing equations three more be added:

$$\mathrm{A} + \mathrm{D} \overset{K_3}{\Longleftrightarrow} \mathrm{B} + \underset{\mathrm{E}}{\mathrm{Et[OSi(OEt)_2]_5OEt}} \tag{2.16}$$

$$\mathrm{A} + \mathrm{E} \overset{K_5}{\Longleftrightarrow} \mathrm{C} + \mathrm{D} \tag{2.17}$$

$$\mathrm{C} + \mathrm{E} \overset{K_6}{\Longleftrightarrow} 2\mathrm{D} \tag{2.18}$$

the following equilibrium constants correspond to them:

$$K_3 = \frac{[\mathrm{B}][\mathrm{E}]}{[\mathrm{A}][\mathrm{D}]} \quad (2.19); \qquad K_5 = \frac{[\mathrm{C}][\mathrm{D}]}{[\mathrm{A}][\mathrm{E}]} \quad (2.20); \qquad K_6 = \frac{[\mathrm{D}]^2}{[\mathrm{C}][\mathrm{E}]} \quad (2.21)$$

As may be seen from Table 3 statistical equilibrium constant calculated from formulas (2.13–2.15) and (2.19–2.21) with use of the equilibrium concentrations calculated from equation (2.4) and equilibrium constants obtained experimentally agree within limits of experiment error.

Equality of these constants indicates that disproportionation reactions oligoethoxysiloxanes follow Flory statistical theory. It is evident from Table 2 and 3 that values of equilibrium concentrations and equilibrium constant remain valid at various temperatures. Enthalpy of equilibrium reactions under consideration is practically equal to zero and the equilibrium is completely statistical.

The investigation on the disproportionation reactions in the presence of HCl, H_3PO_4, HNO_3 showed that these acids couldn't catalyze the processes of disproportionation of oligoethoxysiloxanes. On the base of obtained results the conclusion may be made that during the process of hydrolytic TES condensation, the presence of nucleophilic reagents may influence the disproportionation reaction of formed oligoethoxysiloxanes. At catalysis of hydrolytic polycondensation by acids the disproportionation reaction mustn't markedly influence product composition since it

TABLE 3
Equilibrium constants of disproportionation reaction of oligoet hoxysiloxanes.

Equilibrium constant	Statistical constant	Average value of constant	Experimental constant of equilibrium									
			Disproportionation $Et[OSi(OEt)_2]_2OEt$								Disproportionation $Et[OSi(OEt)_2]_3OEt$	
			KF	Me_4NOH			Me_4N	Me_3SiONa			KF	Me_4NOH
			100°	19°	60°	100°	100°	35°	70°	108°	160°	19°
K_1	1.56	1.52	1.54	1.51	1.51	1.51	1.61	1.53	1.49	1.49	1.50	1.49
K_2	1.76	1.74	1.59	1.69	1.68	1.78	1.78	1.71	1.81	1.79	1.81	1.79
K_3	2.06	2.03	—	—	—	—	—	—	—	—	2.01	2.04
K_4	0.89	0.90	0.92	0.90	0.99	0.94	0.91	0.94	0.79	0.84	0.84	0.79
K_5	0.73	0.66	—	—	—	—	—	—	—	—	0.64	0.68
K_6	0.89	0.90	—	—	—	—	—	—	—	—	0.92	0.88

isn't catalyzed by acids. The disproportionation of products of hydrolytic polycondensation of TES obtained at different values of molar $n = [H_2O]_0 : [TES]_0$ ratio:

$$q_1(EtO)_4Si + nq_1H_2O \Longleftrightarrow q_iEt[OSi(OEt)_2]_{m+1}OEt + 2nq_1EtOH \qquad (2.22)$$

Study of composition of obtained products and reaction rate at products disproportionation with a different extent of TES polycondensation and correlation of this process with a disproportionation of individual ethoxysiloxanes has been conducted.

In the process of TES hydrolytic polycondensation at different $\langle\langle n\rangle\rangle$ linear and cyclic ethoxysiloxanes are formed and linear ethoxysiloxane contents is statistical, estimated from Flory equation (2.4), where x—number of silicon atoms in molecule of linear ethoxysiloxanes, $f = 4$, $P = n/2$, q_0—initial TES concentration. This deriviation was attributed to the absence of equilibrium reactions at hydrolytic polycondensation and formation of ethoxysiloxanes that is disregarded by the Flory theory. The products of TES polycondensation, obtained at ratios $n = 0.2$–1.2 in the presence of 0.005 mol/l HCl were choosen as starting oligoethoxysiloxanes for study of disproportionation.

The disproportionation was carried out in the presence of Me_4NOH in amounts of 0.01 mol/l at 20°C. The process running is controlled by GLC method through determination of content of TES and ethoxysiloxanes with number of silicon atoms from 2 to 5. For products of hydrolytic TES polycondensation, obtained at different $\langle\langle n\rangle\rangle$ values the disproportionation is.characterized by TES concentration increasing and its formation in that products wherein it was absent, by L_2, L_4 and L_5 appearing in the products wherein they are absent and L_2, L_3, L_4 and L_5 redistribution finally. At the disproportionation of product of hydrolytic TES polycondensation, obtained at $n = 0.2$ TES concentration increases from 1.4 up to 1.5 mol/l with simultaneous decreasing of L_2 and L_3 content from 0.3 to 0.25 and from 0.1 to 0.06 mol/l, respectively. At the same time L_4 and L_5 formation is observed with concentration increasing from 0.02 and 0.006 mol/l respectively. In the case of disproportionation of hydrolytic polycondensation product obtained at $n = 1.2$ TES L_2 and L_4 are formed with concentration increasing up to 0.06; 0.01 and 0.001 mol/l, respectively. Content of L_3 and L_5 is diminished from 0.03 up to 0.003 and from 0.01 up to 0.0004 mol/l, respectively. With n rise the time of reaction system transition into equilibrium state (from 2 hr at $n = 0.2$ to 24 hr at $n = 1.2$) is also increased, that is more likely connected with activity change of ammonium catalysts at growth of OH-group content (from 0 at $n = 0.2$ up to 27% at $n = 1.2$), because it is known[32] that activity of tetraalkylammonium catalysts is reduced in the presence of hydroxyl containing compounds. This is also supported by that time of equilibrium reaching in the process of disproportionation of the product of TES hydrolytic polycondensation at $n = 1.0$ in which HO-groups were preliminary condensated is reduced by two times. In all instances equilibrium composition found experimentally in accordance with composition calculated from formula (2.4). In this way the process of disproportionation of products of TES hydrolytic polycondensation is not different from the disproportionation of individual ethoxysiloxanes. As a result of the disproportionation the consumption also takes place up to full exhausting of cyclic ethoxysiloxanes: hexaethoxycyclotrisiloxane (S_3), octaethoxycyclotetrasiloxane (S_4), decaethoxycyclopentasiloxane (S_5), which enter into reactions of polymerization and disproportionation. This is demonstrated in the example of S_4 that in ethanol medium and in the presence of ammonia (ammonia doesn't cause the ethoxysiloxane disproportionation) at room temperature is polymerized up to 100% conversion without formation of low molecular ethoxysiloxanes. Reaction rate adheres to the equation of the first order with constant rate of $1.85{\cdot}10^{-4}\,s^{-1}$. In the absence of alcohol NH_3 doesn't cause polymerization that is why it may be believed that at interaction with alcohol it gives ammonium base:

$$NH_3 + EtOH \Longleftrightarrow EtONH_4 \tag{2.23}$$

which leads to polymerization according to scheme (2.24, 2.25):

$$m[(EtO)_2SiO]_4 + EtONH_4 \Longleftrightarrow EtO[(EtO)_2SiO]_4NH_4 \tag{2.24}$$

$$EtO[(EtO)_2SiO]_4NH_4 \Longleftrightarrow EtO[(EtO)_2SiO]_4H + NH_3 \tag{2.25}$$

In presence 0.01 mol/l of Me_4NOH in amount 0.01 mol/l of S_4 enteres immediately into disproportionation reaction with formation TES and linear ethoxysiloxanes. Content of TES and linear ethoxysiloxanes with numbering of silicon atoms from two up to five also corresponds the statistical estimated from formula (2.4) at $P = 0.5$ equal in conversion. At initial S_4 concentration 1 mol/l 0.4 (0.38) mol/l TES was formed; 0.11 (0.095) mol/l L_2, 0.04 (0.035) mol/l L_3; 0.01 (0.016) mol/l L_4; 0.007 (0.008) mol/l L_5.

Equilibrium diethoxycyclosiloxanes concentration is near to the zero. However this doesn't exlude a possibility of cyclic fragment content in the formed polymeric chain.

2.3 Characteristic Properties of Cooligomerization of Dimethylcyclosiloxanes with Tetraethoxysilane at Catalysis with Nucleophilic Reagents

The reactions of organosiloxanes with organoalkoxysilanes of different functionality and tetraalkoxysilanes catalyzed by nucleophilic and electrophilic reagents and proceeding with redistribution of alkoxy-groups and siloxane bonds are of interest for directed synthesis of a variety monomeric and oligomeric compounds.[33–37] These reactions permit us to change over a wide range the product compositions versus the organoalkoxysilane functionality, substituent nature at silicon, reagent ratios, catalyst and conditions of reaction performing.

The present investigation deals with study on features of co-oligomerization of TES with hexamethylcyclotrisiloxane (D_3) and octamethycyclotetrasiloxane (D_4), catalyzed by nucleophilic reagents: polydimethylsiloxane-α,ω-diolatetetramethylammonium (TMAS), KOH and Me_4NOH (TMAH). At the D_3 interaction with equimolar TES quantities in the presence of TMAS ($[D_3]_0 = [TES]_0 = 0.6$; $[TMAS]_0 = 0.0017$ mol/l over temperature range 20–40°C D_3 is consumed rather faster than TES. Thus if D_3 is fully consumed for 15 min (at 20°C), TES consumes at the same time by 25%. The higher rates of D_3 consumption are possible due to telomerization involving the interaction upon some TES ethoxy groups and extending of dimethylsiloxane chains:

$$a\mathrm{Si(OEt)_4} + mn[\mathrm{Me_2SiO}]_3 \xrightleftharpoons{\text{Cat.}} (\mathrm{EtO})_{4-m}\mathrm{Si}[(\mathrm{OSiMe_2})_{pn}\mathrm{OEt}]_m \tag{3.1}$$

where $p = 3, 4$; $m = 1–4$.

Consumption of D_3 is of the first order according to given concentration D_3

$$W_{\text{Д}\text{р}} = -k^1_{\text{Д}_3}[\text{Д}_3] \tag{3.2}$$

and for TES—the second summable total order according to given concentration of D_3 and TES:

$$W_{\mathrm{TES}} = -k^1_{\mathrm{TES}}[\mathrm{D_3}][\mathrm{TES}] \tag{3.3}$$

Values of effective k_{D_3} and k_{TES} constants are presented in Table 4. The obtained relationships confirmed the assumption of D_3 and TES consumption from equation (3.1) in accordance to which the consumption rate of D_3 is dependent only on given concentration of D_3. On the exposure of the reaction mixture under given conditions after consuming of D_3 the formation 0.067 mol of dimethyldiethoxysilane (DMDS) per 1 mol of taken TES was observed. Formation of DMDS and simultaneous slightly decreasing of TES concentration demonstrate the TES interaction with telomerization products upon terminal ethoxydimethylsiloxy group. However, DMDS low concentration and some change in TES concentration allows to conclude that the product compositions is little affected by this reaction. The major products are tetrafunctional compounds, forming according to equation (3.1). At 100°C D_3 enters into reaction within 1–2 min at concentratration twice as much than of TES ($[D_3]_0 = 1.2$; $[TES]_0 = 0.6$; $[TMAS]_0 = 0.0017$ mol/l); TES is consumed much lower and reaction rate is independent of given D_3 concentration since TES is consumed after D_3 vanishing. In this occasion D_3 consumption rate is described by the equation (3.2). For TES reaction order is changed in comparison with the process at temperatures 20–40°C. The reaction rate is presented by the equation of the first order according to given TES concentration:

$$W_{\mathrm{TES}} = -k''_{\mathrm{TES}}[\mathrm{TES}] \tag{3.4}$$

TABLE 4

Constants of D_3 and TES consumption rates at their cooligomerization catalyzed by TMAS ($[D_3]_0 = [TES]_0 = 0.6$; $[TMAS]_0 = 0.0017$ mol/l).

t,°C	$k_{D3}\cdot10^4$ s^{-1}	$k_{TES}\cdot10^4$ s^{-1}	[DMDS], l/mol
21	5.6	2.0	0.020
28	3.4	4.4	0.025
30	7.5	5.3	0.027
40	56.7	12.7	0.040

This allows to make assumption that in this case TES is actively consumed not only through interaction with D_3 but as well as with linear siloxane fragments of the products obtained according to the equation (3.1)

$$
\begin{aligned}
(\sim Me_2SiO \sim)_x + Si(OEt)_4 &\xrightleftharpoons{\text{Cat.}} (\sim Me_2SiO-)_{x-z}Et \\
&\quad + (EtO)_3Si(OSiMe_2 \sim)_z \sim
\end{aligned}
\tag{3.5}
$$

In contrast to D_3 at D_4 interaction with TES catalyzed by TMAS or TMAH $[D_4]_0 = 1.8$, $[TES]_0 = 1.2$; $[TMAS]_0 = 0.0017$ or $[TMAH]_0 = 0.0034$ mol/l at 80°C coreagents are completely consumed and simultaneously. Consumption rate of D_4 and TES are presented by the equations of the first order (3.2) and (3.4), respectively. From this it follows that at D_4 interaction with TES the reagents consumption proceeds at the expense of reactions, described by the equations (3.1) and (3.5). Close values of effective consumption rate constants of D_4 and TES show that the reactivity of Si—O bond in siloxanes and TES is identical. The comparison of polymerization processes of D_3 and D_4 and their co-oligomerization with TES, catalyzed by TMAS shows that in the presence of TES the catalytic activity of TMAS towards D_3 decreases and increases towards D_4. Thus, if on D_3 polymerization at 40°C ($[D_3]_0 = 0.6$; $[TMAS]_0 = 0.0017$ mol/l) a value of effective constant $k_{D_3} = 10.9 \cdot 10^{-3}\,sec^{-1}$. On D_4 polymerization at 80°C ($[D_4]_0 = 1.8$; $[TMAS]_0 = 0.0017$ mol/l) a value of $k_{D_4} = 4.72 \cdot 10^{-5}\,sec^{-1}$ and on introduction of 1.2 mol/l TES it increases up to $68.5 \cdot 10^{-5}\,sec^{-1}$. At TES interaction with D_3 in the presence and with D_4 in the presence of TMAS or TMAH at 80–100°C the formation of large quantities of DMDS and tetramethyldiethoxydisiloxane (TMDDS) was observed at the expense of redistribution of ethoxy group and siloxane bonds in telomerization products (forming according to the equation (3.1)) or their interaction with TES according to the equation (3.5). Thus, in reaction of D_4 with TES the content of DMDS amounted to 0.45 mol/l, TMDDS—0.27 mol/l at 100°C, 0.4 and 0.18 mol/l at 90°C, 0.26 and 0.18 mol/l at 80°C, respectively that is the same as the participation of 30, 26 and 20% ethoxy groups, introduced with TES ($[D_4]_0 = 1.8$, $[TES]_0 = 1.2$; $[TMAS]_0 = 0.0017$ mol/l). During the reaction proceeding the TMDDS increases gradually and DMDS passes the maximum: 0.53 mol/l at 100°C, 0.45 mol/l at 90°C and 0.32 mol/l at 80°C. Higher rates of content growth of DMDS than of TMDDS and its concentration passing the maximum allows to suppose that DMDS is predominantly produced at the expense of TES interaction with end ethoxydimethylsiloxy group of telimerization products:

$$
\begin{aligned}
&(-O)_3SiO(Me_2SiO-)_n-SiMe_2(OEt) + Si(OEt)_4 \longrightarrow \\
&\qquad (-O)_3SiO(Me_2SiO-)_mSi(OEt)_3 + Me_2Si(OEt)_2
\end{aligned}
\tag{3.6}
$$

This leads to possible formation of DMDS under the reaction running in the quantity more than equilibrium one. At the expense of the subsequent reactions of ethoxy groups and siloxane bonds redistribution with DMDS participation the decreasing of its concentration takes place after passing the maximum up to the equilibrium. As is seen on the base of obtained results at the TES interaction with D_3 and D_4 in the presence of TMAS and TMAH the functionality (active ethoxy group contents) of reaction products could change from 2 up to 6 and over at the average functionality of four. At D_4 interaction with TES in the presence of KOH ($[D_4]_0 = 1.8$, $[TES]_0 = 1.2$; $[KOH]_0 = 0.1$ mol/l) consumption of the reagents is observed with marked rates at 140°C and over. TES enters into reaction considerably faster than D_4. When TES enters almost completely into reaction D_4 is consumed only by 30% (140°C). However D_4 consumption is continued and after TES vanishing up to fully exhausting. Fast consumption of TES at low D_4 consumption demonstrates that telomerization rate according to the equation (3.1) is much below than at ethoxy groups and siloxane bonds redistribution at the expense of telomerization products interaction with TES according to the equations (3.5) and (3.6). The conversion depth by D_4 increases up to 70% by the moment of full TES exhausting at increasing of TES concentration from 1.2 up to 2.2 mol/l and D_4 concentration decreasing from 1.8 to 1.2 mol/l. In reactions catalyzed by KOH the formation of DMDS and TMDDS is also observed, They consist 0.35 (maximum 0.40) and 0.12 mol/l at $[D_4]_0 = 1.8$, $[TES]_0 = 1.2$ mol/l) as well as 0.9 (maximum 1.0) and 0.14 mol/l at $[D_4]_0 = 1.2$, $[TES]_0 = 2.2$ mol/l), respectively. The ethoxy group consumption introduced with TES for formation DMDS and TMDDS accounts for 26% of total quantity. The comparison of D_4 consumption with amount of dimethylsiloxy groups spent for DMDS and TMDDS formation shows that at the initial stage of the reaction a high destruction of the telomerization products takes proceeds with formation predominantly DMDS and TMDDS. This is supported by hexaethoxydisiloxane formation as a results of limiting destruction of the telomerization products. At the prolonged reaction times when D_4 is the practically vanished, decreases of DMDS and TMDDS content to the equilibrium level is observed. There with it approximates to the content of these products in reactions catalysed by TMAS or TMAH. Noted features of D_4 interaction with TES in the presence of KOH are consistent with data given in [37]; wherein the reaction between TES and D_4 in the presence of KOH (at distillation of produced DMDS and TMDDS) formation of silicon dioxide may occur, that is a limiting case of TES ethoxy groups used for the production of these products. In this manner, the conducted investigation indicates that for considered reactions of dimethylcyclosiloxanes with TES three types of processes may be pointed out: telomerization taking place at the initial stages; TES interaction with the telomerization products and redistribution of ethoxy groups and siloxane bonds in the products formed at the expense of the processes of two previous types. The contribution of these processes may be changed with changing in activities of dimethylcyclosiloxane and catalyst, temperature and time of reaction performing. Thus, on use of highly active D_3 and TMAS as catalyst at temperatures over 20–40°C telomerization process is predominant. At D_4 cooligomerization with TES in the presence of KOH at 140°C and higher at the initial reaction stage the processes of cleavage the telomerization products by tetraethoxysilane are dominant. In the case of TES cooligomerization with D_3 and D_4 in the presence of TMAS or TMAH at temperatures over 80–100°C all the processes under consideration proceed at with high rates.

2.4 Investigation on the Regularities of Organosilsesquioxane Interactions with Tetraethoxysilane

The regularities of interaction of organosilsesquioxanes $(RSiO_{1.5})_n(T_n^R)$ where R = Me, Vi, Ph with tetraalkoxysilanes (TAS), tetramethoxysilane (TMS), tetraethoxysilane (TES) and tetrapropoxysilane (TPS) in the presence of nucleophilic catalyst—KOH have been investigated. During the reaction proceeding TAS interaction with T_n^R with redistribution of alkoxy groups and siloxane bonds. The distribution of alkoxy groups and ≡Si—O— bonds between $Si(OR')_4$ and structural units $RSi(O—)_3$ may be presented by the equation:

$$(R'O)_4Si + RSi(O—)_3 \overset{KOH}{\Longleftrightarrow} (—O)_aSi(R'O)_{4-a} + R(R'O)_bSi(O—)_{3-b} \quad (4.1)$$

where a may be changed from 0 to 4 and b from 0 to 3.

The redistribution reaction may be presented most simply as follows:

$$\equiv Si—OR' + =(R)Si^*—O— \Longleftrightarrow \equiv Si—O— + =(R)Si^*—O—R' \quad (4.2)$$

where ≡Si— designated tetrafunctional and $=(R)Si^*$— designated trifunctional units.

Due to the equilibrium character of the process the reaction products must contain the following tetra- and trifunctional units $(R'O)_4Si$(TAC), $(R'O)_3SiO$ (I), $(R'O)_2Si(O—)_2$ (II), $(R'O)Si(O—)_3$ (III), $Si(O—)_4$ (IV), $RSi(O—)_3$ (V), $R(R'O)Si(O—)_2$ (VI), $R(R'O)_2SiO$ (VII), and in the limiting case organotrialkoxysilanes —$RSi(OR')_3$ (VIII). The combination of units containing siloxane bond leads to formation oligoalkoxysiloxanes of different composition and structure, they may be present only as brutto-formula displaying the content of different units. The reaction scheme with regard to formed monomeric and oligomeric products may be given as the following equation:

$$\begin{aligned} d[RSiO_{1,5}]_n + q(R'O)_4Si \overset{KOH}{\Longleftrightarrow} & \; cRSi(OR')_3 + z[(R'O)_3SiO_{0,5}]_f - \\ & [(R'O)_2SiO]_s[(R'O)SiO_{1,5}]_g[SiO_2]_m[(R'O)RSiO]_h[RSiO_{1,5}]_k[R(R'O)_2SiO_{0,5}]_j \\ & + p(R'O)_4Si \end{aligned} \quad (4.3)$$

Organotrialkoxysilanes VIII were obtained in the pure state for their identification and quantitative determination in the reaction products identification was carried out by methods of GLC, NMR ^{29}Si, ^{13}C, ^1H spectroscopy. Analysis of NMR ^{29}Si spectra of the starting compounds and reaction products at the different reagent ratios allowed to identify the signals applying to silicon atoms in TAS, units I–III, V–VIII. Silicon signals for TAS and VIII are singlet and for I–III and V–VII—widened complicated multiplets resulting from their inclusion into various types of structural fragments. Chemical shifts of ^{29}Si signals do not significantly depend on alkyl group in alkoxy substituent and have the following values:

δ^{29}Si TAS 0 (−78) – (−82) ppm; δ^{29}Si I (−85) – (−90) ppm;
δ^{29}Si II (−95) – (−97) ppm; δ^{29}Si III (−101) – (−105) ppm;

δ^{29}Si V (−67) – (−80) ppm; (R = Me); (−77) – (−85) ppm (R = Ph, Vi);
δ^{29}Si VI (−56) – (−60) ppm; (R = Me); (−71) – (−74) ppm (R = Ph, Vi);
δ^{29}Si VII (−45) – (−51) ppm (R = Me); (−62) – (−67) ppm (R = Ph, Vi)
δ^{29}Si VIII (−38) – (−44) ppm (R = Me); (−53) – (−58) ppm (R = Ph, Vi).

Integral intensity ratios of silicon signals for T_n^R and TAS in the initial mixture as well as integral intensity sum of TAS, tetrafunctional units I–IV and for trifunctional units V–VIII in finished products correspond to the taken reaction mixture composition. Units IV and V were the most difficult to identify. Thus, IV could be identified in neither reaction product and V was identified only at molar ratio $[T_n^R]_0 : [TAS]_0 = 1 : 0.5$. Good agreement of molar ratio of rated values for tetrafunctional and trifunctional units found with experimentally from integral intensity ratios of ^{29}Si signals allowed to find out that ^{29}Si NMR can by used for quantitative determination of TAS, VIII, units I–III and V–VII in the reaction mixture with an accuracy of 10%. This also indicates the absence or low content of unit IV under chosen ratios of the reagents. Mole fraction of each unit was determined for TAS and I–IV on the base of ^{29}Si NMR spectra by a formula:

$$S'_n \Big/ \sum_{n=0}^{n=4} S'_n \quad (n = 0\text{–}4) \tag{4.4}$$

and for V–VIII by a formula

$$S''_m \Big/ \sum_{m=0}^{m=3} S''_m \tag{4.5}$$

where S'_n—integral intensity of silicon signals for tetrafunctional units, S''_m integral intensity of silicon signals for trifunctional units.

It was proved by means of GLC method and by TAS and VIII content change that on various TAS interaction with T_n^{Ph} at $[T_n^{Ph}]_0 = 0.33$ mol/l, $[TAS]_0 = 1$ mol/l, $[KOH]_0 = 0.008$ mol/l and $t = 70$°C, TMS was the most reactive (65% conversion was achieved during 3 min), then follows TES (25 min). The growth of TAS reactivity as alkyl substituent content is decreased agress well with nucleophilic character of the reaction and drop of alkyl group steric effect. The higher is TAS reactivity the more is $RSi(OR')_3$ formation rate. The reactivity of T_n^R with different "R" does not change significantly. Under the chosen ratio of reagents and after reaction of TAS with T_n^R is in the equilibrium TAS content was 0.37–0.42 mol. fr. (in regard of $[TAS]_0$ and VIII—0.40–0.50 mol.fr. (in regard of $[T_n^R]_0$). On the ground of reaction product chromatography analysis for the content of $(R'O)_4Si$ and $RSi(OR')_3$ balanced amounts one can come to the conclusion that the nature of a substituent at silicon in T_n^R or alkoxy group does not greatly affect them. The study of T_n^R reaction with TAS at temperatures of 40, 50, 60 and 70°C ($[T_n^R]_0 = 0.33$ mol/l, $[KOH]_0 = 0.008$ mol/l) proved that balanced content of TAS and VIII does not depend on temperature. It is demonstrated by the example of T_n^{Ph} reaction with TMS. On the ground of analysis of silicon signal integral intensity ratios in ^{29}Si NMR spectra by equations (4.4) and (4.5), equilibrium content in molar fraction of TAS, I–IV (in regard to $[TAS]_0$) and

V–VIII (in regard to $[T_n^R]_0$) with $[T_n^R]_0$ and $[TAS]_0$ molar ratios (in terms of one unit)—1:0.5; 1:1.5; 1:3; 1:4.5; 1:6 was found. With the purpose to find general regularities of alkoxy groups distribution by units experimental data comparison with possible statistic content of various units in the reaction product equilibrium mixture was carried out. Thus molar fractions of alkoxy groups (a_0) related to initial TAS and siloxy bonds (b_0) related to T_n^R were calculated in regard to total sum of reactive groups by formulas (4.6, 4.7):

$$a_0 = 4[TAC]_0 : (4[TAC]_0 + 3[T_n^R]_0) \tag{4.6}$$

$$b_0 = 1 - a_0 \tag{4.7}$$

The sum of molar fractions of R′O-groups and siloxy bonds, participating in the exchange is assumed as 1. Equilibrium constant K_e can be calculated on the ground of reaction equation (4.5) by formulas (4.8) and (4.9):

$$K_e.a_e.b_e = (a_0 - a_e)^2 \tag{4.8}$$

$$b_e = (1 + a_e - 2a_0), \text{ to } K_e = (a_0 - a_e)^2/(a_e)\cdot(1 - 2a_0 + a_e) \tag{4.9}$$

Where a_e is an equilibrium molar fraction of alkoxy groups, related to tetrafunctional units, b_e—is an equilibrium molar fraction of siloxy bonds, related to trifunctional units; a_e/a_0 ratio can be determined on the base of ^{29}Si signal integral intensities in NMR-spectra of equilibrium mixture by the following formulas:

$$a_e/a_0 = \sum_{n=0}^{n=4} S'_n \Big/ \left(\sum_{n=0}^{n=4} S'_n + \sum_{m=0}^{m=3} S''_m\right) = y \tag{4.10}$$

$$\sum_{n=0}^{n=4} S'_n = 4S'_{TAC} + 3S'_I + 2S'_{II} + S'_{III} \tag{4.11}$$

S'_{TAS}, S'_I, S'_{II} and S'_{III} are areas of silicon signals in tetrafunctional units, involving 4-1 ethoxy groups at silicon respectively

$$\sum_{m=0}^{m=3} S''_m = 3S''_{VIII} + 2S''_{VII} + S''_{VI} \tag{4.12}$$

S''_{VIII}, S''_{VII}, S''_{VI} are areas of silicon signals in trifunctional units, involving 3-1 ethoxy groups at silicon. "K_p" value can be determined by formula (4.13):

$$K_e = (a_0 - a_0y)^2/a_0y(1 + a_0y - 2a_0) = a_0(1-y)^2/(y\cdot[1 - a_0(2-y)]) \tag{4.13}$$

It was found that "K_e" values for TAS reaction with T_n^R were equal to 1–0.1, i.e. functional group distributions between tetra- and three functional units are proportional to molar fraction of the functional groups, related to these units and are statistic ones. Formulas of statistic distribution were used to determine equilibrium quantities of $[TAS]_e$, $[VIII]_e$ and units $[I]_e - [VI]_e$ at statistic content. The contents of each type units provided by tetrafunctional silicon atoms (in mol. fract.) can be calculated by thc following equation:

$$[\mathrm{TAC}]_e = (a_e)^4/(a_0)^4 \tag{4.14}$$

$$[\mathrm{I}]_e = 4(a_e)^3(a_0 - a_e)/(a_0)^4 \tag{4.15}$$

$$[\mathrm{II}]_p = 6(a_e)^2(a_0 - a_e)^2 0/(a_0)^4 \tag{4.16}$$

$$[\mathrm{III}]_e = 4(a_e)(a_0 - a_e)^3/(a_0)^4 \tag{4.17}$$

$$[\mathrm{IV}]_e = (a_0 - a_e)^4/(a_0)^4 \tag{4.18}$$

The content of various types of trifunctional units can be calculated by the equations:

$$[\mathrm{VIII}]_e = (a_0 - a_e)^3/(1 - a_0)^3 \tag{4.19}$$

$$[\mathrm{VII}]_e = 3(a_0 - a_e)^2(1 - 2a_0 + a_e)/(1 - a_0)^3 \tag{4.20}$$

$$[\mathrm{VI}]_e = 3(a_0 - a_e)(1 - 2a_0 + a_e)^2/(1 - a_0)^3 \tag{4.21}$$

$$[\mathrm{V}]_e = (1 - 2a_0 + a_e)^3/(1 - a_0)^3 \tag{4.22}$$

Hence on the ground of equations (4.14–4.22) statistic equilibrium contents of all unit types were calculated spectroscopy and GLC for TAS. Change of calculated and experimental values of various type unit content in regard of reagent ratios are shown in Tables 5 and 6. On the ground of equation (4.9) and value of $K_e = 1$ follows that $a_e = a_0^2$. Comparison of calculated and experimental data for tetrafunctional

TABLE 5
Unit equilibrium contents during TMS reaction with T_n^{Me} (1–4), T_n^{Vi} (5–8) and T_n^{Ph} (9 – 12), TPS with T_n^{Me} (13–15), T_n^{Ph} (16–18) at various temperatures and theoretically calculated ones (19) at initial reagent ratios $[T_n^R]_0$:$[TAS]_0$ = 1:3.

N	t°C	a_0	$[TAC]_0$	$[I]_e$	$[II]_e$	$[III]_e$	$[IV]_e$	$[V]_e$	$[VI]_e$	$[VII]_e$	$[VIII]_e$
1	70	0.80	0.38	0.45	0.15	0.02	—	—	0.12	0.43	0.45
2	60	-//-	0.39	0.47	0.13	0.01	—	—	0.10	0.45	0.44
3	50	-//-	0.38	0.45	0.16	0.01	—	—	0.12	0.44	0.44
4	40	-//-	0.37	0.47	0.16	—	—	—	0.11	0.44	0.45
5	70	-//-	0.36	0.46	0.15	0.03	—	—	0.14	0.44	0.42
6	60	-//-	0.35	0.47	0.18	—	—	—	0.12	0.46	0.42
7	50	-//-	0.35	0.46	0.19	—	—	—	0.17	0.45	0.38
8	40	-//-	0.37	0.47	0.16	—	—	—	0.12	0.44	0.44
9	70	-//-	0.34	0.47	0.19	—	—	—	0.06	0.47	0.47
10	60	-//-	0.35	0.48	0.17	—	—	—	0.15	0.46	0.39
11	50	-//-	0.36	0.47	0.17	—	—	—	0.17	0.44	0.41
12	40	-//-	0.37	0.46	0.16	—	—	—	0.21	0.44	0.35
13	70	-//-	0.41	0.46	0.13	—	—	—	0.19	0.48	0.33
14	60	-//-	0.37	0.45	0.18	—	—	—	0.21	0.47	0.32
15	50	-//-	0.39	0.45	0.16	—	—	—	0.17	0.46	0.37
16	70	-//-	0.38	0.47	0.15	—	—	—	0.12	0.48	0.40
17	60	-//-	0.38	0.47	0.15	—	—	—	0.13	0.49	0.38
18	50	-//-	0.38	0.46	0.16	—	—	—	0.13	0.44	0.43
19	—	-//-	0.41	0.46	0.15	0.03	$1 \cdot 10^{-4}$	$8 \cdot 10^{-3}$	0.10	0.38	0.51

TABLE 6

Equilibrium unit contents on T_n^{Me} reaction with TES (1, 4, 12, 20) and TPS (5, 13, 21), T_n^{Ph} with TMS (6, 14, 22), TES (2, 7, 15, 23) and TPS (8, 16, 24), T_n^{Vi} with TMS (9, 17, 25) and TES (10, 18, 26) and theoretically calculated ones (3, 11, 19, 27)

N	t°C	a_0	$[TAC]_0$	$[I]_e$	$[II]_e$	$[III]_e$	$[IV]_e$	$[V]_e$	$[VI]_e$	$[VII]_e$	$[VIII]_e$
1	70	0.40	0.05	0.13	0.35	0.47	—	0.27	0.43	0.25	0.25
2	-//-	-//-	0.04	0.12	0.38	0.46	—	0.26	0.45	0.23	0.06
3	—	-//-	0.03	0.15	0.35	0.35	0.13	0.22	0.43	0.29	0.06
4	70	0.67	0.18	0.40	0.26	0.16	—	—	0.32	0.48	0.20
5	-//-	-//-	0.22	0.47	0.31	—	—	—	0.29	0.51	0.20
6	-//-	-//-	0.14	0.39	0.33	0.14	—	—	0.23	0.50	0.27
7	-//-	-//-	0.15	0.34	0.33	0.18	—	—	0.27	0.51	0.22
8	-//-	-//-	0.18	0.42	0.30	0.10	—	—	0.28	0.51	0.21
9	-//-	-//-	0.17	0.42	0.30	0.11	—	—	0.25	0.49	0.26
10	-//-	-//-	0.17	0.40	0.35	0.08	—	—	0.24	0.55	0.21
11	—	-//-	0.20	0.40	0.29	0.10	—	—	0.22	0.44	0.30
12	70	0.86	0.49	0.38	0.13	—	—	—	0.22	0.39	0.39
13	-//-	-//-	0.51	0.40	0.09	—	—	—	—	0.35	0.65
14	-//-	-//-	0.48	0.42	0.10	—	—	—	0.13	0.37	0.50
15	-//-	-//-	0.48	0.41	0.11	—	—	—	—	0.50	0.50
16	-//-	-//-	0.47	0.43	0.10	—	—	—	—	0.39	0.61
17	-//-	-//-	0.50	0.41	0.09	—	—	—	0.12	0.40	0.48
18	-//-	-//-	0.48	0.42	0.10	—	—	—	—	0.53	0.47
19	—	-//-	0.55	0.36	0.09	0.01	$4{\cdot}10^{-4}$	$3{\cdot}10^{-3}$	0.05	0.31	0.64
20	70	0.89	0.60	0.35	0.05	—	—	—	—	0.47	0.53
21	-//-	-//-	0.59	0.34	0.07	—	—	—	—	0.37	0.63
22	-//-	-//-	0.57	0.37	0.06	—	—	—	0.11	0.33	0.56
23	-//-	-//-	0.59	0.35	0.06	—	—	—	—	0.39	0.61
24	-//-	-//-	0.58	0.36	0.06	—	—	—	—	0.39	0.61
25	-//-	-//-	0.56	0.37	0.07	—	—	—	0.09	0.34	0.57
26	-//-	-//-	0.58	0.34	0.08	—	—	—	—	0.40	0.60
27	—	-//-	0.63	0.31	0.06	0.005	$1{\cdot}10^{-4}$	$1{\cdot}10^{-3}$	0.03	0.26	0.70

units (Table 6) demonstrated their good agreement on recording by both ^{29}Si NMR spectoscopy and GLC for TAS.

Deriviations are in the range of determination error. General regularity of threefunctional unit content change tends to decline from statistic data regarding organotrialkoxysilanes VIII and to increase regarding units VI, VII (Table 6). Deriviations from the calculated data may result from insignificant equilibrium shift among of trifunctional units towards mixed alkoxysiloxane units.

Thus, on the ground of ^{29}Si NMR spectroscopy it was found that on TAS interaction with T_n^R alkoxy-groups distribution between trifunctional and tetrafunctional units as well as various type tetrafunctional unit contents in equilibrium products of catalytic rearrangement were close to statistic one, but increased content of alkoxysilane units was typical for trifunctional ones.

The study of various unit equilibrium contents at temperature range of 40–70°C by ^{29}Si NMR spectroscopy shows that they do not depend on temperature (Table 5). These agree with GLC data and leads to the conclusion that enthalpy factor slightly effects equilibrium composition of catalytic rearrangement reacion on alkoxy group interaction with siloxane bond.

Study of equilibrium composition of various type units, TAS and VIII on TAS interaction with T_n^R demonstrates that enthalpy factor slight dependence on rearrangement process is similar to that of organosilixane catalytic polymerization process.[36]

2.5 Study of Equilibrium Reactions at Organosiloxane Interaction with Hydrogen Chloride

Hydrolysis reactions of various organochlorosilanes constantly attract attention of researches, as they are the basic means for various organosiloxane production. Hydrogen chloride gas or hydrochloric acid which can significantly effect reaction direction are formed as a rule at organochlorosilane hydrolysis. Thus, it was shown in [38] that in the presence of 29 and 34% hydrochloric acid 1,1,1,3,3,5,5,7,7,7-decamethyltetrasiloxane undergoes catalytic rearrangement with the formation of hexamethyldisiloxane, octamethylcyclotetrasiloxane and linear siloxane with various molecular mass due to siloxane bond cleavage.

The higher is hydrocloric acid concentration the deeper are conversions. The study of trimethylchlorosilane co-hydrolysis with organochlorosilanes of various functionality showed that co-hydrolysis product compositions depended on siloxane backbone catalytic rearrangement under hydrochloric acid effect.[8,9] According to [40] organochlorosilane hydrolysis is reversible. Values of equilibrium constant of R_3SiCl hydrolysis reaction taking place by equation (5.1) are the same in the studied range of hydrochloric acid concentrations (from 26 to 42%) and can be calculated by formula (5.2):

$$R_3SiCl + H_2O \Longleftrightarrow R_3SiOSiR_3 + 2HCl \tag{5.1}$$

$$K_1 = [B(A + B)a]/(Aa) \tag{5.2}$$

where A—R_3SiCl concentration and B—$(R_3Si)_2O$, a_1—activity of H_2O, a_2—activity of HCl. However, taking into consideration the values of a_1 and a_2, given in[39] and,[40] we have found that K_1 values increased several times when hydrochloric acid concentration changes from 26 to 42%. Along with hydrochloric acid HCl_{gas} also efficiently cleaves siloxane bond when it is bubbled through organosiloxane. There is a number of patents[41–43] where problems of organochlorosilane cleavage by HCl_{gas} are highlighted. Results given in these works do not allow to identify general regularities of HCl interaction with siloxanes.

The effect of HCl, dissolved in water or water salt solutions as well as in gaseous condition on monofunctional organochlorosilane hydrolysis reversibility is investigated in this paper. The composition study of Me_3SiCl and HMe_2SiCl water hydrolysis products demonstrated close relationship between hydrolysis products and final concentration of formed hydrochloric acid when hydrochloric acid concentration was 25% initial organochlorosilanes were found in reaction products along with $(Me_3Si)_2O$ and $(HMe_2Si)_2O$. Their content increases as hydrochloric acid concentration grows. Maximal content of Me_3SiCl and HMe_2SiCl in hydrolysis products achieved 84% from the primary amount at 20°C and hydrochloric acid concentration—42.4 and 42.6% respectively. According to the reversible character of the process, and when contact time is long enough, $(Me_3Si)_2O$ and $(HMe_2Si)_2O$ interact with hydrochloric acid with the formation of balanced amounts of related organochlorosilanes and water in R_3SiCl—$(R_3Si)_2O$—HCl—H_2O system. R_3SiCl content is determined by hydrochloric acid final concentration. On $(Me_3Si)_2O$ and $(HMe_2Si)_2O$ interaction with HCl_{gas} the degree of cleavage results from the balanced character of the process and is related to maximal concentration of hydrochloric acid, produced in the reaction. Thus, maximal cleavage of $(Me_3Si)_2O$ and $(HMe_2Si)_2O$ achieved at HCl_{gas} bubbling at the pressure of 1 atm and 20°C is 84%. 42.4% hydrochloric acid concentration for HMe_2SiCl and 42.6% for Me_3SiCl correspond to this cleavage degree. Hydrogen chloride concentration in organic and water phases and consequently $(Me_3Si)_2O$ cleavage depth can be increased due to temperature drop. Maximal cleavage degree of $(Me_3Si)_2O$ and $(HMe_2Si)_2O$ (99%) was achieved at the temperature of −14°C, when formed aqueous phase was hydrochloric acid of 50% concentration. This explains the choice of temperature ranges for $(Me_3Si)_2O$ cleavage from +10 to −15°C.[44–46] The increase of $(R_3Si)_2O$ cleavage degree can be also achieved without temperature drop due to HCl pressure increase as it also resulting in the growth of its concentration in organic acid aqueous phases.

It was found that in the presence of hydrochloric acid solution $(Me_3Si)_2O$ cleavage by HCl gas is much faster than in its absence. This allows to suppose that $(Me_3Si)_2O$ cleavage takes place not only in organic phase and in aqueous one or in the interface, in the latter cases the reaction is faster thereby. Comparison of $(Me_3Si)_2O$ and $(HMe_2Si)_2O$, $[(ClCH_2)Me_2Si]_2O$ and $(Et_3Si)_2O$ with 40.6% hydrochloric acid taken in such ratio that final concentration of hydrochloric acid is 40% demonstrated that balanced content of $(R_3Si)_2O$ and R_3SiCl depends on substituent type at silicon. Product compositions at $(R_3Si)_2O$ cleavage by hydrochloric acid (in terms of taken $(R_3Si)_2O$) is given below:

$$\underset{63.7\%}{HMe_2SiOSiMe_2H} \underset{H_2O}{\overset{2HCl}{\rightleftharpoons}} \underset{36.3\%}{2HMe_2SiCl} \qquad (5.3)$$

$$\underset{62.1\%}{Me_3SiOSiMe_3} \underset{H_2O}{\overset{2HCl}{\rightleftharpoons}} \underset{37.9\%}{2Me_3SiCl} \qquad (5.4)$$

$$\underset{86.7\%}{(ClCH_2)Me_2SiOSiMe_2(CH_2Cl)} \underset{H_2O}{\overset{2HCl}{\rightleftharpoons}} \underset{13.3\%}{2(ClCH_2)Me_2SiCl} \qquad (5.5)$$

$$\underset{90.2\%}{Et_3SiOSiEt_3} \underset{H_2O}{\overset{2HCl}{\rightleftharpoons}} \underset{9.8\%}{Et_3SiCl} \qquad (5.6)$$

Balanced content of $(R_3Si)_2O$ increases with the growth of the size of substituents at silicon in the following sequence:

$$(Et_3Si)_2O > [Me_2(ClCH_2)Si]_2O > (Me_3SiO)_2 \cong (HMe_2Si)O_2$$

This also occurs on Me_3SiCl, HMe_2SiCl, Et_3SiCl and $(ClCH_2)Me_2SiCl$ hydrolysis with water at such reagent ratios that hydrochloric acid final concentration is 40%, which points to the balanced character of reaction mixture composition both under organosiloxane cleavage by hydrochloric acid and R_3SiCl hydrolysis.

Decrease of the organochlorosilane balanced with growth of the size of substituents on silicon was observed on $(R_3Si)_2O$ cleavage by HCl_{gas}. Interaction with HCl_{gas} at $-10°C$ conversion for $(Me_3Si)_2O$ and $(HMe_2Si)_2O$ was 98%, for $[(ClCH_2)Me_2Si]_2O$—20% and for $(Et_3Si)_2O$—14% in a similar sequence the organodisiloxane cleavage rate decreases. $(R_3Si)_2O$ balanced content increases may result from the growth of intermediate R_3SiOH stability and their content in an organic phase as the size of substituents on silicon increases. R_3SiOH effect on the process can be shown as follows:

$$R_3SiOSiR_3 + 2HCl \Longleftrightarrow R_3SiOH.HCl + R_3SiCl \Longleftrightarrow 2R_3SiCl + H_2O \quad (5.7)$$

Dependence of product composition on R_3SiCl hydrolysis and hydrochloric acid interaction with $(R_3Si)_2O$ on final concentration of the produced hydrochloric acid is the result of hydrogen chloride activity change when bonded by water with formation of hydrate complexes. The lower the hydrochloric acid concentration the lower is HCl reactivity, as with the degree of hydration growth energy consumption for complex destruction increases. R_3SiCl absence in hydrolysis products at hydrochloric acid low concentrations (below 25%) and shows that at molar ratio of H_2O to HCl equal to 6 or higher the process is actually irreversible. Molar ratio of H_2O to HCl equal to 6 corresponds to $HCl.6H_2O$ complex and maximal saturation of the first hydrate layer for oxonium complex $[H_3O^+5H_2O]Cl$. When hydrochloric acid concentration is more than 25% hydration degree is below maximal, which results in HCl reactivity increase in regard of siloxane bond. Thus, saturated solution of hydrochloric acid with 36.6% concentration (at 20°C and atmospheric pressure) corresponding to average composition of hydrate complex $HCl.3{,}5H_2O$ demonstrated high activity to $(Me_3Si)_2O$ and $(HMe_2Si)_2O$. Unlike HCl water reactivity drops with the increase of hydrochloric acid concentration as energy consumption necessary for destruction of hydrate complexes with HCl. Hydration influence on hydrolysis is clear from various heat effects on Me_3SiCl hydrolysis with great excess of water and concentrated hydrochloric acid. At Me_3SiCl hydrolysis with hydrochloric acid in conditions providing HCl_{gas} formation the process is endothermal (reaction mixture temperature decreases). This results from low heat effect of hydrolytic reaction with HCl_{gas} production ($\Delta H(1)$— $+11.7\,kJ/mol$); calculated on the base of Me_3SiCl, $(Me_3Si)_2O$, H_2O, HCl_{gas} formation heats, given in [47], and it does not compensate energy spent on HCl hydrate complex destruction. Me_3SiCl hydrolysis by large excess of water is accompanied by significant heating of the reaction mixture, as high energy of HCl hydration ($-75.2\,kJ/mol$) provides exothermal effect. Me_3SiCl—H_2O—HCl—$(Me_3Si)_2O$ system balanced composition dependence on solvation process at HCl and H_2O interaction is evident from reaction (5.1) thermodynamics with regard of reagent conditions.

$$2Me_3SiCl_I + H_2O_I \Longleftrightarrow Me_3SiOSiMe_{3I} + 2HCl_{aq} \quad (5.8)$$

where the following record can be made

$$\Delta G\ (298\,\mathrm{K}) = \Delta H\ (298\,\mathrm{K}) - 293.15\Delta S\ (298\,\mathrm{K}) \tag{5.9}$$

Here

$$\Delta H = \Delta fH(\mathrm{Me_3SiOSiMe_{3l}}) - 2\Delta fH(\mathrm{Me_3SiCl_l}) - \Delta fH(\mathrm{H_2O_l}) + 2\Delta fH(\mathrm{HCl_{aq}}) \tag{5.10}$$

Enthalpy of HCl_{aq} formation depends on a number of water moles accounted for HCl mole in water solution. According to [45] this dependence can be expressed by a formula:

$$\Delta fH(\mathrm{HCl_{aq}})\,\mathrm{kJ} = -126.6 - 9.3366\,\mathrm{M} + 6.84218\,\mathrm{M}^2 \tag{5.11}$$

Other formation enthalpies were taken from [45]. Then

$$\Delta H = 239.1 + 2\Delta fH(\mathrm{HCl_{aq}})\,\mathrm{kJ} \tag{5.12}$$

ΔS value is determined by reaction (5.9) component entropies; HCl_{aq} entropy can be found from HCl vapor pressure above hydrochloric acid aqueous solution, taken from,[46] enthalpies of HCl vapor from HCl aqueous solution, calculated by equation (5.11) and absolute entropy of HCl_{gas} equal to 186.8 J/(mol.K).[47] Other component entropies were taken from [48]. Then

$$\Delta S = -186.4 + 2S(\mathrm{HCl_{aq}})\,\mathrm{J/K} \tag{5.13}$$

Combining equations (5.9, 5.12, 5.13) we'll have:

$$\Delta G = -RT\ln K = 294 + (2\Delta fH(\mathrm{HCl_{aq}}) - 0.29315S(\mathrm{HCl_{aq}})\,\mathrm{kJ} \tag{5.14}$$

"K" value can be calculated by experimental data regarding organic and aqueous phase compositions (see Table 7)

$$K = n_1(\mathrm{Me_3SiOSiMe_3})(n_2(\mathrm{HCl}))^2/n_3(\mathrm{H_2O})(n_4(\mathrm{Me_3SiCl}))^2 \tag{5.15}$$

Here $n_1(\mathrm{Me_3SiOSiMe_3})$, $n_2(\mathrm{HCl})$, $n_3(\mathrm{H_2O})$, $n_4(\mathrm{Me_3SiCl})$—number of moles of each component.

$RT\ln K$ value was converted to the total number of moles equal to 6, conventional value, chosen in regard of reaction (5.10) stoichiometry Experimental data are described by equation (5.16).

$$\begin{aligned}-RT\ln K &= 299.7 \pm 7 + (1.987 \pm 0.05)5.\Delta fH(\mathrm{HCl_{aq}})\\ &\quad - 0.29315\mathrm{S}(\mathrm{HCl_{aq}})\,\mathrm{kJ}, \quad r = 0.998\end{aligned} \tag{5.16}$$

Agreement of theoretical and found by the least squares method coefficients of equations (5.14) and (5.16) testifies to the actual equilibrium between aqueous and organic phases. Equation (5.15) advantage against equation (5.2) is its better suitability for calculations. More over on the ground of equation (5.16), we can determine reaction (5.8) enthalpy from equilibrium data at the same temperature due to the relationship between $\Delta fH(\mathrm{HCl_{aq}})$ and hydrochloric acid concentration.

TABLE 7
Balanced Compositions and Aqueous Phase Properties in $Me_3SiCl—H_2O—HCl—Me_3SiOSiMe_3$ system.

Balanced Compositions (experimental) HCl mol, (%)	H_2O mol	$(Me_3Si)_2O$ mol	Me_3SiCl mol	ΔG^b kJ	ΔG^c kJ (on 6 mols)	Index ΔfH (HCl_{aq})	$p(HCl)^a$ mm.Hg	$S(HCl_{aq})$ J mol.k
0.686 (25)	4.162	0.343	0.0026	−21.1	−24.4	−157.7	1.5	19.2
0.823 (30)	3.885	0.412	0.019	−12.9	−15.1	−155.2	10.6	11.5
0.933 (34)	3.663	0.467	0.0775	−7.11	−8.28	−152.5	50.5	7.3
0.987 (36)	3.552	0.494	0.163	−3.97	−4.60	−151.2	105	5.8
1.042 (38)	3.441	0.521	0.402	−0.04	−0.04	−149.8	210	4.6
1.097 (40)	3.330	0.549	0.595	1.41	1.52	−148.6	399	3.5
1.114 (40.6)	3.296	0.557	0.832	2.91	3.01	−148.2	475^a	3.4
1.152 (42)	3.219	0.576	2.451	7.87	6.38	−147.2	709	3.1
1.168 (42.6)	3.185	0.584	4.583	10.8	6.80	−146.9	832^a	3.0

Notice: a) Pressure of HCl vapor over hydrochloric acid with concentration of 40.6 and 42.6 was calculated by the equation $\ln p(HCl)$ mm. Hg $= -19.851 + 9.7425\,(c/10) - 0.8375\,(c/10)^2$, found for concentration range of 38–42%; b) Calculated; c) Experimentally found.

This possibility was not noticed by the authors.[39] Who had determined reaction (5.8) enthalpy by measuring balanced composition dependence on temperature.

R_3SiCl hydrolytic reaction and $(R_3Si)_2O$ cleavage by hydrogen chloride are possible in any of available phases (gas, organic, aqueous) as well as on their interface as each component is in the equilibrium with each phase. The possibility of all components of the reaction system presence in each phase is confirmed by GLC method. When the reaction system composition was studied on Me_3SiCl hydrolysis with water and dioxane mixture with toluene, providing homogenity (Me_3SiCl—2.5%, H_2O—0.8%, dioxane—91.2%, toluene—5.5 wt%) simultaneous presence of significant amounts of $(R_3Si)_2O$, Me_3SiCl, Me_3SiOH and HCl was shown.

Hydrochloric acid analysis formed on Me_3SiCl hydrolysis demonstrated organosilicone product presence in it, their total content was 0.007 mol/l in terms of Me_3SiCl (determined by atomic adsorption spectroscopy by silicon content). Relationship between HCl and water activity under hydrolysis and hydration processes is still more evident under hydrolysis by salt solutions. On Me_3SiCl hydrolysis by NaCl, KCl, NH_4Cl, $CaCl_2$, LiCl solutions, HCl effect on hydrolysis products composition depended critically on the strength of hydrate complexes, formed by these salts. On Me_3SiCl hydrolysis by NaCl, KCl, NH_4Cl saturated solutions at hydrochloric acid concentration higher than 25%, Me_3SiCl and $(Me_3Si)_2O$ ratio in reaction products is actually the same as under hydrolysis by water. In the presence of $CaCl_2$ and LiCl saturated solutions hydrolysis is inhibited. Thus, if under hydrolysis by water the balanced composition of Me_3SiCl and $(Me_3Si)_2O$ is achieved very quickly after the reagents have been mixed, in $CaCl_2$ and LiCl presence period when the equilibrium is achieved increases several times. In organic phase increased content of Me_3SiCl which gradually decreased to equilibrium. Period of system balancing increases several times on $CaCl_2$ solution transfer to LiCl solutions of similar concentrations and with the increase of relative share of organic phase. Increase of period for system balancing at Me_3SiCl hydrolysis by $CaCl_2$ and LiCl solutions results from the activity decrease of water bonded to hydrate complexes with salts.

The other peculiarity of Me_3SiCl hydrolysis in the presence of $CaCl_2$ and LiCl saturated solutions is in the presence of Me_3SiCl balanced amounts in reaction products already at low HCl concentration in the aqueous phase. Me_3SiCl balanced content achieves 60% on Me_3SiCl hydrolysis by LiCl saturated solution at HCl concentration in aqueous phase—7%, $CaCl_2$—26% and by water—42%. The equilibrium in Me_3SiCl—$(Me_3Si)_2O$ system is shifted towards Me_3SiCl as HCl concentration increases in aqueous-salt phase. With the decrease of salt concentration the present in Me_3SiCl—$(Me_3Si)_2O$ composition is achieved at higher HCl concentrations. Comparison of hydrolytic product composition at similar concentrations of $CaCl_2$ and LiCl solutions demonstrated that in the case of LiCl the equilibrium is shifted towards higher Me_3SiCl content. Thus for 42% $CaCl_2$ and LiCl solutions involving 9% HCl, molar ratio of $[Me_3SiCl] / [(Me_3Si)_2O]$ is 0.01 and 8.5 respectively. Large efficiency of HCl effect in aqueous solutions of metal chlorides is the result of solution ion strength increase and decrease of HCl dissociation degree in a solution.

Study of $(Me_3Si)_2O$ interaction with HCl gas in the presence of $CaCl_2$ solution showed that $(Me_3Si)_2O$ cleavage is faster than in hydrochloric acid presence. An induction period is observed on the initial stage in the same way as the course of $(Me_3Si)_2O$ cleavage in salt absence which is evidently due to the necessity of aqueous-salt phase formation, promoting process activation. Water bonding to strong hydrate complexes in $CaCl_2$ presence results in more considerable degree of $Me_3SiOSiMe_3$ cleavage. It agrees with data[42] proving that at reagent ratios providing that maximum hydration degree of water-formed salts does not exceed 6 molecules of water per 1 molecule of salt, $Me_3SiOSiMe_3$ qualitative cleavage is possible at 20°C in the presence of water-free $ZnCl_2$, $CaCl_2$ and $MgCl_2$ salts. The salts move the equilibrium towards Me_3SiCl.

Investigation results of Me_3SiCl hydrolysis by salt solutions prove that salt effect on the process is determined by hydration energy. HCl slightly decomposes hydrate complexes of the considered salts due to high energy of $CaCl_2$ and LiCl hydration. HCl solubility in $CaCl_2$ and LiCl solutions is lower than in water but low degree of HCl hydration in these salt solutions promotes its high activity in siloxane bond cleavage reaction which agrees with the experiment. HCl concentration in LiCl solutions is lower than in $CaCl_2$ solutions at similar salt concentrations. This is because LiCl molar concentration increase in comparison with $CaCl_2$ and H_2O bonding degree in hydrate complexes is higher. For 42% $CaCl_2$ solution molar ratio of water and salt is 8.5 and for LiCl—3.2. Taking into account that coordination number for inside hydrate sphere for Ca^{+2} is 6 and for Li^{+1} is 4.[49,50] at the closen concentration in LiCl solution water is bonded much stronger than in $CaCl_2$ solution. This results in LiCl more profound effect on Me_3SiCl hydrolysis than that of $CaCl_2$.

2.6 Study of Catalytic Rearrangement of Organosiloxanes at Interaction with Organochlorosilanes

α,ω-Dichloroligodimethylsiloxane synthesis is of practical and theoretical interest. Such compounds are widely used to produce organosiloxanes of tailor-made composition and structure[6] and block-copolymers.[51] Study of equilibrium and unequilibrium regularities of α,ω-dichloroligodimethylsiloxanes also allows to appreciate the peculiarities of Si—O and Si—Cl bond mutual effect on their reactivity. Basic method of said oligomer synthesis can be a reaction of dimethyldichlorosilane (DMDCS) partial hydrolysis or catalytic rearrangement on DMDCS interaction with dimethylcyclosiloxanes.[52] Regularities of octamethylcyclotetrasiloxane (D_4) catalytic telomerization reaction with DMDCS in the presence of electrophilic catalysts such as Lewis acids ($FeCl_3$, $AlCl_3$, $ZnCl_2$), their hydrates ($FeCl_3.6H_2O$, $AlCl_3.6H_2O$, $Al_2(SO_4)_3.18H_2O$, $ZnCl_2.4H_2O$), inorganic acids (H_2SO_4, H_3PO_4), aromatic sulfuric acids ($PhSO_3H$,(4-Me)$C_6H_4SO_3H$, (4-Me)(3-NO_2)$C_6H_3SO_3H$) and their mixtures with H_3PO_4. Catalytic rearrangement reaction on D_4 interaction with DMDCS can be shown in the following equation:

$$a\,[Me_2SiO]_4 + b\,Me_2SiCl_2 \overset{Cat.}{\Longleftrightarrow} c\,Cl[Me_2SiO]_{4n}SiMe_2Cl + d\,[Me_2SiO]_m \quad (6.1)$$

Study of various catalysts relative activity in the process of rearrangement was carried out at molar ratio of Me_2SiCl_2:$D_4 = 1{:}10$. When Lewis acid hydrates were used DMDCS quantity was taken in excess in regard of water involved in catalysts. Study of anhydrous $FeCl_3$, $AlCl_3$, $ZnCl_2$ activity demonstrated that reaction rate is very low in their presence. At the same time their hydrates showed high catalytic activity and fast consumption of D_4 and DMDCS is observed. As water in hydrate complexes interacts with DMDCS with hydrogen chloride isolation hydrate complex catalytic activity is determined by the activity of hydrogen chloride complex with Lewis acid. This is also confirmed by high catalytic activity of anhydrous Lewis acid when hydrogen chloride is passed through the reaction mass or on water introduction into reaction system involving anhydrous Lewis acid.

Comparison of activity of catalysts based on Lewis and organic acid in terms of time of D_4 50% conversion at 1% catalyst concentration showed the activity decrease in a series

$$FeCl_3.6H_2O > H_3PO_4 > H_2SO_4 > AlCl_3.6H_2O > ZnCl_2.2H_2O$$

Study of DMDCS and D_4 conversion dependence on time in the presence of 1% series of Lewis acid and inorganic acid hydrate complexes was carried out. The obtained data testifies that there is an induction period on D_4 conversion kinetic curves which is absent on DMDCS conversion curves. It should be mentioned that telomerization in the presence of the studied catalysts allows us to bring the reaction to the equilibrium (>0.5% DMDCS and 5% D_4).

The investigation of catalytic activity of H_2SO_4/H_3PO_4 binary mixture (1% + 1%) proved that its activity exceeded the activity by either component at 2% concentration. However in this case the induction period of the reaction is long because of binary catalyst low solubility in the reaction mixture. In this regard sulfuric acid-based catalysts, soluble in the studied reaction mixture are of significant interest. Benzenesulfuric acid, *p*-toluensulfuric acid, 4-methyl-3-nitrobenzenesulfoacid were studied as arylsulfuric acids. In the presence of 1% aromatic sulfoacids the process induction period is long, and their activity is a bit lower than that of phosphoric acid. DMDCS is completely consumed within 1–1.5 hours and the equilibrium in D_4 process is achieved within 8–10 hours. When aromatic sulfoacids in mixture with

H_3PO_4 are used, the induction period is several times reduced and reaction rate increases. In terms of D_4 consumption catalytic system activity changes in a series

$$(4\text{-Me})(3\text{-NO}_2)C_6H_3SO_3H/H_3PO_4 > PhSO_3H/H_3PO_4$$
$$> (4\text{-Me})C_6H_4SO_3H/H_3PO_4 > H_2SO_4/H_3PO_4$$

The induction period for these systems reduces in the same sequence. High activity of acid mixture can be explained by multistage telomerization. The possible pathway of telomerization process can be demonstrated as a series consecutive-parallel reactions

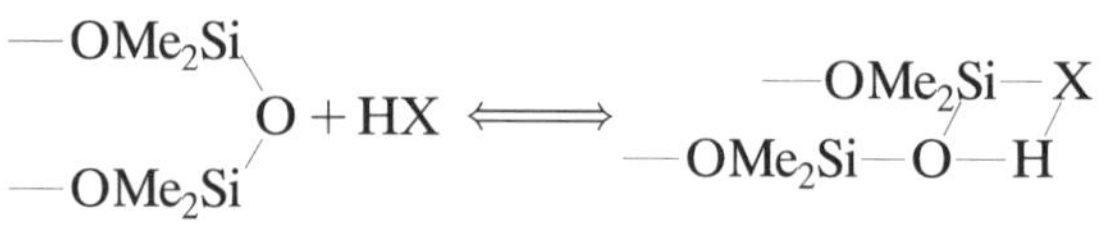

(6.2)

$HX = HX_1$ or HX_2—acid catalysts used

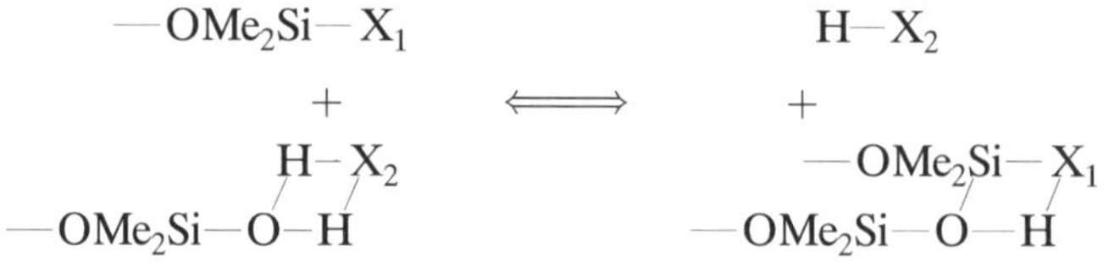

(6.3)

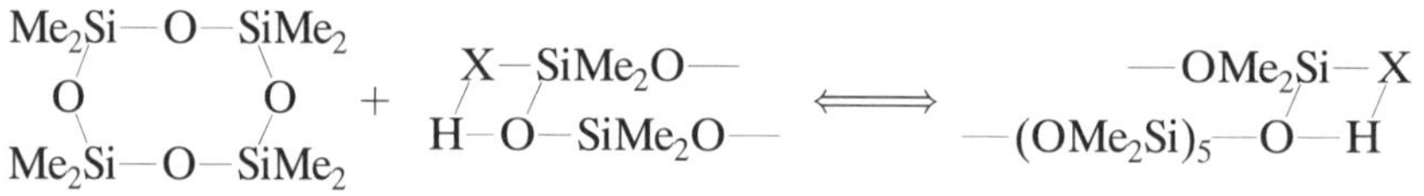

(6.4)

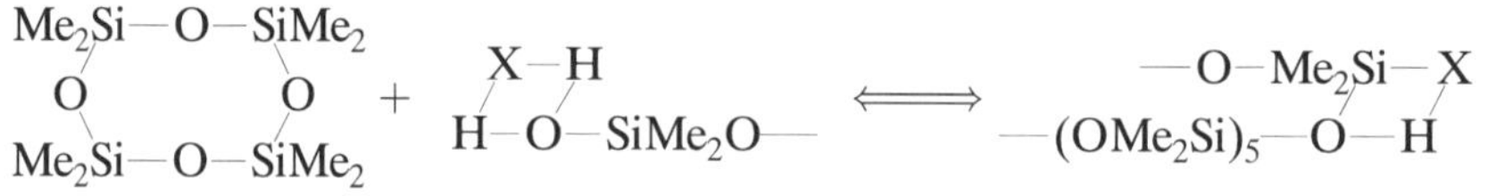

(6.5)

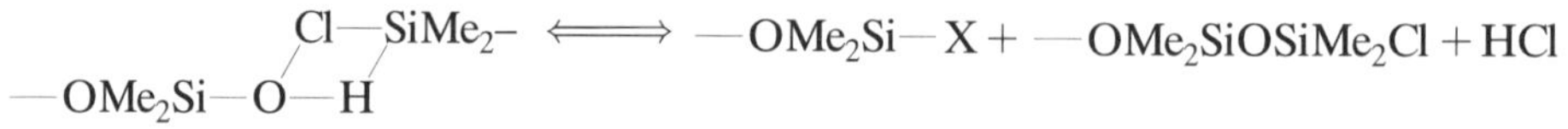

(6.6)

$$\text{—}(OMe_2Si)_nOMe_2Si\text{—}X + HCl \Longleftrightarrow \text{—}(OMe_2Si)_nMe_2SiMe\text{—}Cl + HX \quad (6.7)$$

There are differences in activity on the stage of the reaction centre formation (equation 6.2) and its reactions by siloxane bond (equation 6.4 and 6.5) for each catalyst. However the exchange reaction (equation 6.3) may result in total increase of reaction rate as the rates of reaction centre formation and its interaction with siloxane bond can increase. Rate constant of DMDCS and D_4 consumption were calculated in terms of reversible reactions of the first order. Constant values are given in Table 8. For mixed catalysts based on aromatic sulfo and phosphoric acids

TABLE 8
Values of DMDCS and D_4 consumption rate constants in the reactions catalyzed by complex catalysts based on aromatic sulfoacids and H_3PO_4.

Catalyses $ArSO_3H/H_3PO_4$ (0.1 mol/l:0.046 mol/l)	k_{DMDCS}, s^{-1}	k_{D4}, s^{-1}
$PhSO_3H/H_3PO_4$	$(0.60 + 0.038)\cdot 10^{-2}$	$(1.84 + 0.05)\cdot 10^{-3}$
$(4\text{-Me})C_6H_4SO_3H/H_3PO_4$	$(1.67 + 0.017)\cdot 10^{-2}$	$(1.77 + 0.05)\cdot 10^{-3}$
$(4\text{-Me})(3\text{-NO}_2)C_6H_3SO_3H/H_3PO_4$	$(3.14 + 0.060)\cdot 10^{-3}$	$(2.72 + 0.04)\cdot 10^{-3}$

each reagent consumption rate on kinetic sites of the curves does not depend on current concentration of other reagent and the reaction is the first order one for each reagent. This leads to the conclusion that in the course of telomerization each reagent enters into a number of independent reactions determining the observed kinetic peculiarities, and observed order of the reaction is imagined and constant values are conditional. Reactions with DMDCS, with end dimethylchlorosilane group in linear chain and with the growing polymer siloxane chain are possible for D_4. Higher rate constants of DMDCS consumption in comparison with D_4 show that along with dimethylsiloxane cycle opening (equation 6.8) DMDCS simultaneously reacts by siloxane chain with formed α,ω-dichloroligodimethylsiloxane (equation 6.9)

$$[Me_2SiO]_4 + Me_2SiCl_2 \xrightleftharpoons{\text{Cat.}} Cl(Me_2SiO)_5SiMe_2Cl \tag{6.8}$$

$$Me_2SiCl_2 + Cl(Me_2SiO)_5Me_2SiCl \xrightleftharpoons{\text{Cat.}} \begin{array}{l} Cl(Me_2SiO]_nMe_2SiCl \\ + Cl(Me_2SiO]_{5-n}Me_2SiCl \end{array} \tag{6.9}$$

In order to find out the reaction rate effect on catalyst component concentration D_4 telomerization with DMDCS by $(4\text{-Me})(3\text{-NO}_2)C_6H_3SO_3H/H_3PO_4$ catalytic mixture was carried out at various catalyst component ratios. Analysis of relationship between rate constant k_{D_4} values and catalyst component concentration showed that total reaction order in terms of catalysts was 3, order in terms of H_3PO_4 was 1 in terms of $(4\text{-Me})(3\text{-NO}_2)C_6H_3SO_3H$-2. Thus, the equation of D_4 consumption rate looks as follows.

$$W_{D_4} = k_{D_4}[D_4][H_3PO_4][Me(NO_2)C_6H_3SO_3H]^2 \tag{6.10}$$

TABLE 9
Values of D_4 consumption constant at various concentrations and component ratios of the catalytic mixture. $Me(NO_2)C_6H_3SO_3H/H_3PO_4$

H_3PO_4 mol/l	$(4\text{-Me})(3\text{-NO}_2)C_6H_3SO_3H$ mol/l	Constant of D_4 consumption rate, s^{-1}
0.17	0.023	$106\cdot 10^{-5}$
0.10	0.046	$272\cdot 10^{-5}$
0.05	0.023	$35.5\cdot 10^{-5}$
0.025	0.012	$4.4\cdot 10^{-5}$
0.10	0.023	$66\cdot 10^{-5}$

TABLE 10
Values of D_4 consumption rate constant in the course of catalysis by mixture of $Me(NO_2)C_6H_3SO_3H$ and H_3PO_4 (0.025 mol/l: 0.012 mol/l).

DMDCS:D_4 ratio	K_{D_4}, C^{-1}
1:10	$(4.38 + 0.2) \cdot 10^{-5}$
1:2	$(30.6 + 0.4) \cdot 10^{-5}$
1:1	$(72.2 + 0.4) \cdot 10^{-5}$

Study of DMDCS:D_4 initial ratio effect on telomerization reaction rate was carried out. Reaction pathway at initial ratios of DMDCS:D_4 = 1:10, 1:2 and 1:1 with H_3PO_4 (0.25 mol/l), and $Me(NO_2)C_6H_3SO_3H$ (0.012 mol/l) mixture grows as DMDCS content increases. Values of D_4 consumption rate constant are shown in Table 10.

Change of ratio DMDCS:D_4 in 10 times the value of rate constant k_{D_4} increases more 16 times.

3 CONCLUSION

In the result of the investigations we can formulate a number of general regularities for reaction study.

1. For rearrangement reactions with ≡Si—O—Si≡ or ≡Si—O—Si≡ and ≡Si—OR bond participation equilibrium constant does not depend on temperature, which indicates that reaction enthalpy is close to zero.
2. The studied reactions are enough described by kinetic equations for reversible reactions with the identical constant values up to a high level of conversion.
3. The initial concentration effect of all magnets on reaction rate constants was observed for all studied reactions. This effect is determined by the formation of several type reaction centres with various reactivity catalysts.

REFERENCES

1. V.M. Kopylov, C.P. Agashkov, A.M. Mosin and M.A. Gluchova, *Zh. Obshchei Khimii.*, 1989, **59**(5), p. 1065.
2. V.M. Kopylov, A.F. Fedotov, M.I. Shkol'nik and I.M. Raigorodskij, *Zh. Obshchei Khimii.*, 1989, **59**(11), p. 2515.
3. V.M. Kopylov, P.L. Prichod'ko, V.V. Kireev, N.G. Glasunova and I.M. Hasanov, *Vysokomolekularnye Soedineniya. B.*, 1988, **30**(12), p. 898.
4. V.M. Kopylov, I.S. Shragin, T.I. Ribkina, A.I. Chernishov, M.I. Shkol'nik and E.N. Uhina, *Zh. Obshchei Khimii.*, 1984, **54**(2), p. 359.
5. V.M. Kopylov, A.G. Voronkov, G.M. Zietlin, V.V. Kireev and S.K. Zinovich, *Vysokomolekularnye Soedineniya. A.*, 1984, **26**(8), p. 1706.
6. V.M. Kopylov, L.M. Hananashvili, M.I. Shkol'nik and A.G. Ivanov, *Vysokomolekularnye Soedineniya. A.*, 1995, **37**(3), p. 394.
7. V.M. Kopylov, A.G. Voronkov, G.M. Zietlin, V.V. Kireev and S.K. Zinovich, *Vysokomolekularnye Soedineniya A.*, 1984, **T26**(10), p. 789.

8. V.M. Kopylov, S.P. Agashkov, V.V. Kireev and M.E. Krilova, *Vysokomolekularnye Soedineniya. A.*, 1987, **29**(7), p. 1465.
9. V.M. Kopylov, S.P. Agashkov, V.V. Kireev and M.E. Krilova, *Deponente*, 1985, ONIITECHIM, Cherkassi, pp. 642–85.
10. I.V. Saharova, D.F. Yakovenko, T.V. Yakovenko and V.M. Kopylov, in book Chemistry of Organosilicon Compounds. Collection of scientific articles, 1988, Moscow: GNIIHTEOS. NIITECHIM., p. 135.
11. R.H. Krible and J.R. Elliot, *J. Am. Chem. Soc.*, 1945, **67**, p. 1813.
12. Pat. 3312737, 1983, BRD *R.J. Chim.*, 1985, 21H127.
13. Pat. 217520, 1983 DDR *R.J. Chim.*, 1985, 16H94.
14. N.M. Emanuel and D.G. Knorre, The Course of Chemical Kinetic, 1984, Moscow: Visshaja Shkola, p. 205.
15. L.M. Khananaschvili and V.M. Kopylov, Advance in Organosilicon Chemistry. Chemistry Series, Moscow: MIR Publishers, **985**, p. 91.
16. M. Edelmen, *Amer. Chem. Phys.*, 1846, **16**(1), p. 16.
17. A.W. Dearing and E.E. Keid, *J. Am. Chem. Soc.*, 1928, **50**(21), p. 3058.
18. K.A. Andrianov, *Organosilicon Compounds*, 1955, Moscow: Geochimizdat, p. 161.
19. K.A. Andrianov and M.V. Sobolevskiy, *Highermolecular Organosilicon Compounds*, 1949, Moscow: Oborongiz, p. 170.
20. M.G. Voronkov and L.A. Jagata, *Izvest. AN Latv. SSR. Ser. chim.*, 1967, 4, p. 452.
21. M.G. Voronkov and L.A. Zhagata, *Zh. Obshchei Khimii.*, 1967, **37**(11), p. 2551.
22. V.A. Vehov and E.P. Rudnik, *Zh. Neorganicheskoyi Khimii.*, 1965, 10, p. 2359.
23. M.G. Voronkov, *Zh. Prikladnoy Khimii.*, 1970, **43**, p. 611.
24. S. Dhar and V.J. Daran, *J. Am. Chem. Soc.*, 1959, **81**(23), p. 6372.
25. T.J. Tatakani, *J. Chem. Soc. Japan Pure Chem. Sec.*, 1953, **74**(4), p. 974.
26. Yu.I. Rastorguev and A.I Kusnezov, *Zh. Prikladnoy Khimii.*, 1981, **54**(9), p. 2111.
27. Yu.I. Rastorguev and A.I. Kusnezov, *Zh. Prikladnoy Khimii.*, 1982, **55**(10), p. 218.
28. M.G. Voronkov and L.A. Zhagata, *Zh. Obshchei Khimii.*, 1967, **37**(5), p. 1156.
29. Pat. 2909549 USA *Ref. Zh. Khimii.*, 1962, 5, pp. 5–162.
30. H. Mark and A.W. Tobolsky, Physical Chemistry and High Polymeric Substances, 1950, N.Y.-L.: Interscience Publ. Inc., Chap. IX, p. 61.
31. K.A. Andrianov, L.M. Tartakovskaja and V.M. Kopylov, *Izvest. AN USSR. Ser. chim.*, 1975, 6, p. 1443.
32. V.M. Kopylov, D.Ya. Jinkin, P.L. Prihod'ko, A.M. Gasanov and V.A. Kovjazin, *Vysokomolekularnye Soedineniya. A.*, 1981, **23**(3), p. 651.
33. M.G. Voronkov, V.P. Mileshkevich and Yu.A. Jujelevskij, *Siloxane bond*, 1976, Novosibirsk, Nauka, p. 413.
34. Pat. 2909549 USA *Ref. Zh. Khimii.*, 1962, 5, pp. 5–162.
35. G.F. Sablina and B.G. Zavin, VI All Union Conference on Organosilicon Compounds Chemistry and use. *Abstracts. Riga*, 1986, p. 33.
36. M.G. Voronkov, Heterolitic Decomposition Reactions of Silicon Bond, 1961, Moscow, Nauka, p. 48.
37. M.G. Voronkov, *Zh. Obshchei Khimii.*, 1959, **29**(3), p. 907.
38. F.R. Mayo, *J. Polymer Sci.*, 1961, **5**(1), p. 57.
39. J.F. Hyde, P.L. Brown and A.L. Smith, *J. Am. Chem. Soc.* 1960, **82**(11), p. 5854.
40. J. Akelof and J.W. Teare, *J. Chem. Soc.*, 1937, **59**(3), p. 1855.
41. Pat. 3013920. BRD C.A. 1982, **96**, p. 6864p.
42. Pat. 3151677. BRD C.A. 1983, **99**, p. 19521v.
43. Pat. 3303707. BRD C.A. 1985, **102**, p. 6796k.
44. J.B. Pedley and J.N.P.L. Rylance, Computer analysed thermochemical Data, Univ. Sussex, 1974.
45. Technical Note 270–1. *National Bureau of Standards*, 1965.
46. Chemist Reference Book, 1965, Moscow: Khimija, **3**, p. 337.
47. V.A. Rjabin, M.A. Ostroumov and T.F. Svit, Thermodynamic Properties of Substances. Reference book. L. Khimija., 1977.
48. V.G. Genchel, R.M. Golosova, V.N. Kostrjukov, A.M. Mosin, O.P. Samorukov and I.I. Skorohodov, Thermal Properties of Organosilicon Compounds, 1973, GNIIHTEOS. Moscow. NIITECHIM, p. 168.
49. V.A. Rabinovich, Thermodynamic activity of ions in solution of electrolytes, 1985, Leningrad. Chimija, p. 176.

50. A.F. Cotton and G. Wilkinson, Advanced inorganic chemistry. N.Y. Interscience Publisher a Division of John Willey & Sons, 1967, part. 2. p. 494.
51. A. Noshay and J. McGrath, lock Copolymers, 1977, Academy Press, N.Y.
52. Yu.A. Jujelevskij, N.G. Sviridova and G.I. Karpov, *Zh. Obshchei Khimii.*, 1981, **51**(6) p. 1342.

Some Peculiarities of Phenolic Stabilisers Consumption and Role of their Transformation Products in the Oxidation Process

E.L. SHANINA and G.E. ZAIKOV

Institute of Biochemical Physics, Russian Academy of Sciences

Most stabilisers—substances which are able to react with peroxy radicals of substrate, transforming them into inactive species. Substituted phenols have these properties. These stabilisers are efficient and have low toxicity and can be used for example on stabilisation of polymer wrapping in food industry. There are a large number of phenolic stabilisers and the best are hindered phenols (with bulk substituents in the *o*-position), their chemical properties and stabilising abilities are described in many books and reviews.[1,2] Accumulated information facilitates choice of specific stabiliser for given material in the given processing or service conditions, but often process of selection is empirical and such situations make difficult development of new compositions.

Choice of the optimal stabiliser is the problem that arises very often. In principal this is a problem of selection of inhibitor with following properties:

a. full compatibility with polymer,
b. rather slow consumption rate, which enables sufficient stability during processing and exploitation.

High consumption rate does not always indicate low inhibiting activity, sometimes it is a result of physical losses, but usually it is an indication of inhibitor participation in the side chemical reactions. As a result kinetic curve of inhibitor consumption, reflecting all processes in the oxidising system and is the only reliable basis for its efficiency evaluation. Comparison of different curves for different stabilisers, polymers, oxidation conditions give information about consumption mechanisms. Some problems connected with the kinetics of phenol antioxidant consumption and the role of their transformation into products are considered in this article in relation to the inhibited oxidation of polyolefins.

KINETIC SCHEME OF INHIBITED OXIDATION BY PHENOLS

At high oxygen pressures, the phenols inhibited oxidation of polyolefins can be described as follows:

$$(0)\quad \text{initiation} \xrightarrow{+O_2} RO_2^{\bullet} \qquad W_i$$

$$(2)\quad RO_2^{\bullet} + RH \xrightarrow{+O_2} ROOH + RO_2^{\bullet} \qquad k_2$$

$$(3)\quad ROOH \xrightarrow{+O_2} 2\delta\, RO_2^{\bullet} + \text{products} \qquad k_3$$

$$(7)\quad RO_2^{\bullet} + PhOH \longrightarrow PhO^{\bullet} + ROOH \qquad k_7$$

$$(8)\quad RO_2^{\bullet} + PhO^{\bullet} \longrightarrow QP(\text{quinolide peroxide}) \qquad k_8$$

$$(9)\quad PhO^{\bullet} + PhO^{\bullet} \longrightarrow \text{products (methylenquinones etc)} \qquad k_9$$

The more complete scheme should be supplemented with the following reactions;

$$(-7)\quad PhO^{\bullet} + ROOH \longrightarrow PhOH + RO_2^{\bullet} \qquad k_{-7}$$

$$(10)\quad PhO^{\bullet} + RH \longrightarrow PhOH + R^{\bullet} \qquad k_{10}$$

$$(12)\quad PhO^{\bullet} \longrightarrow r^{\bullet} + \text{products} \qquad k_{12}$$

$$(13)\quad PhOH + ROOH \longrightarrow PhO^{\bullet} + RO_2^{\bullet} + \text{products} \qquad k_{13}$$

In this simplified scheme the alkyl radicals reactions are not taken into consideration in spite of the fact that in solid polymer unlike the liquid hydrocarbons radical concentrations ratio $[R]/[RO_2]$ can be high even at high oxygen pressures.[3,4]

In the reaction scheme direct oxidation of phenol with atmospheric oxygen is also absent. For a number of years this reaction was considered to occur only at temperatures higher than 200°C. However recently data has been obtained, which indicates the necessity of consideration of this reaction at lower temperatures. Studies of three phenols in solid polypropylene and in inert solvents indicate, that the initial consumption rates for each phenol in both media are practically equal. Therefore, at 130°C the inhibitor consumption rate is controlled predominantly by oxidation of phenol itself.[5] Results, obtained in other experiments showed, that even at the much lower temperatures oxidation of inhibitor in the blend PE–PP is to be taken into account.[6]

The possibility of ignoring the phenol oxidation reaction is usually based on the thermochemical calculation for the simple reaction

$$PhOH + O_2 \rightarrow PhO^{\bullet} + HO_2^{\bullet}$$

This reaction is strongly endothermic. Its thermal effect can be calculated using equation

$$q_1 = D_{OH}(HO_2^{\bullet}) - D_{OH}(PhOH)$$

where $D_{OH}(HO_2^{\bullet})$ and $D_{OH}(PhOH)$ are the energies of O—H bonds in the $HO_2^{\bullet}$ radical and in phenol. Rate constant can be estimated assuming that the activation energy can not be lower than the value of $-q$, and supposing that the preexponential factor has normal value $\approx 10^9$ l/mole sec. Such estimation results in the value of the rate constant a few orders lower than experimentally observed. This discrepancy indicates the complex nature of phenol oxidation process, which most likely proceeds via phenoxy radical formation and its reaction with oxygen. Such a scheme works in the case of the model substance—2,6-di-tert-butyl-*p*-quinone oxidation with oxygen.[7]

The above reaction can be regarded as part of the chemical process called inhibited autooxidation. Another step is necessary to take into account reactions of molecular products arising as a result of the first group of reactions and reactions of substances with pro- or antioxidative activity: quinones, methylenequinones, quinolide peroxides.

However step by step expansion taking into account additional reactions makes kinetic description of the overall process difficult or even impossible. Therefore it is necessary to limit the set of reactions in each case in order to simplify calculations.

Nevertheless it is necessary to understand clearly the consequences of such simplification and exclusion of some reactions.

In the accessible reviews[7–10] quantitative data which could characterise the activity of the above mentioned products are practically absent.

QUINOLIDE PEROXIDES

During inhibition with phenols quinolide peroxides (QP) can be formed as a result of reactions of phenoxy radicals with oxygen or with peroxy radicals. In the first case so called symmetric QP of I, II types are formed, in the second case the asymmetric QP III and IV are formed.

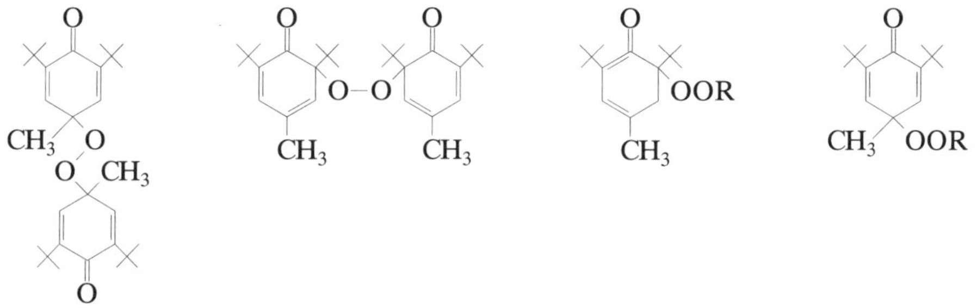

I II III IV

Taking into consideration the simple scheme of inhibited oxidation (initiation and reactions (7), (8) and (9)) the probability of QP formation can be found from equation (1):[11]

$$\alpha^2(1+\alpha) - A(1-\alpha)/k_9 = 0$$

where

$$A = \frac{k_8^2 W_i}{k_7^2 [\text{PhOH}]^2} \tag{1}$$

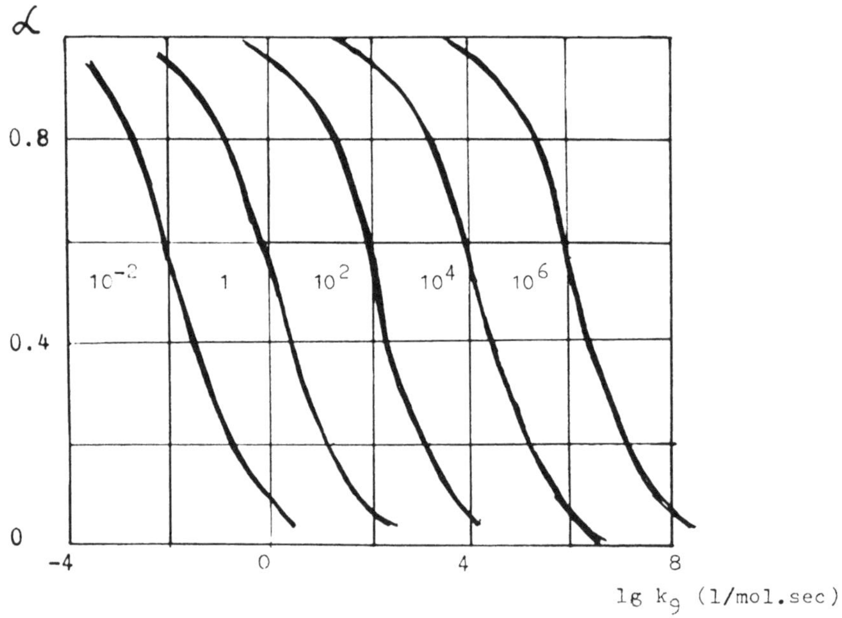

Figure 1 Dependence of k_9 on α for different values of parameter A (values of A are given in the figure).

This probability depends on the phenol structure and conditions of the process. For the very stable 2,4,6-tri-tert-butylphenoxy radicals this probability is always equal to 1. The numerical solutions of (1) at different values of parameter A are shown on Figure 1.[12]

Since other peroxide substances QP are capable of O—O bond rupture and their decomposition process leads to the formation of two active radicals.

Decomposition kinetics of tri-tert-butylphenol (TTBP) was studied[13] by two different methods: ESR—stable nitroxyl radical consumption rate measurement and spectrophotometry—measurement of QP consumption rate. First of these two methods gave information about initiation rate and second—about rate of dissociation. It was shown, that QP decomposition followed a first order kinetics with activation energy values of 29–35 kcal/mole. Some of the kinetic parameters for QP decomposition are given in Table 1. From these data it can be seen, that the thermal stability of QP is practically independent on the nature of the tert-alkyl substituent bonded with the cyclohexadiene fragment by the O—O bridge. Decomposition rate constants of p-QP depend on the nature of α-substituent and are much lower then for corresponding o-isomers. Decomposition rate constants of different QP are practically independent of concentration. Oxygen does not influence the decomposition rate but changes the assortment of products.

Comparison of two set of data—decomposition and initiation rate constants allow calculation of the initiation efficiency (cage effect). In the liquid phase these values are close to 1, in the polymer matrix (polypropylene) they are lower.*

* Low molecular peroxide was added to the polymer and its consumption rate was studied.

TABLE 1
Kinetic Parameters of QP Decomposition.[1]

Substance	Solvent	Pre-exponent sec^{-1}	Activation Energy kcal/mole	Lgk (90°)	Method[1]
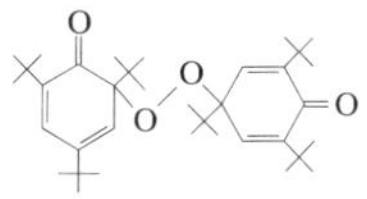	n-decane	15.4	32.2 ± 1.0	−3.85	A
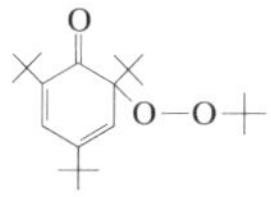	solid PP	—	—	−3.54 ± 0.1 (102°)	B
	solid PP	16.65	35.5 ± 1.5	−4.54	A
	n-decane	14.05	30.5 ± 1.0	−4.18	A, B
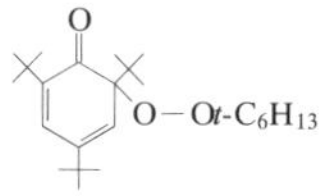	n-decane	14.07	30.6 ± 1.0	−4.2	A, B
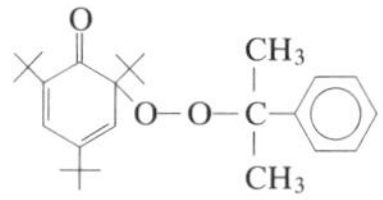	n-decane	15.53	32.2 ± 1.0	−3.72	A
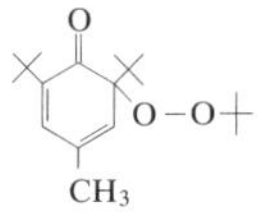	n-decane	—	—	−3.83 ± 0.5	B
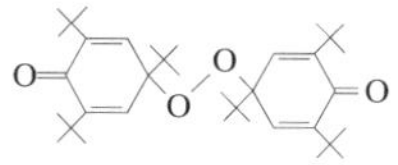	n-decane	14.55	32.2 ± 1.0	−4.77	A, B
	chlorobenzene	—	—	— −3.05 ± 0.2 (115°C)	
	cumene	13.46	29.5 ± 1.0	−3.48	
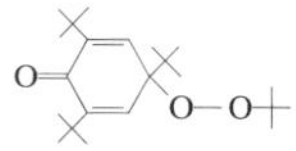	solid PP	—	—	−6.24	A
	n-decane	13.99	33.0 ± 2.0	−5.74	A
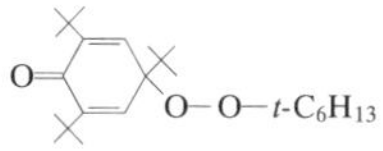	n-decane	13.52	35.4 ± 2.0	−5.73	A
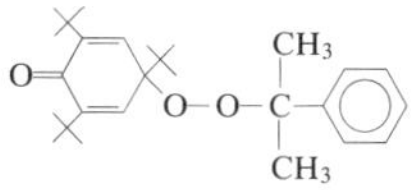	n-decane	15.69	35.0 ± 2.0	−5.17	A
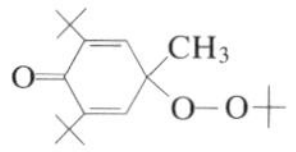	n-decane	13.58	33.0 ± 2.0	−6.18	A
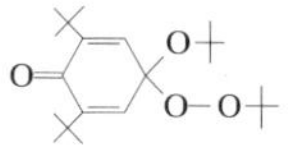	n-decane	12.81	29.0 ± 2.0	−4.6	A
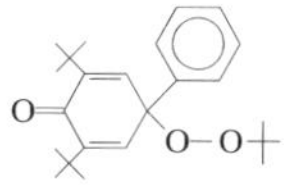	n-decane	14.4	31.5 ± 2.0	−4.45	A
QPPP	solid PP	—	—	−4.5 (115°)	B

[1] A-measurements of active radicals generation (ESR)
B-measurements of QP consumption rate (spectrophotometry)

It is important to note, that the QP decomposition constants, especially the ones for the *o*-isomers, are much higher then the rate constants of hydroperoxide decomposition.

QP bonded to polymer chain were synthesised.[11] Authors proved, using different methods, that the cyclohexadiene fragment was really bonded to the polymer. Thermal decomposition of this QP was studied and the main product of this process—quinone was identified.

In the other work[14] ionol was added to the oxidised PP. Hydroperoxide acts as an initiator and as a result QP was formed. Bonding was proved using UV and ESR spectroscopy.

Calculations made for oxidation of PP inhibited with TTBP showed that for three initiation rates—W_1 for hydroperoxide, W_2 for *o*-QP and W_3 for *p*-QP—the following dependence is correct:

$$W_1{:}W_3{:}W_2 = 1{:}0.3{:}3.5(90^\circ\text{C})$$

Decomposition of bonded to polymer QP leads to destruction of the polymer chain. After 96 hours of photooxidation the tensile strength of the IPP film, containing QP, was twofold lower then of the free of QP film.[11]

It is obvious, that QP can act as an initiator, but sometimes situation becomes more complicated, because in the process of QP decomposition strong inhibitors can be formed. As a result of QP V decomposition, two phenols are formed—2,6-di-tert-butyl-1,4-benzoquinone VI and 4-tert-butoxy-2,6-di-tert-butylphenol VII.[2] Formation of inhibitors from QP explains some pecularities of oxidation process. In [15] the influence of some nonsymmetrical QP (VIII and IX) on the oxidation of atactic PP (APP) at 120° was studied.

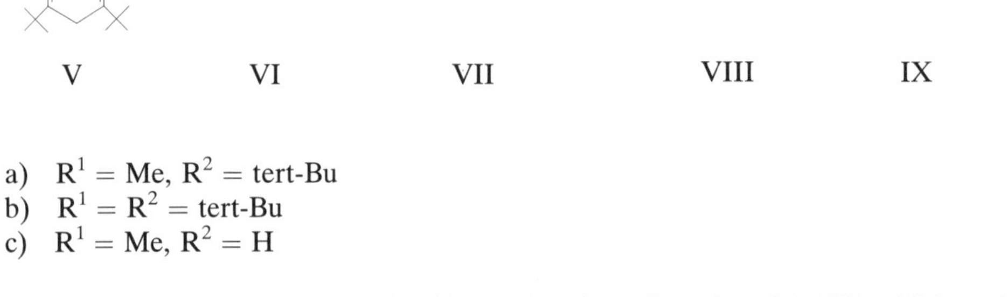

V VI VII VIII IX

a) $R^1 = Me$, $R^2 =$ tert-Bu
b) $R^1 = R^2 =$ tert-Bu
c) $R^1 = Me$, $R^2 = H$

Of these substances the most noticeable accelerating effect gives QP VIII, addition of 2×10^{-3} mole/kg of this QP led to oxidation of polymer with a constant rate without an induction period. At the same time IX a, b and c acted as inhibitors of APP oxidation and inhibiting effect of IXb was stronger than of IXa but the strongest inhibitor was IXc. Induction period of oxidation of APP with 5×10^{-4} mole/kg of QP

IXc was 6.6 times longer than for the pure polymer. This result most probably is connected with the formation of such strong inhibitor as ionol from QP IXc.

Some differences in behaviour of QP in the process of polymer and liquid hydrocarbon oxidation were observed.[11,15] For example, QP IXc inhibits APP oxidation but accelerates oxidation of tetralin. The same behaviour was observed for QP IXa, but the efficiency of the last is lower in both substrates[15] and were explained by different oxidation rates of the polymer and hydrocarbon. But could be explained by different cage effects. If quinone is formed as a product, its inhibition activity may be much higher in the polymer because of a higher concentration of alkyl radicals. Another possible reason could be different products of QP decomposition in different media. For example, decomposition of QP V in the melt in the absence of solvents leads to phenol and quinone in practically equal quantities.[16]

METHYLENEQUINONES

Formation of the methylenequinones (MQ) is possible in the process of inhibited phenol oxidation as a result of reaction between two phenoxy radicals. The key condition for their formation is the existence of at least one hydrogen atom at the carbon atom of *o*- or *p*-position relative to the OH-group. The structure of these substances are similar to those of quinones but one of the oxygen atoms is substituted by a methylene group. For MQ formed from hindered phenols the following structures are possible:

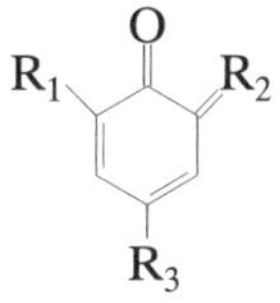

I (*o*-MQ)

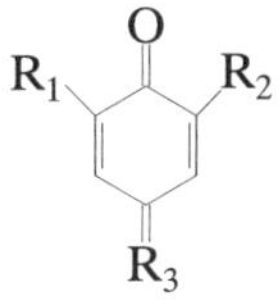

II (*p*-MQ)

Methylenequinones have high chemical activity. For example, formed from the ionol, MQ spontaneously dimerises with formation of stilbenquinone and bisdihydroxyphenylethan even in dilute solutions.[17] Nevertheless MQ inhibits decene oxidation.[18]

Similar to other substances MQ quinones effectively react with alkyl radicals. Parameters of this process were measured[19] and some of them are given in Table 2. Alkyl radicals react with the double bond of MQ and this mechanism was confirmed by the absence of activity in the case of MQ III. This substance does not inhibit styrene polymerisation even at concentration of 10^{-2} mole/l (60°, initiation rate 2.5×10^{-7} mole/l.sec). Having strongly hindered double bond substance IV is also inactive in this process.

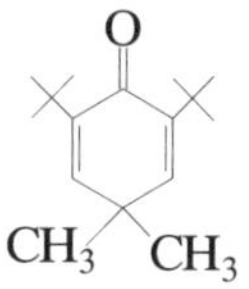

III

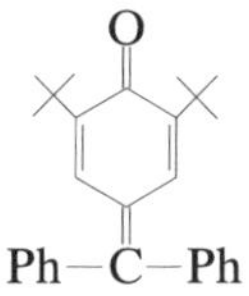

IV

TABLE 2

Rate Constants of some Methylenequinones in the Reactions with Alkyl (k_3) and Peroxy (k_7) Radicals.[19,20]

Substance	$k_3 \times 10^5$, l/mole.sec	$k_7 \times 10^4$, l/mole.sec	k_3/k_7	Method
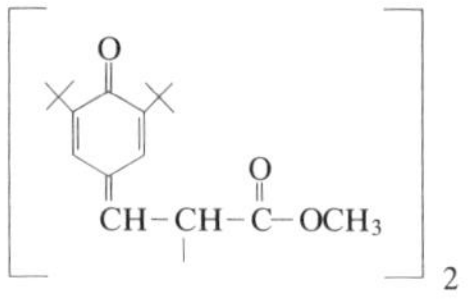	1.3 0.9	0.14 0.058	93 150	A B
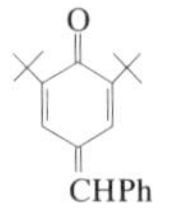	0.18	2.0	0.9	A
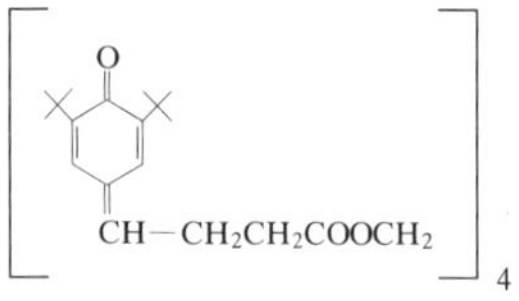	0.08	0.018	45	A
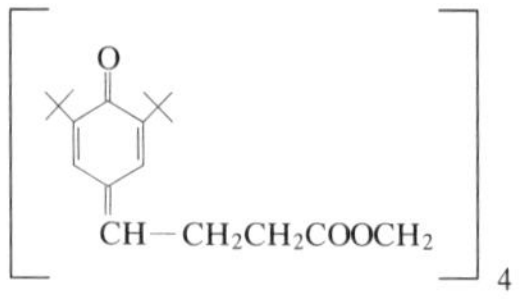	0.03	0.018	17	B
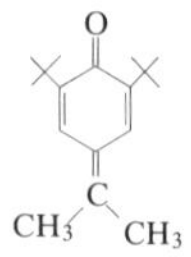	—	1.6	—	A
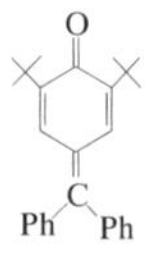	doesn't inhibit styrene polymerisation	doesn't inhibit cumene oxidation	—	

A—styrene polymerisation
B—cumene oxidation

Significant feature of MQ is their ability to react not only with alkyl, but also with peroxy radicals. For example all MQ (except α,α'-disubstituted) studied[20] inhibited cumene oxidation. Termination of almost all chains took place on the inhibitor molecules. Independence of the oxygen pressure was also proof of reaction with peroxy radicals. Mechanism of termination seems to be the same as for alkyl radicals—addition to the double bond. This mechanism is in agreement with experimental data about the nonreactivity of substance without double bond outside the ring. This substance doesn't inhibit cumene oxidation similar to IV with strongly hindered double bonds. Absence of phenols in all these experiments was proved by special experiments.

In a number of cases k_7 values for phenol and corresponding MQ are rather close one to another but the stoichiometric coefficient of the inhibition is lower for MQ and equal to 1.* Measured values of k_7 do not depend on the concentration of MQ over a wide range of concentration values, this fact is evidence of low activity from MQ formed radicals. Also it was shown that the phenoxy radical formed as a result of reaction between MQ and the peroxy radical was inactive in chain propagation.

Certain advantages of MQ as an inhibitor in comparison with phenols is the absence of hydroperoxide—chain branching product—among the products of reaction with peroxy radicals. Rate constants of MQ reactions with peroxy radicals usually are 1–2 orders of magnitude lower, than with alkyl radicals, Table 2, but some MQ exhibit equal activity for both types of radicals, for example, V.[19]

Such activity towards both the alkyl and peroxy radicals ensures high efficiency of MQ as a stabiliser. For example, the transformation products of Irganox 1010 and silanophenol inhibit thermooxidative destruction of PP almost as strongly as the starting phenols.[21] Quantitative data about some MQ as PP oxidation inhibitors are presented in Table 3.[22] In the solid polymer the concentration of alkyl radicals is higher, than in the liquid phase and the activity of MQ is determined by a combination of reactions with both types of radicals. Simultaneous progress of these two reactions leads to a dependence of the effective k_7 value on oxygen pressure, for example it can be seen for MQ VIII. This MQ has a 20–40 times higher rate constant for reaction with alkyl radicals in comparison to peroxy. For MQ VI such a dependence of the stoichiometric coefficient of inhibition on O_2 pressure does not exist, because this MQ efficiently terminates the kinetic chains via reaction with peroxy radicals.

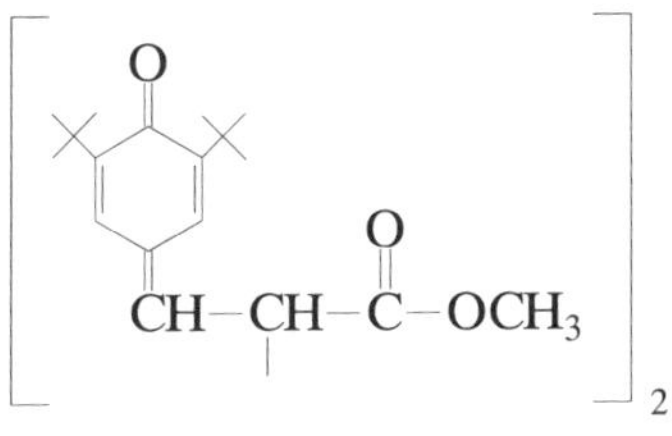

V

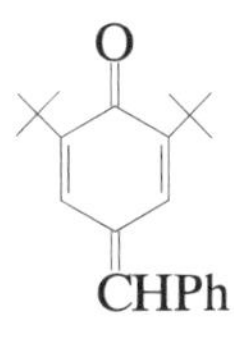

VI

For most of the methylenequinones the stoichiometric coefficients of inhibition in air are higher than in oxygen. This fact can be explained by the following reaction:[22]

$$\text{MQ} \longrightarrow \text{PhO}^\bullet \xrightarrow{+\text{R}^\bullet} \text{PhOH}$$

* These measurements were made in the presence of initiator. For autoxidation term "stoichiometric coefficient of inhibition" is rather senseless.

TABLE 3
Stoichiometric coefficients of Inhibition and k_7/k_2 Values for MQ in the Process of with Dicumene Peroxide Initiated Polypropylene Oxidation.[22]

Substance	Gaseous Phase	$k_7/k_2 \times 10^3$	f_{02}^1
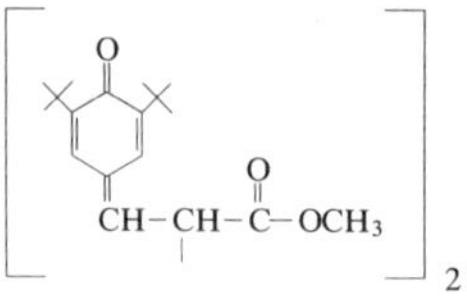	oxygen air	1.6 1.6	0.9 0.9
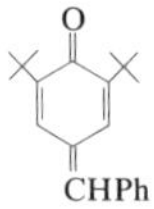	oxygen air	0.73 0.44	1.8 2.4
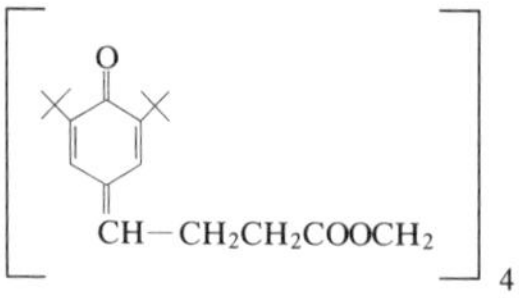	oxygen air	14.0 9.0	1.3 2.1
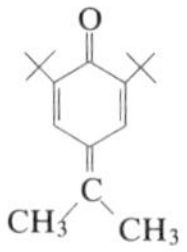	oxygen air	1.8 1.8	3.0 3.0
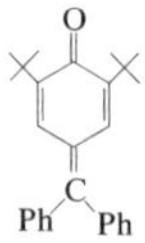	does not inhibit	oxidation process	

[1] These values were found from equation $f = w_i\,\tau_{ind}/[MQ]_0$

Dependence of the antioxidative activity of MQ with the following structure

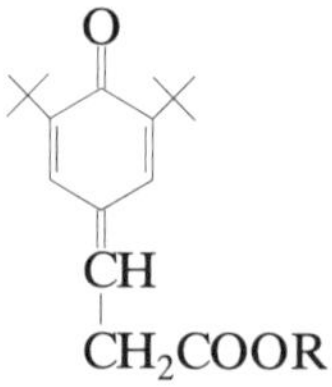

VII

$R = CH_3;\ C_{18}H_{37}$

on temperature in tetralin oxidation initiated with azo-bis-isobutronitrile was observed.[23] At 65°C in the chlorobenzene (initiator concentration—5×10^{-3} mole/l) both methylenequinones slightly deaccelerated oxidation, but without initiator at 120°C (autoxidation of tetralin in the trichlorobenzene solution) they behaved as initiators. It is interesting to note the same behaviour of the non-identified product of ionol transformation in PP (130°C, air).[24] In the initiated process of PP oxidation it acted as an inhibitor (80°C), but did not inhibit autoxidation of this polymer at 100°C.

MQ VIII efficiently stabilises the PP melt.[25] Its activity stays the same even after double extrusion. MQ must possess volatility close to one of the ionol and preservation of its activity implies chemical bonding of MQ to the polymer chain. Formation of the products IX and X in the model reaction of MQ VIII with ethyl radicals demonstrates successful competition of this MQ with O_2 for these radicals and confirms high activity of MQ towards alkyl radicals.

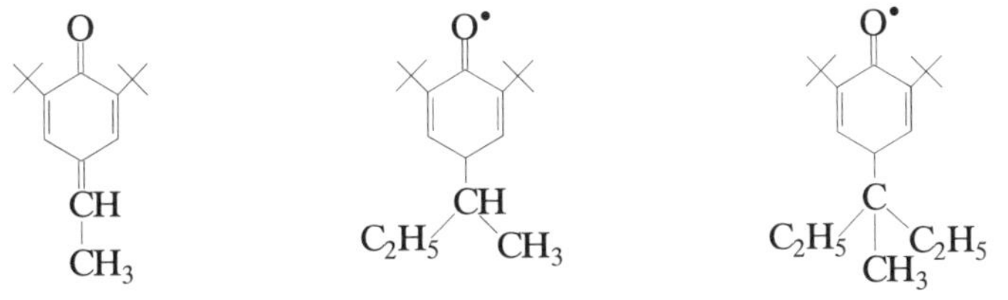

VIII IX X

Besides their own activity in the radical processes MQ are intermediate products in the processes of formation of other compounds with inhibitor ability. Dimerization of MQ XI can be considered as a possible mechanism of formation of four-nuclear derivative of 2,2′-methylenebis-(4-methyl-6-tertbutylphenol):[26]

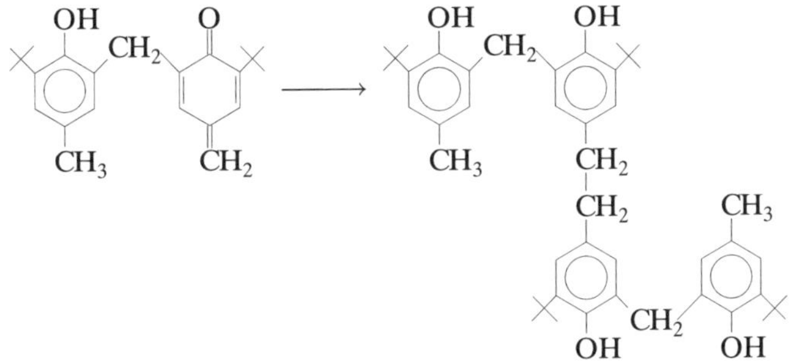

XI

It is necessary to mention however that this dimer can also be the product of benzyl radical XII dimerization:

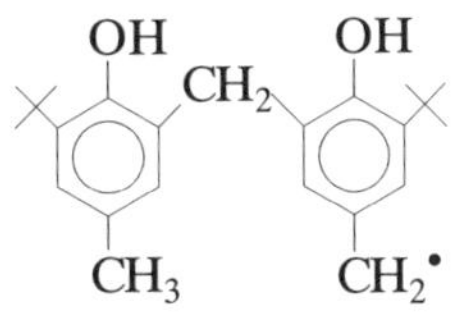

XII

Hypothesis about possible rearrangement of the aryloxyradical to the benzyl was stated in a number of papers, but direct evidences of such a process was not obtained until now. As a result of dimerization of methylenequinone—ionol radicals disproportionation to stilbenequinone is formed, but the inhibiting activity of this compound is rather low.[27]

One of the products of Phenol XIII transformation is MQ XIV (hydrogalvinoxyl) which is a very active inhibitor comparable with ionol. This MQ gives very stable radical product—galvinoxyl XV.

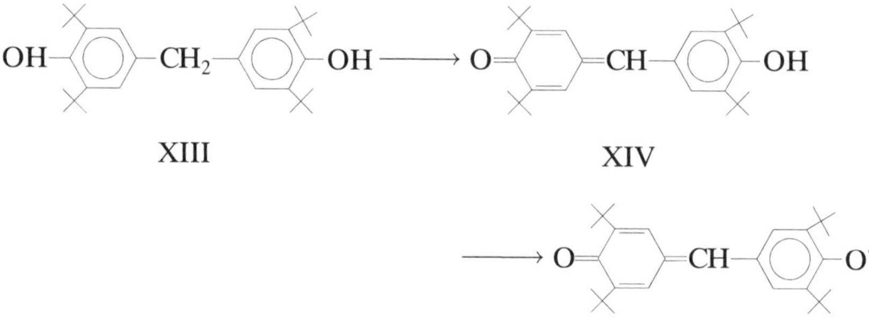

XIII XIV XV

Galvinoxyl is an effective stabiliser of PP melt under conditions of limited oxygen access, when competition with oxygen for alkyl radical is not possible.[28,29] In this process regeneration arises, because galvinoxyl gives hydrogalvinoxyl that again gives radicals. Relative concentrations of galvinoxyl and hydrogalvinoxyl depend on the ratio of the alkyl and peroxy radicals concentrations.[28]

Transformations of Phenol XIII can be used as an illustration of the sequence formation of substances with pro- and antioxidative activity. For example, able to stabilise the melt in the absence of oxygen galvinoxyl is rather easy oxidised with oxygen, giving quinolide peroxide—initiator, accelerating oxidation of galvinoxyl itself[30] as well as oxidation of the polymer. At the same time among the galvinoxyl transformation products are phenol and quinone capable of inhibiting oxidation and stabilise the polymer. Such transformation sequences are typical for phenol antioxidants and can be responsible for the different efficiency of phenol antioxidants depending on process conditions (temperature, initiation rate etc.).

QUINONES

Formation of quinones as the products of different phenol antioxidant transformations in the inhibited oxidation process is quite usual. These substances are able to efficiently bond to alkyl radicals with π-bond systems. Usually quinones do not react with peroxy radicals. For example, in decene in the presence of initiator (50°C, quinone concentration—10^{-6}–5×10^{-5} mol/l, initiator—dicyclohexylperoxydicarbonate) quinones I–IV* are being consumed only in the absence of oxygen.[31]

* Namely these quinones were chosen because they were transformation products of corresponding 2,6-di-tert-butyl- and 2,6-diphenylphenoles when these phenols were used as inhibitors.

p-Benzoquinone deaccelerates initiated oxidation of isooctane at 60°C only if its concentration is higher, than 3×10^{-2} mole/l.[32]

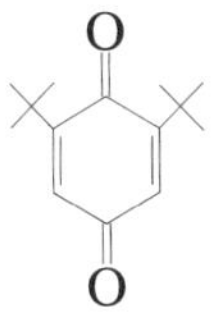

I

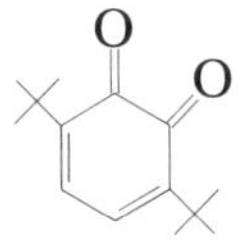

II

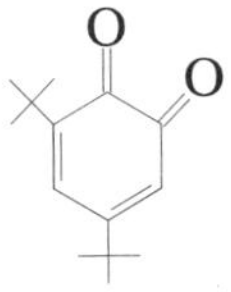

III

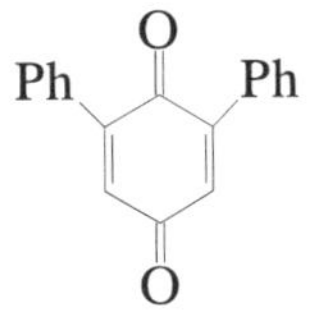

IV

Nevertheless in some cases, for example during oxidation of isopropanol[33] quinones can react with peroxy radicals and such reactions are possible if the corresponding radicals possess reducing power. Reaction with such radicals in a solid polymer enables quinone regeneration in the inhibition process.

Directly roles of quinone I and stilbenequinone V in the APP oxidation were investigated:[14]

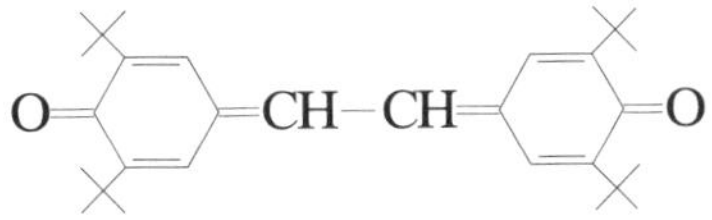

V

At 120°C both substances inhibited APP oxidation, addition of each of them to polymer in 5×10^{-4} mole/kg concentration led to an increase of the induction period correspondingly 2.2 and 3.4 times. In the solid polymer the ratio of alkyl to peroxy radicals concentrations is higher than in the liquid phase as a consequence, of diffusion limitations and some substances that do not behave as stabilisers in the liquid phase can manifest such properties in the solid polymer. The higher are the diffusion limitations the higher has to be inhibiting activity of such substances.

Interesting data dealing with inhibitor regeneration were obtained during investigation IPP oxidation inhibited with bisphenols.[34,35] It was shown that bisphenols VI and VII terminate chains with stoichiometric inhibition coefficients (2.5–3.6) if benzoyl peroxide was used as an initiator. If preliminary accumulated polymer hydroperoxide was used as an initiator in the same conditions the stoichiometric inhibition coefficients became several times higher.

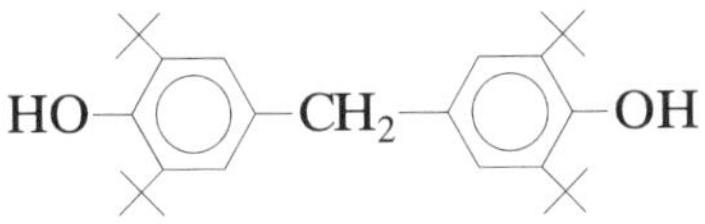

VI

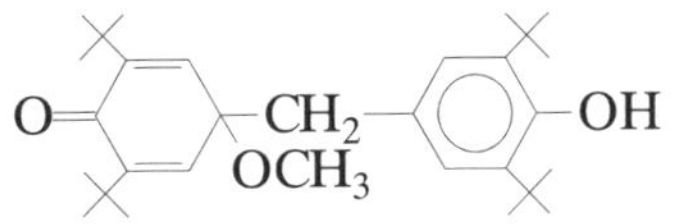

VII

This effect has been related to formation of quinones in the oxidation process of PE and IPP oxidation. Values of the stoichiometric inhibition coefficients for some quinones are presented in Table 4. Repeated termination takes place by phenol as well as quinone addition to polymer. Experiments showed that a necessary condition

TABLE 4
Inhibition Parameters for some Phenols and Quinones in the Reactions of Inhibited Oxidation of PE and IPP (93°C).[34,35]

Substance	Polymer	Initiator	f	$(2k_7/k_2) \times 10^3$	$2K_A/K_P$
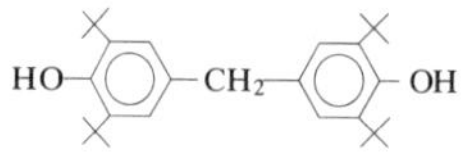	IPP	Benzoyl peroxide	2.5	—	—
	HDPE	Benzoyl peroxide	2.6	—	—
	HDPE	POOH	2.9	—	—
	IPP	POOH	27	—	—
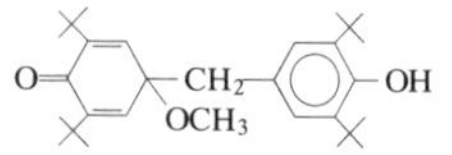	HDPE	Benzoyl peroxide	1.8	—	—
	IPP	POOH	33	—	—
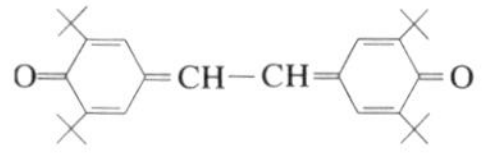	IPP	Benzoyl peroxide	—	0.5	0.093
	IPP	POOH		5.0	0.68
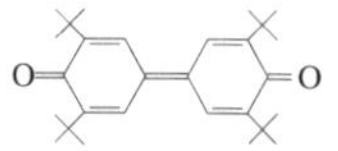	IPP	Benzoyl peroxide	—	0.38	0.018
	IPP	POOH		1.0	0.2

[1] Ratio of constants of reactions with alkyl and peroxy radicals.

for the regeneration process is building a block hydroperoxide. This phenomenon is characteristic of PP oxidation. In oxidised PE where predominantly isolated hydroperoxide groups are formed regeneration is impossible. Regeneration did not occur if in PP artificially isolated hydroperoxide groups were formed. In the block hydroperoxides IPP chains, termination on the quinone molecules proceeds more intensively and not only through reaction with alkyl radicals but with peroxy. Quinones can react with peroxy radicals possessing reducing power. Such a radical is $HO_2^\bullet$ which formation is a result of hydrogen peroxide decomposition. Hydrogen peroxide can be formed in the process of polymer oxidation during hydroperoxide decomposition. Interaction of $HO_2^\bullet$ radical with quinone can lead to inhibitor regeneration. For example:

$$Q + HO_2^\bullet \longrightarrow PhO^\bullet + O_2$$
$$PhO^\bullet + RO_2^\bullet \longrightarrow ROOH + Q$$

Experiments with PP added to a chlorobenzene hydrogen peroxide system confirmed the validity of the hypothesis about the $HO_2^\bullet$ radicals part in the quinones regeneration process. In this case repeated termination took place. The total regeneration cycle can be described as a sequence of reactions:

$$ROOH \longrightarrow H_2O_2 \xrightarrow{RO_2^\bullet} HO_2^\bullet \xrightarrow{Q} QH \xrightarrow{RO_2^\bullet} Q \xrightarrow{HO_2^\bullet} QH \text{ and so forth.}$$

From the standpoint of polyolefins stabilisation this result is not very useful, because all these effects arise in the rather deeply oxidised polymer, containing significant concentrations of hydroperoxide. But it is possible that these data could be useful for

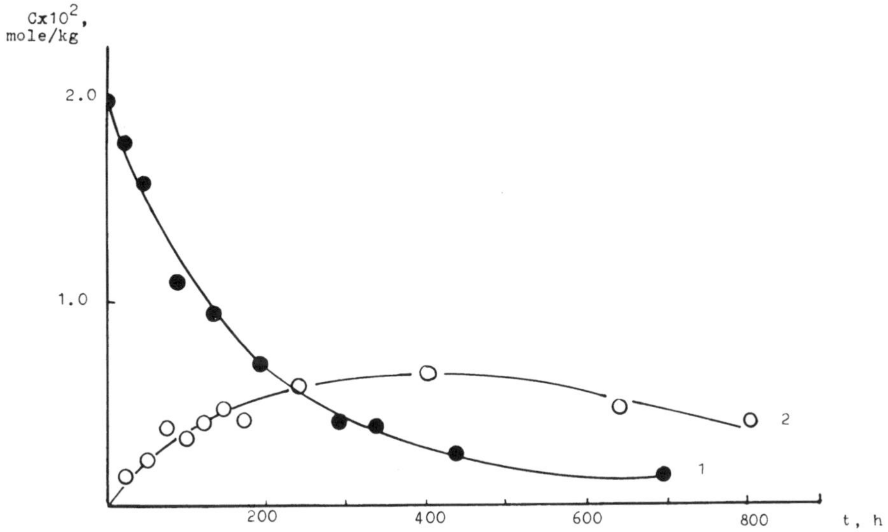

Figure 2 The kinetics of bisphenol consumption (1) and diphenoquinone accumulation (2) in the oxidizing polypropylene (130°, air).

choice of the stabilising composition for polymers of more complex chemical structure.

Interesting results were obtained during investigation of inhibition with 4,4′-bis(2,6-di-tert.butylphenol) oxidation at 130°C in air.[36] Product of this phenol transformation—quinone—shows synergy effect with the parent phenol. The kinetic curves (Figure 2) indicate that a certain amount of phenol consumption becomes slower and the concentration of quinone reaches maximum and then begins to fall, quinone behave as typical intermediates in the process. Experiments with specially made mixtures of phenol and quinone confirmed the existence of a synergy effect. One of the possible reactions able to explain this effect is the reaction between phenol and quinone with formation of active phenoxy radicals:

$$PhOH + Q \longrightarrow PhO^{\bullet}$$

In the process of autoxidation where values for the stoichiometric inhibition coefficients can be very far from the theoretical values can give this synergy effect.

INHIBITORS CONSUMPTION IN THE OXIDISING POLYMER

All processes of inhibitor consumption can be roughly divided in to two groups; firstly—direct inhibition consumption and secondly—through side reactions. In the absence of these side reactions inhibitor consumption would proceed with a constant rate and than decrease sharply till the end of the IP. In such a situation the value of IP would be proportional to the initial inhibitor concentration. Such ideal cases are very seldom observed in the autoxidation process. Only in the initiated process with a high initiation rate can side reactions be suppressed and it is possible to obtain a linear dependence of IP on the concentration of inhibitor and constant a consumption rate equal to the initiation rate is observed.*

Such an effect was observed in the oxidised PP (PP hydroperoxide acted as initiator) inhibited with TTBP.[37]

Among the physical processes, leading to the losses of inhibitor, evaporation is the most important one. If consumption of inhibitor is connected with its evaporation, the concentration is changing proportional to the square root of time and the rate of the process is controlled by the rate of inhibitor diffusion towards the surface. If the diffusion does not control the process, it can be described by a first order kinetic law.

Among the most important side chemical processes of phenol inhibitor consumption, is oxidation with oxygen. This problem has been partially considered above, but because of its great importance it is useful to discuss further oxidation of inhibitor with air oxygen. This process is especially important at high inhibitor concentrations. Of the many phenolic inhibitors the lowest oxidation rate (experiments with chlorobenzene solution of the inhibitor) is observed in Irganox 1010 (tetrakis[methylene(3,5-di-tert-butyl-4-hydroxyhydrocinnamate) methane). Inhibitors consumption in the interval of concentration 2×10^{-3}–10^{-2} proceeds with a constant rate (2×10^{-9} mole/kg sec at 140°).**

As a rule the kinetic curves for inhibitor consumption are very complicated reflecting variation of the reactions in this process. Accumulation and consumption of different active products of phenol transformation and hydroperoxide formation make their contribution to the process.

Some examples of inhibitor consumption curves are given in Figure 3. Variant (*a*) is a variant for an "ideal" inhibitor with constant consumption rate and distinct transient region. Different intermediate maximums and minimums on the consumption curves (b) usually are due to formation of different products and sometimes maybe to regeneration of inhibitor. Such curves are usual for polymer melts, where the concentration is high and the contribution of side reactions is especially significant.[39] First order kinetics of inhibitor consumption (c) can be a result of evaporation as well as of oxidation. Experiments with three different hindered phenols gave evidence, that oxidation of all of them in the liquid phase (chlorobenzene solution) proceeds in accordance with this kinetic law.[5] Measured effective constants of this process were 8.0×10^{-7} (TTBP), 4.86×10^{-6} (ionol), 5.81×10^{-7} (bis-phenol 2246) sec^{-1}. In PP only consumption of TTBP follows first order kinetics with a rate constant 1.15×10^{-6} sec^{-1}.*** Comparison of consumption processes in

---

* In the most common case when side reactions are suppressed τ_{ind} depends on the inhibitor concentration C_0 linearly:

$$\tau_{ind} = kC_0 + \tau'$$

where τ'—independent on C_0 time, corresponding to the transient period from inhibited to uninhibited oxidation. At the high initiation rates this term can be omitted and proportional dependence can be obtained as in [37].

**As was reported in [38] at 120° and initial concentration 8.5×10^{-4} mole/kg.sec consumption rate for this inhibitor is 7×10^{-11} mole/kg.sec.

*** Phenoxy radical from TTBP does not enter the disproportionating reaction, may be because of this reason such simple kinetics is possible.

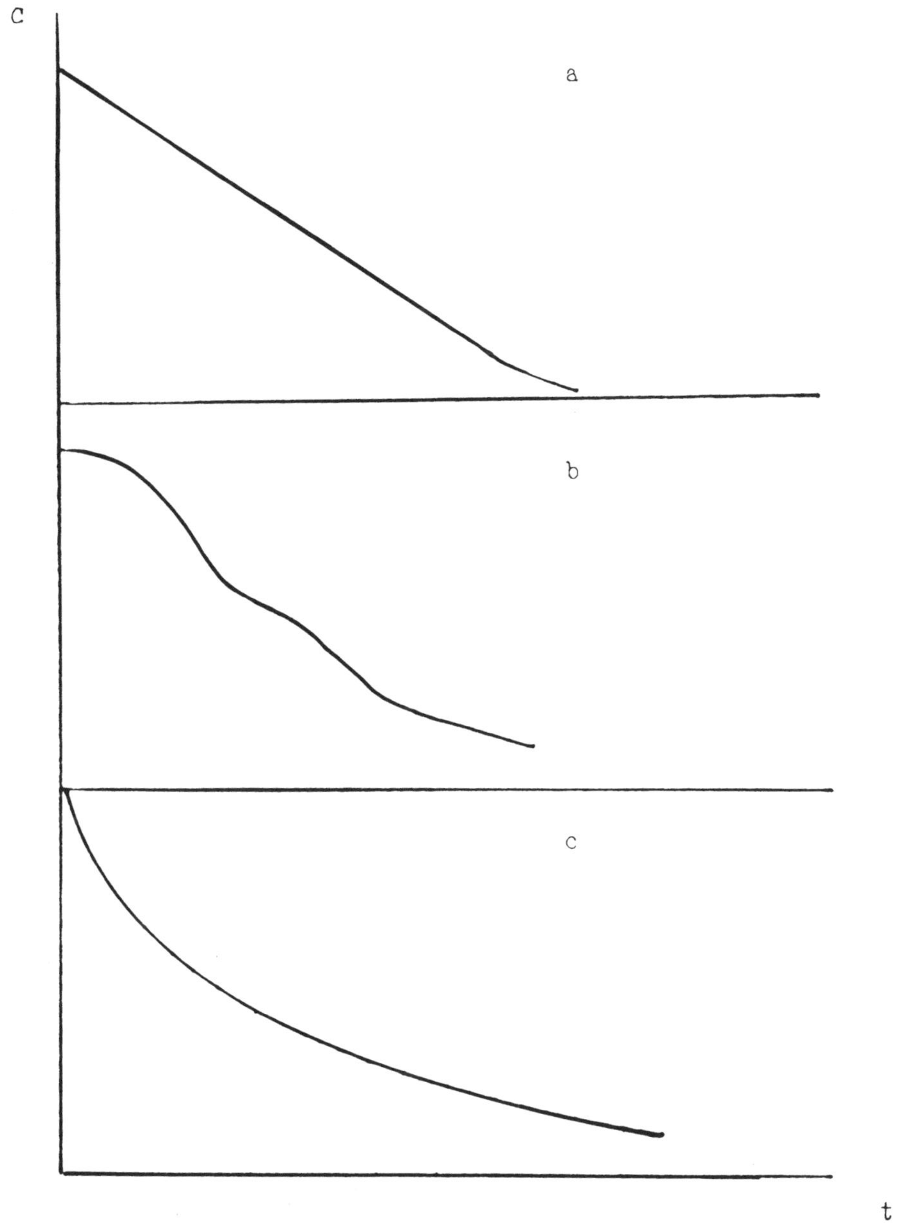

Figure 3 Different types of phenols consumption curves in the oxidizing polymer.

the liquid phase and polymer showed that the initial parts of corresponding curves are practically coincident. This fact indicates the primary role of phenol oxidation at least in the beginning of the process when concentrations are high. For deeper levels of conversion inhibitor consumption rates in PP become faster then in chlorobenzene because besides oxidation of phenol itself other inhibition process occur.

It is possible to evaluate at least approximately the contribution of inhibitor oxidation to the total rate of consumption. The initial rate of TTBP consumption in PP at 130° is about 10^{-8} mole/kg sec.[5] Assuming that the consumption of Irganox 1010 in the same polymer is controlled only by "useful" processes and taking a value of 4×10^{-10} mole/kg sec for its consumption rate it is possible to predict the same value for TTBP as 1.6×10^{-9} mole/kg.sec. The "useful" value for TTBP is then only 16% of the total consumption rate. This is a very rough evaluation because it is necessary to take into account that the contribution of the oxidation rate is significantly lower at lower inhibitor concentration, and depends on temperature.

Phenol oxidation undoubtedly proceeds as a radical process and can contribute to the initiation process as a result of $HO_2^\bullet$ radical formation. In turn this process has to accelerate inhibitor consumption. Lately we studied oxidation of 2,6-di-tert-butylhydroquinone in the liquid phase and successfully described this process with a scheme in which reaction of phenoxy radicals with oxygen was included.[7]

Among other side reactions the following

$$PhOH + ROOH \longrightarrow PhO^\bullet + RO_2^\bullet$$

is worth mentioning. Its contribution can be seen at high inhibitor concentrations.

The problem of side reactions in inhibited oxidation and criteria for taking these reactions into consideration is analysed in detail.[1]

Formation of new inhibitors in the process of the initial inhibitor consumption leads to the appearance of so called secondary IP after removal of the starting inhibitor from the polymer. After removal of ionol during oxidisation at 200° and oxygen pressures of 300 mm, PP secondary IP was observed,[44] and leads to the conclusion that the new inhibitor is more active than the starting one.[24] After extraction of low molecular substances from polymer oxidised with ionol (oxidation at 130°, air, initial ionol concentration 10^{-2} mole/kg) besides ionol at least one more inhibitor is found to be present in the solution. Rate constant of reaction with peroxy radical of cumene for this inhibitor is 2.7×10^3 l/mole.sec (60°), for the ionol corresponding value is 1.48×10^4 l/mole.sec.

Secondary IP were observed also after elimination of a non-reacted inhibitor 2246 in a number of polymers: polyethylene (PE), PP, polyisobutylene (PIB), butyl rubber (BR).[40] The longest values were observed in PE and PIB, the shortest—in PP. In all polymers values of IP went through a maximum. All results were qualitatively similar, any correlation with polymers oxidability was absent. In the inhibitor consumption process at least two pathways for active product formation exist; inhibited oxidation itself and oxidation of inhibitor. The second is unlike, the first one seems to be practically independent on the nature of polymer, the more so since all four polymers are non-polar hydrocarbons. Proportion of products for every polymer is different even if each set of such products is the same in every polymer. Apparently, search for a correlation with some property of the polymer is hopeless.

Secondary IPs were observed also after washout of low molecular products from PP oxidised at 130°.[24] Polymer was thoroughly washed with benzene but even after this operation some inhibitor stayed in it raising the possibility that the inhibitor which gave this secondary IP is bound to the polymer chain. Such chemically bound inhibitors have been observed.[41] A number of facts lead to the hypothesis of a quinomethide structure for these inhibitors bound to the polymer chain. A similar supposition was made in,[41] where authors supposed that bounding proceeds via reaction with the hydroperoxide group of the polymer. In the case of polynuclear phenols, formation of products with high molecular weight is possible. Elimination of these products is very difficult in the washout process and also by evaporation.

Addition of synergist—hydroperoxide decomposer—di-laurylthiodipropionate did not influence the consumption rate of the three phenolic antioxidants, studied in [23] indicating that the stationary concentration of PP hydroperoxide in the induction period is low and coincides with theory.[1] In this connection it is useful to return to the data about the synergist influence on the induction periods of PP oxidation for two antioxidants—Irganox 1010 and EC 63 (octadecyl 3-(3,5-di-phenyl-4-hydroxy phenyl)-propionate).[36] From these data it is well seen that the addition of synergist significantly increases the situation for EC 63 and only slightly for Irganox 1010 and as a result the efficiency of both inhibitors becomes comparable. Thus the influence of the synergist is only noticeable for a bad inhibitor which can not maintain a stationary character for the process.

In conclusion it is necessary to analyse one more problem inhibitor concentration measurement. Usually spectrophotometry is used, after elimination of inhibitor from the polymer. Measurement of the band at 270–280 nm is used with an extinction coefficient $\varepsilon \cong 2 \times 10^3$ l/mole.cm. It is however necessary to take into account that the adsorption band of these phenols products lie in the same region. For example,[17] the characteristic adsorption bond for methylenequinones lies at slightly long-wave lengths for different MQ between 270 and 310 nm,* but the extinction coefficients for MQ are practically an order of magnitude higher, than for phenols. Position of adsorption maximums for QP depend on their structure, for *o*-peroxides λ_{max} is near to 315 nm (($\varepsilon \cong 3 \times 10^4$ l/mole.cm), for *p*-peroxides—230–240 nm (($\varepsilon \cong (1\text{–}2) \times 10^4$ l/mole. cm). Thus it is possible to make a mistake in the measurement of the phenol concentration. Molecular weights of these products are close to these of phenols and during *in vacuo* evaporation volatilites of these compounds are extracted. Besides, some phenols with more than one phenol ring in molecule can give products with partially quinoid and partially phenolic structure. It is rather difficult to resolve this problem studying UV spectra. Of course all these difficulties become negligible if conversion of starting phenol is low.

Results of kinetic method of phenols concentration measurements can also be attributed to the starting phenol only at low conversions. This method includes the following operations: extraction of phenol with chlorobenzene, adding of this extract to a mixture of cumene (substrate) and initiator—azo-bis-isobutironitrile, measurement of the induction period of cumene oxidation in standard conditions and calculation of phenol concentration using known values of initiation rate and stoichiometric coefficient of inhibition.[5] Possible source of error in this case are—phenol transformation products which inhibit or initiate cumene oxidation. The number of products which distort the result in this case are less than for spectrophotometry.

---

* For ionol $\lambda_{max} = 278$ nm and for corresponding MQ—285 nm.[2]

In theory, the ideal method of following the inhibitor concentration is liquid chromatography. But in the process of inhibited oxidation the number of products is high and it is especially true for stabilisers with more than one phenolic *nucleus*.

CONCLUSIONS

In the most cases only part of inhibitor is consumed efficiently. Even if physical losses are absent significant decrease of antioxidative activity of inhibitor takes place as a result of its participation in the side chemical processes, primarily in reaction with oxygen.

Phenol transformation products, mainly methylenequinones, quinolide peroxides are able to contribute to the process of inhibited oxidation. Among the products of QP decomposition, inhibitors can be formed and these inhibitors can balance the initiating effect of peroxides and even lead to resulting inhibition of processes. Yield and products ratio depend on conditions and this is the reason for the observed dependence on oxidation temperature and substrate type.[14,42,43]

The same difficulties arise from evaluation of the role of MQ, its behaviour can be different depending on oxidation conditions.[22] As a result of reaction with $R^\bullet$ or $RO_2^\bullet$ radicals MQ transform to phenoxy radicals with ill defined properties. It is known that these radicals do not participate in chain propagation reactions and apparently do not react with peroxy radicals, because stoichiometric inhibition coefficients for MQ are close to 1.[19] This indicates low activity of phenoxy radicals. It is necessary to take into account the ability of methylenequinones to dimerisation, that can lead to formation of phenols with significant inhibiting effect.

REFERENCES

1. V.A. Roginskii, *Phenol'nye Antioksidanty. Reaktsionnaya sposobnost I effektivnost.* (Phenolic Antioxidants. Reactivity and efficiency). 1988, Nauka, Moscow.
2. V.V. Ershov., G.A. Nikiforov and A.A. Volod'kin., *Prostranstvenno-zatrudnennye fenoly.* (Sterically hindered phenols), 1972, Khimiya, Moscow.
3. E.T. Denisov., *Uspekhi khimii*, 1978, **47**, p. 1090.
4. E.T. Denisov and N.M. Emanuel, *Kinetika i kataliz*, 1973, **14**, p. 823.
5. E.L. Shanina, V.A. Roginskii and G.E. Zaikov, *Vysokomol. Soedinen.*, 1986, **A28**, p. 1971.
6. E.L. Shanina and G.E. Zaikov, *Plasticheskie massy*, 1994, **N3**, p. 78.
7. E.L. Shanina and V.A. Belyakov, unpublished results.
8. J. Pospišil, *Developments in Polymer Stabilization*, 1979, Applied Science Publishers Ltd., **1**, p. 1.
9. J. Pospišil, *Degradation and stabilization of polymers*, 1983, Elsevier, Amsterdam etc., **1**, p. 193.
10. a. J. Pospišil, *Adv. Polym. Sci.*, 1980, **36**, p. 69.
    b. J. Pospišil, *Polym. Degr. & Stab.*, 1993, **40**, p. 217, ibid, 1993, **39** p. 103.
11. V.Z. Dubinskii, Dissertation. *Quinolide peroxides in the inhibited by phenols oxidation.* 1978, Ufa.
12. V.A. Roginskii, V.Z. Dubinskii, I.A. Shlyapnikova and V.B. Miller, *Europ. Polym. J.*, 1977, **13**, p. 1043.
13. V.A. Roginskii, L.G. Plekhanova, V.Z. Dubinskii, G.A. Nikiforov, V.B. Miller and V.V. Ershov, *Izv. AN SSSR Ser. Khim.*, 1975, **N6**, p. 1327.
14. J. Kovarova-Lerchova, J. Pilar, G. Samay and J. Pospišil, *Eur. Polym. J.*, 1978, **14**, p. 601.
15. I. Buben and J. Pospišil, *J. Polym. Sci., Polym. Symp.*, 1976, **N57**, p. 261.
16. C. Cook, R. Woodworth and P. Fianu, *J. Am. Chem. Soc.*, 1956, **78**, p. 4159.
17. A.A. Volod'kin and V.V. Ershov, *Uspekhi Khimii*, 1988, **N4**, p. 590.

18. G.S. Popova, Dissertation. *Investigation of the mechanism of the antioxidative action of 2,6-di-tert-butyl-4-methylphenol*, 1975, Leningrad.
19. N.V. Zolotova, M.B. Tokareva, E.T. Denisov, A.A. Volod'kin and V.V. Ershov, *Kinetika i Kataliz*, 1979, **20**, p. 56.
20. N.V. Zolotova, F.A. Galieva, M.B. Tokareva, E.T. Denisov, A.A. Volod'kin and V.V. Ershov, *Kinetika i Kataliz*, 1979, **20**, p. 48.
21. A.A. Volod'kin, V.V. Ershov, N.N. Gorodetskaya, N.A. Tupikina and L.I. Kudinova, *Dokl. AN SSSR*, 1976, **227**, p. 896.
22. N.V. Zolotova, E.T. Denisov, A.A. Volod'kin, V.V. Ershov and F.A. Galieva, *Vysokomol. soed.*, 1981, **A23**, p. 145.
23. J. Lerchova, G.A. Nikiforov and J. Pospišil, *J. Polym. Sci., Simposium*, 1976, **N57**, p. 249.
24. E.L. Shanina, V.A. Belyakov and G.E. Zaikov, *Vysokomol. Soedinen.*, 1989, **B31**, p. 86.
25. T.J. Henman, *Developments in Polymer Stabilization*, 1979, Applied Science Publishers LTD., London, p. 39.
26. L. Taimr and J. Pospišil, *Angew. Makromolek. Chemie*, 1973, **39**, p. 189.
27. I. Buben and J. Pospišil, *J. Polym., Sci., Simposium*, 1976, **N57**, p. 255.
28. R. Bagheri, K.B. Chakraborty and G. Scott, *Polym. Degr. & Stab.*, 1983, **5**, p. 197.
29. R. Bagheri, K.B. Chakraborty and G. Scott, *Polym. Degr. & Stab.*, 1983, **5**, p. 145.
30. V.Z. Dubinskii, V.A. Belyakov, V.A. Roginskii and V.B. Miller, *Izv. AN SSSR, Ser. Khim.*, 1975, **N1**, p. 51.
31. I.A. Shlyapnikova, V.A. Roginskii and V.B. Miller, *Izv. AN SSSR, Ser. Khim.*, 1978, **N11**, p. 2487.
32. Yu.B. Shilov and E.T. Denisov, *Vysokomol. Soedinen*, 1974, **A16**, p. 1736.
33. E.T. Denisov, *Izv. AN SSSR, Ser. Khim.*, 1969, **N2**, p. 328.
34. Yu.B. Shilov and E.T. Denisov, *Vysokomol. Soedinen*, 1982, **A24**, p. 837.
35. Yu.B. Shilov and E.T. Denisov, *Vysokomol. Soedinen*, 1985, **A26**, p. 1751.
36. E.L. Shanina, G.E. Zaikov and N.A. Mukmeneva, *Polym. Degr. & Stab.*, 1996, **51**, p. 51.
37. V.A. Roginskii, E.L. Shanina, V.I. Rubtsov and V.B. Miller, *Kinetika i Kataliz*, 1977, **N6**, p. 1576.
38. E.A. Giezen, Proceedings of the first conference on degradation and stabilisation of polymers. AKZO res. lab. and Inst. of Chem. Phys. of the Acad. of Sci. of the USSR, 1975, Moscow, p. 91.
39. L.L. Yasina, B.A. Gromov, V.B. Miller and Yu.A. Shlyapnikov, *Vysokomol. Soedinen*, 1966, **A8**, p. 1411.
40. I. Gomory, *Eur. Polym. J.*, 1970, **6**, p. 1047.
41. J. Koch, *Angew. Makromolek. Chemie*, 1971, **20**, p. 35; ibid, **20**, p. 21.
42. I. Buben and J. Pospicil, *Coll. Czech. Comm.*, 1975, **40**, p. 987.
43. I. Buben and J. Pospicil, *Coll. Czech. Comm.*, 1975, **40**, p. 977.

Definition of Terms and Classification of Processes Relating to Aging Polymers

N.M. EMANUEL, V.Ya. SHLYAPINTOKH, O.N. KARPUKHIN, Yu.V. MOISEEV, T.V. POKHOLOK, G.E. ZAIKOV and K.Z. GUMARGALIEVA

N.N. Semenov Institute of Chemical Physics, Russian Academy of Sciences, 4, Kosygin st., Moscow, 117334, Russia

In the former USSR, a unified system of standards relating to protection from corrosion and aging is being developed.

There are three standards related to the subject in question: "Stareniye Polimernykh Materialov. Terminy 1 Opredeleniya. GOST 17050–71 / Polymer Aging. Terms and Definitions. GOST 17050–71"; "Plastmassy. Stareniye i Stabilizatsiya. Terminy i Opredeleniya. RS 5029–75 / Plastics. Aging and Stabilization. Terms and Definitions"; and "Standard Definitions of Terms Relating to Plastics. ANSI/ASTM D 883–78".

The first two standards have become obsolete in many respects. The last one is too general and contains practically no definitions dealing specifically with polymer aging.

The present work is an attempt by a research team of the Institute of Chemical Physics, the USSR Academy of Sciences, who have spent many years investigating the problems of polymer aging and stabilization, to develop a list of standard terms and definitions of concepts used in association with aging processes.

AGING OF POLYMER MATERIALS

During treatment, processing, storage and use, polymeric materials are exposed to multiple factors provoking or promoting various chemical and physical transformations, which affect the properties of polymeric material. Since such changes develop in time and usually result in deterioration of properties, the term "aging" appears to be quite relevant for characterization of the processes involved. Stuart was probably the first to use in polymers the term "aging" which had yet earlier been borrowed by certain branches of science and technology from biology. However, its use in many standard situations has not been governed by strict definitions.

The term aging is applied broadly to processes that are spontaneous and result in deterioration of the properties of material.

It should be remembered that there are certain physical and chemical processes that improve the properties of polymeric materials. However, such processes are normally carried out to deliberately modifying the properties, and should not be included under the term “aging”. In biology, aging is understood as a sequence of irreversible transformations.

Aging of a polymeric material, is a series of physical and chemical processes in a polymer material which brings about a spontaneous variation of its composition and structure.

Most of the following definitions relate to polymeric materials.

1 AGING OBJECTS

Aging object refers to polymers, polymer materials and items manufactured from them.

Polymers are high-molecular compounds whose molecules consist of a large number of identical units held together by chemical bonds.

Polymers consisting of molecules having a high molecular mass retain their individuality in various phase transitions and dissolution. This distinguishes polymers from molecular and ionic crystals which also consist of recurrent atomic groups.

Oligomers are the members of the homological series occupying a place between monomers and polymers.

Prepolymers are oligomers or polymers containing reactive groups and are used for the production of polymeric materials.

A polymeric material may include other ingredients, e.g.: fillers, pigments, plasticizers, stabilizers, etc.

Material may also contain undesirable impurities, e.g.:—residues of catalyst, monomer, etc.

Polymer materials may be classified according to composition, morphology and use.

Secondary polymeric material are materials produced by processing of used materials or items of industrial waste.

2 POLYMER MATERIAL PROPERTIES

Aging affects the properties of polymeric materials.

Properties of materials are assessed in terms of property indices and aging monitored by the variation of some property index.

Property index is a parameter characterizing qualitatively or quantitatively, the polymer material property in question.

Characteristic index is a parameter which most adequately characterizes the applicability of the aging object for some particular use, Appendix I.

3 AGING FACTORS AND CONDITIONS

Aging of polymeric materials takes place under conditions determined by various factors which may be divided into internal and external ones.

External factors are environmental factors including heat, light, ionizing radiation, physically or chemically active media, living organisms and their metabolism products, various mechanical loads, electric, electromagnetic, ultrasonic fields, etc.

In the course of aging, a material is often subject to the combined effect of many external factors, e.g., heat and light, radiation and oxygen attack.

Internal factors are the structure, composition, manufacturing process and other internal conditions promoting and/or otherwise influencing the aging of polymeric materials. Internal factors may include the presence of residues of catalyst and initiating agent, internal stresses in the material, cracks, weak bonds in macromolecules, reactive groups in macromolecules, etc. Internal factors, reflect, the prehistory. Internal factors such as cracks, local stresses, etc., may arise in material during the aging process and may be promoted by external factors. Depending on the processes involved, aging factors may be divided into physical, chemical and biological effects.

Aging conditions are the factors, acting on the material during processing, working, storage and use.

There has been an earlier definition of the term "service of item": according to GOST 21964–76, "the service of an item is the sum of the production and use of the item for an intended purpose, maintenance, storage, transportation as well as all forms of repair carried out by the user." Here, the term signifies the lifetime of an item from the moment of manufacture to the end of service. According to this Standard, storage and transportation of items are just special cases of their use. What differentiates the use of a material from the use of an item is that after the item as a whole can no longer perform its function (fails), its parts may still be usable and may be re-processed for re-utilization.

Processing means a series of steps needed to convert a polymeric material into an item or one item into another.

Storage is the keeping of a polymeric material under conditions known to prevent deterioration of its properties.

4 PROCESSES INVOLVED IN AGING

The processes occurring during aging are of chemical, physical and physico-chemical nature.

Chemical transformations involve alteration of the chemical structure of polymer or other than polymeric components of a polymer composition. The chemical processes which accompany aging of a polymeric material usually comprise three major stages:

—initiation (formation of active sites);
—development stage;
—decay of active sites.

Active sites are chemically active species such as free radicals, active atoms and molecules.

At the development stage the dominant processes are degradation, cross-linking and polymer-analog reactions of macromolecules.

Degradation is the process leading to breaking of chemical bonds in the main macromolecular chain which results in reduction of the degree of polymerization of the plastic.

The composite process of degradation may include the following sub-processes.

decomposition is the breaking of chemical bonds of the main macromolecular chain.

depolymerization is separation of the terminal monomer molecules from the macromolecule.

cross-linking is formation of chemical bonds between neighbor macromolecules.

polymer-analogous reactions is the transformation of a group of atoms in a macromolecule with the degree of polymerization remaining the same.

The physico-chemical processes include such processes that cause a change of the composition of polymeric material.

Sorption is any process of absorption of a substance by a polymeric material.

Adsorption is surface sorption.

Absorption is sorption in the bulk of material.

Desorption is the process of liberation of the sorbed substance by polymeric material.

Diffusion is directional transfer of matter under the effect of a gradient of chemical potential due to the thermal motion of particles. Diffusion processes play a very important role in the interaction of polymeric material with aggressive media, gaseous (O_2, O_3, SO_2, NO_2, etc.) and liquid (acids, bases, etc.). Diffusion is responsible for the migration of additives or impurities in a polymeric material. Examples are the sweating and washout of additives.

Plasticization is an increase of elasticity or plasticity of a polymeric material during the processing stage achieved by addition of special agents (plasticizers). Low-molecular aging products may also have a plasticizing effect.

Physical transformations involve changes in the physical structure of polymer materials. The most important of them are phase transitions, change of the physical state and submolecular structure.

Crystallization is the first-kind phase transition resulting in spatial ordering of macromolecules in material.

Amorphization is the first-kind phase transition resulting in spatial disordering of macromolecules in material.

Polymorphic transformation is the first-kind phase transition of one crystalline form to another.

Glass transition is the transition of polymer to a glassy state (i.e. the state in which segmental motion of macromolecules is frozen).

Orientation is rearrangement of the structural elements of a polymeric material under effect of a directed internal or external stress causing the macromolecular axes to assume predominantly the directions along the reference axes.

Relaxation processes are the changes of properties of polymeric material in the course of physical transition from a nonequilibrium to equilibrium state.

Submolecular structural changes are variations of the physical structure of polymeric material characterized by various forms of mutual ordering of its macromolecules.

The basic submolecular structural elements are glubules, fibrils, spherolites and crystallites.

Physical and chemical transformations bring about changes in the physical and chemical structure of polymeric material which manifest themselves macroscopically in:

Crazing is the violation of material continuity either on the surface or in the bulk.

Fatigue is a change of polymeric material properties under effect of multiple cyclic loading.

Creep is the time-dependent increase of strain of a polymeric material under effect of a constant mechanical stress.

Fracture is the loss of integrity of material under the effect of mechanical stresses.

5 BASIC TYPES OF AGING

Aging processes may be classified according to the major aging factor.

Thermal aging is the aging under the effect of heat and in the absence of effects from other factors.

Light (photo) aging is the aging under the effect of UV or visible light.

Chemical aging is the aging under the attack of chemically active agents.

Since aging in oxygen and ozone are very common types of aging, they are defined as independent entries.

Oxidative aging (or thermooxidative aging) is the aging under oxygen attack.

Ozone aging is the aging under ozone attack.

Radiation aging is the aging under the attack of an ionizing radiation.

Biological aging is aging under the effect of living organisms and products of their metabolism.

Electric aging is aging in an electric field.

Ultrasonic aging is aging in an ultrasonic field.

Ablation is aging in a hot stream of gas and solid particles.

Aging under mechanical loading is under effect of static and/or dynamic mechanical loads.

In practice, aging is normally stimulated by a set of factors, e.g., light plus heat, heat plus oxygen, etc.

Aging processes may be classified according to the environmental conditions.

Artificial weathering is aging of polymeric material under conditions created artificially to imitate the natural conditions or accelerate the aging process.

Natural weathering is aging under the effect of the complex of natural environmental factors.

Natural weathering is divided into several distinct types, viz. aging on an open platform, shelf aging, aging in a heated or unheated room, etc.

Aging in the cosmos is aging in the outer space.

Aging in the living body is aging incorporated in the tissues (organs) of the living body.

Such terms as "aging in the ground" and "aging in an aqueous medium" are also used at times.

6 METHODOLOGY OF AGING CONTROL

Among the properties of polymeric materials some are fundamental. For example, the chemical composition, molecular mass distribution of each component, the physical structure of material. Other properties are secondary.

In scientific and industrial research certain particular properties of polymeric materials may attract special interest depending on the object of research. The investigators use the time histories of these parameters as indicators of the aging process.

In order to distinguish aging from eventual alterations of a property due to changed external conditions (temperature, humidity, etc.), either the variation of the relevant property index measured under fixed conditions of the variation of some fundamental property itself are used as aging process characteristics.

7 CRITERIA OF RESISTANCE TO AGING

Aging resistance (stability) is the ability of a polymeric material to retain its properties within specified ranges under specified aging conditions.

The polymer may be resistant to some particular aging factor. For instance, light resistance (stability) of a polymer material is determined by its ability to retain properties under the effect of light; chemical resistance (stability) is the resistance of a polymer material to the attack of chemically active agents, etc.

Keeping quality is the property of a polymeric material to remain serviceable during and after storage.

Shelf life time is the time for which a material may be stored under specified conditions until its serviceability is impaired.

Serviceability is the state of a polymeric item in which it is usable for a given function and its performance characteristics are within the specified ranges.

Service life is the time during which a polymeric item is able to perform its function until it becomes unserviceable.

The lifetime of a material of which an item is made may be longer than that of the item itself, since the item may fail because some other component may have failed. Therefore, the lifetime of a material used in an item is usually calculated theoretically rather than experimentally determined.

Guaranteed life is the time over which item performance within the specified limits is guaranteed by the manufacturer.

As a rule the guaranteed life differs from the service lifetime.

Reliability is the property of a polymer item to remain serviceable throughout a specified service lifetime.

Such characteristics as keeping quality, guaranteed life and reliability may be used as special criteria of material resistance to aging.

Quantitatively the material resistance to aging is represented by the aging factor or service lifetime.

Aging factor is the relative variation of a property index at a given moment of time during the aging process. Aging factor is usually defined either as y/y_0 or as $\frac{y-y}{y_0-y}$, where y_0, y and y are the initial, current and final values of the property index.

Aging function is a mathematical representation of the aging kinetics of a polymeric material (item) based on some aging model or experimental data.

The aging function of a material is obtained through generalization of the available data about the material. With its help one may predict variation of the properties of material under any conditions. The question of reliability of such predictions may be answered by carrying out the statistical analysis of the experimental data from which the aging function was derived.

Aging kinetics is the time-dependent variations of material property under specified conditions.

Aging model is a hypothetical mechanism or a procedure for an empirical description of the kinetics of aging of a polymeric material (item).

8 PREDICTIONS

The properties of a polymeric material (item) in storage or service may be forecast and predicted.

Forecast is a scientifically-substantiated conclusion about the expected polymer material (item) properties after a specified period of use or storage.

Prediction is a description of the possible changes of the polymer material (item) properties on the basis of the expertise.

The expected service lifetime and property variations are the characteristics which have to be forecast more often than other characteristics.

The **service lifetime forecast** is the determination of the service lifetime of a polymeric item from the results of preliminary tests.

The **property variation forecast** is the determination of the variation in time of a property index under specified service conditions from the results of preliminary tests. Accelerated tests are most often used for such preliminary testing.

9 TESTS

Tests are operations carried out for the purpose of determining the property indices of a polymeric material.

Tests may have to be used to determine the time-dependent variations (time histories) of the properties of material either under natural or artificial conditions. Tests may have the object of either determining the aging kinetics of a polymeric material or determining its stability under specified conditions.

Test specimen is an object of given dimensions and shape made from a polymeric material specifically for testing purposes.

Accelerated test is the test carried out under conditions and by a method specifically designed to obtain the required data about the aging process.

Test program is the list or sequence of investigatory operations required to achieve the object of the test.

10 AGING PROTECTION

Polymer materials can be protected from the detrimental effects of aging in various ways. The one used most widely is by incorporation of agents which inhibit polymer aging processes. Less common forms of protection are chemical or structural modifications.

Stabilization of polymer materials—improvement of the resistance to aging.

Stabilizers—are the agents incorporated to improve its aging resistance.

Stabilizer effectiveness—a value characterizing the stabilizer's ability to improve the aging resistance.

Stabilizing compositions—mixtures of compounds incorporated to improve their aging resistance.

Synergism—the combined stabilizing effect is greater than or at least equal to the effectiveness of the most active component of the mixture.

Antagonism—is the weakening or loss of the protective effect inherent in a given stabilizer or stabilizing composition as a result of addition of one or more compounds.

Inhibitors—agents incorporated to retard the aging process.

Stabilizers are classified according to the basic aging factor:

Thermostabilizers—the stabilizing agents which improve polymer stability to heat.

Depending on the intended function, thermostabilizers are divided into free radical acceptors and aging product acceptor.

Free radical acceptor—stabilizer which combines with free radicals to form stable products, complexes or radicals.

Aging product acceptor—stabilizer deactivating the catalytically active aging products.

Light stabilizer—stabilizer which improves polymer resistance to

There are two types of light stabilizers:

UV-absorber—uncolored light stabilizer having absorption in the UV region of the spectrum.

Quencher—light stabilizer protecting a polymeric material by physically or chemically quenching the excited electron states of the chromophor groups present in the polymer.

Antioxidants—stabilizers improving resistance of polymeric materials to attack of oxygen.

The broad class of antioxidants includes free radical acceptors, peroxide decomposers, metal deactivators.

Peroxide decomposer—antioxidant which decomposes peroxide without producing free radicals.

Metal deactivator—stabilizer suppressing the catalytic activity of metals and their compounds in processes of oxidation with molecular oxygen.

Antiozonant—stabilizer improving resistance to ozone attack.

Fire retarding agent—stabilizer suppressing combustibility of polymeric materials.

Antirad—stabilizer improving resistance to an ionizing radiation.

Antifatigue agent—stabilizer improving resistance to repeated mechanical loading.

Structure forming agent—compounds capable of affecting the physical structure of a polymeric material.

Protective coatings—coats applied to a surface to protect it from aging.

Sealant compositions—polymer- or oligomer-based compositions applied to surfaces of articles with the purpose of decreasing permeability with respect to different fluids.

Biocides—agents incorporated to protect it from attack of living organisms.

Biocides include:

gicides—biocides protecting polymer materials from attack of microscopic fungi.

Lamicide—biocides protecting polymer materials from the attack of mollusca.

Algocides—biocides protecting polymer materials from the attack of seaweeds.

Bactericides—biocides protecting polymer materials from the attack of bacteria.

REFERENCES

1. N.M. Emanuel, *Some problems of the chemical physics of polymer aging and stabilization*, 1979, **Usp. Khimii, 48**(12), p. 2113.
2. *Encyclopedia of Polymers*, 1977, Moscow, Sovetskaya Entsiklopediya Publishers, pp. 1–3 (in Russian).
3. *Concise Chemical Encyclopedia*, 1961, Sovetskaya Entsiklopedia Publishers, pp. 1–5 (in Russian).
4. *"Bolshaya" Soviet Encyclopedia*, 1970, Moscow, Sovetskaya Entsiklopedia Publishers, (in Russian).
5. *Plastics Manual*, ed. by V.M. Kataev, V.A. Popov and B.I. Sakhin, 1975, Khimiya Publishers, Moscow, pp. 1–2.
6. D.W. Van Krevelen, *Properties of Polymers Correlations with Chemical Structure*, 1972, Elsevier publishing Company Amsterdam–London–New York.
7. GOST 17050–71, *Aging of Polymer Materials. Terms and Definitions.*
8. ANSI/ASTM D 883–78, *Standard Definitions of Terms Relating to Plastics.*
9. RS 5029–75, *Plastics, Aging and Stabilization. Terms and Definitions.*
10. H.A. Stuart, *Physik der Hochpolymeren*, 1955, Springer, Berlin, Bd. 3.
11. R. Gächter and H. Müller, *Taschenbuch der Kunststoff-Additive, Carl Hanser Verlag*, München-Wien, 1979, 571 S.

APPENDIX 1
Properties of Polymeric Materials.

No.	Property	Property Index
	Molecular mass, molecular mass distribution	Mean-numerical molecular mass, $\bar{M}_n$ Mean-mass molecular mass, $\bar{M}_w$ Mean molecular mass, $\bar{M}_z$ Mean-viscosity molecular mass, $\bar{M}_\eta$
I.	*Thermophysical Properties*	
1.	Dimensional characteristics:	
	a) volume and density	$V\left[M^3\right]$ and ρ (kg/m^3)
	b) thermal expansion	Volumetric coefficient of thermal expansion, $\alpha\left[K^{-1}\right]$ Linear coefficient of thermal expansion, $\beta\left[K^{-1}\right]$
	c) expansion in fusion	Increase of molar volume in fusion, ΔV_m
2.	Calorimetric Characteristics	
	a) heat capacity	Specific heat capacity at constant volume, c_v (J/kg.K) Specific heat capacity at constant pressure, c_p (J/kg.K) Molar heat capacity at constant volume, C_v (J/kg.K) Molar heat capacity at constant pressure, C_p (J/kg.K)
	b) heat of fusion (crystallization)	ΔH_m (J/mol)
	c) enthalpy and entropy	ΔH (J/mol), ΔS (J/mol.K)
	d) heat resistance	T (K)
	e) thermal stability	T (K)
3.	Cohesion and Adhesion Characteristics	
	a) molar energy of cohesion	$E_{\rm coh}$ (J/mol)
	b) internal pressure	π (Pa)
	c) surface energy	E_s (J/mol)
	d) Adhesion between polymers	Reversible work of adhesion, $W_{\rm adh}$ (N/m^2)
4.	Transition Temperatures	
	a) glass transition temperature	$T_{\rm g}$ (K)
	b) melting point	$T_{\rm m}$ (K)
5.	(Thermodynamical and Kinetic) Flexibility of Macromolecules	
6.	Solubility	
	a) solubility parameter	δ (J$^{1/2}$/m$^{3/2}$)
	b) solubility limit critical mixing temperature	Flory point, T (K)
II.	*Polymer Properties in Force Fields*	
1.	Mechanical (viscoelastic) Properties	
	a) elastic properties	Bulk modulus, K (N/m^2) Shear modulus (stiffness), G (N/m^2) Young's modulus, E (N/m^2) Poisson's ratio, (ν)
	b) viscoelasticity of resins	Young's modulus, E (N/m^2)
	c) viscoelasticity	Elasticity and viscosity modulus
	d) dynamic mechanical parameters	Mechanical loss tangent, $tg\delta$
	e) stress relaxation and creep	Complex modulus of elasticity, E^*. Relaxation time spectra.

2. Ultimate Mechanical Characteristics	
a) stress-strain curves of solid polymers	Elasticity modulus, E (N/m^2) Yield strength, σ_y (Pa) Breaking stress, σ_b (Pa) Ultimate elongation, ε (%)
b) fatigue strength (breaking stress)	f.s. (Pa)
c) durability	Number of loading cycles to rupture under given mechanical stress, N
d) impact strength (resistance to instantaneous impacts) Izod, Charpy, Distant tests, under tension	I (J/m^2)
3. Long-Term Mechanical Characteristics	
a) durability	τ (sec)
b) deformation at rupture	ε, %
4. Other Fracture Characteristics	
a) hardness (Brinell, Vickers, Rockwell, Shore)	H_B (kg/mm)
b) resistance to scratching (wear)	Wear resistance (mg/1000 cm^3)
c) friction (internal, surface)	Friction coefficient, μ
5. Optical Properties	
a) light absorption	Absorption coefficient, ε (lm/mol.cm) Light transmittance, T (%)
b) light refraction	Refractive index, n; Molar refraction, R
c) dissipation	Haze, turbidity
d) reflection	Refractive index, n
6. Electric Properties	
a) dielectric polarization	Dielectric constant, ε Molar polarization of dielectric, ε_n Dipole moment, μ; loss tangent of dielectric, $tg\delta$
b) static charge accumulation and electric conductivity	Bulk conductivity, γ (1/Ohm m^{-1}) Bulk resistivity, Ω (Ohm/m)
c) ultimate electric characteristics	Dielectric strength (kV/mm) (breakdown voltage) Electric arc resistance
7. Magnetic Properties	
a) magnetic susceptibility	χ
b) magnetic resonance (ESR, NMR)	
III. *Transfer Phenomena in Polymers*	
1. Heat energy transfer	Heat conductivity (J/cm.m.K)
2. Polymer solution viscosity	Ultimate viscosity number (intrinsic viscosity, Staudinger index) (cm^3/g)
3. Polymer melt viscosity	
4. Melt elasticity	
5. Polymer dissolution and melting	
6. Permeability of polymers: Gas, vapor and liquid transfer by diffusion in polymers	Solubility of gases and vapors in polymers, S (cm^3/cm^3 Pa) Permeability for gases and vapors, P ($m^3.m^2/m^3$.Pa.sec)
Diffusion of simple gases, vapors and liquids	Diffusion coefficient, D (m^2/sec)

Physical Chemistry of Topological Disorder: Sorption and Reactions of Low-Molecular Compounds in Polymers.

Yu.A. SHLYAPNIKOV

United Institute of Chemical Physics, 117334, Moscow, Russia

Various topological structures, namely knots, folds and entanglements of the polymer chains, differing from their surroundings in terms of relatively order, play a significant role in many processes taking part in polymers, especially those involving low-molecular compounds.

INTRODUCTION

Some time ago, the author proposed a two-component model of a polymeric substance, which considers the bulk polymer as a solution of various units of disorder (UODs) in a certain ideally ordered substance. These units are formed by topological structures: numerous knots, folds and entanglements of the polymer chains.[1–3] The great lengths of the chains ensure stability of these structures even in the polymeric melt. The model helps us to explain many phenomena in the physical chemistry of polymers.

Begin with polymer crystallinity. Many polymers, including the simplest polyolefins, contain both crystalline and amorphous phases, the ratio of which change with temperature[4] and apparently with pressure. According to the Gibbs Phase Rule:

$$F + P \leq C + 2 \tag{1}$$

where F is the number of freedom degrees, equal to 2 (temperature and pressure), P the number of co-existing phases, also equal to 2 (crystalline and amorphous), and C the number of components, which must be $C \geq 2$. If one component is the polymer, the lacking second component must be the set of structures preventing complete crystallization of the polymer, that is various entanglements of the polymer chains and which are the units of disorder ζ_i[3] (Figure 1).

Considering UODs as mobile molecules of a quasi-compound, the osmotic pressure of which prevents the elements growing to a crystalline phase, the formula of the polymer crystallinity was derived in [1]:

$$(1 - \alpha) = \frac{RT \sum[\zeta_i]}{-\Delta F_{\text{cr}} - \sum \chi_j [X_j]} \tag{2}$$

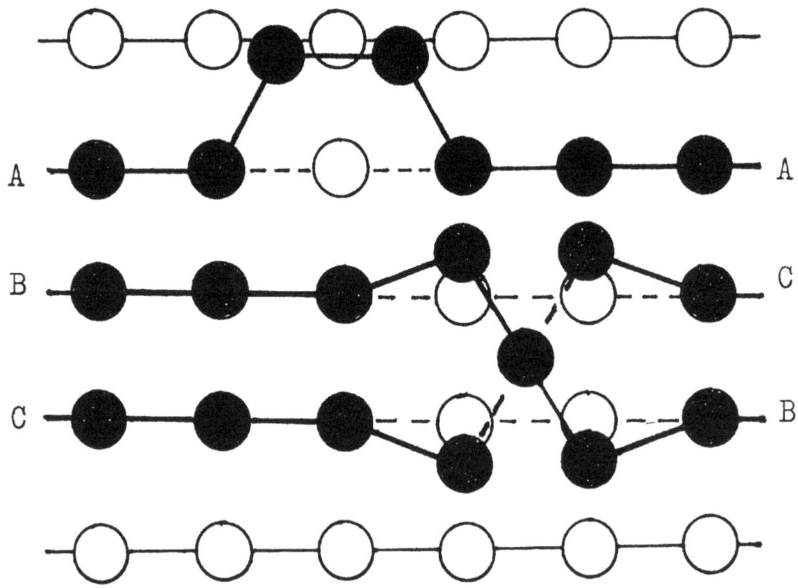

Figure 1 The scheme of the simplest units of disorder: fold (A–A) and interlacement (B–B and C–C).

where ΔF_{cr} is the decrease of free energy on polymer crystallization, calculated for mass unit of the polymer, X_j the various foreign monomeric units in the polymer chains, and χ_j the decrease of free energy of crystallization due to introducing of these units. This formula contains the concentration of UODs, which depends on many factors including the pre-history of the sample, therefore no synonymous expression connecting the polymer crystallinity with content of foreign monomeric unit can exist.

Besides the polymer, polymeric materials may contain various low-molecular compounds as dies, plasticizers, antioxidants, antipyrenes etc. These compounds can react with one another, with polymer and with oxygen. It will be shown below, the factors controlling the reaction of low-molecular compounds in polymers may differ from those in low-molecular solvents.

As shown earlier,[3,5,6] low-molecular compounds dissolved in the polymeric substance can not form the solvent shells in the ordered part of the polymer and penetrate into the pre-existing elements of free volume—the sorption centers based on topological structures: various knots, folds and entanglement of the long polymer chains. For each type of centers Z_i, the equilibrium between molecules A outside the centers and those in the centers (which may be considered as complexes $A \cdot Z_i$) exists:

$$A + Z_i \overset{K_{ai}}{\rightleftharpoons} A \cdot Z_i \tag{3}$$

Following from (1) the relation between $[A]$ and $[A \cdot Z_i]$ for any type of centers will be:

$$[A \cdot Z_i] = \frac{K_{ai}[Z_i][A]}{1 + K_{ai}[A]} \tag{4}$$

The total concentration of A in the polymer $[A]_p$ containing the set of various centers will be the sum:

$$[A]_p = [A] + \sum_i \frac{K_{ai}[Z_i][A]}{1 + K_{ai}[A]} \tag{5}$$

If the medium surrounding the polymer sample contains compound A in concentration $[A]_m$ the relation between these concentration is expressed by Henry Law:

$$[A] = \gamma_a [A]_m \tag{6}$$

The sorption isotherm of A, i.e. the relation between $[A]_m$ and $[A]_p$ following from (5) and (6) is:

$$[A]_p = [A] + \sum_i \frac{K_{ai}[Z_i]\gamma_a[A]_m}{1 + K_{ai}\gamma_a[A]_m} \tag{7}$$

Experiments show that the sorption isotherms for the most compounds with molecular masses between 150 and 2000 obey the simple Langmuir-type law which we will write in the form:

$$[A]_p = \frac{a[A]_m}{1 + b[A]_m} \tag{8}$$

where $[A]_m$ is the concentration of A in surrounding medium. In inverse coordinates ($1/[A]_p$ vs $1/[A]_m$) this relation turns into:

$$\frac{1}{[A]_p} = \frac{1}{b[A]_m} + \frac{b}{a} \tag{9}$$

That is the sorption obeys the Langmuir-type law (4) if the sorption isotherm transforms in inverse coordinates ($1/[A]_p$ vs $1/[A]_m$) into straight lne.

It may be demonstrated that expression (6) virtually coincides with the simple Langmuir law at various assumptions about distribution of $[Z_i]$ over equilibrium constant K_{ai}. Thus taking the ratio $\rho = \Delta[Z_i]/K_i$ to be constant in the range $K_{a1} \leq K_{ai} \leq K_{a2}$:

$$\rho = \Delta[Z_i]/\Delta K_{ai} = [Z_a](K_{a2} - K_1)^{-1} \tag{10}$$

but zero outside this range, neglecting concentration of mobile A compared to $\sum[A \cdot Z_i]$ and substituting the sum (6) with integral, we get:

$$\begin{aligned} [A]_p &= \rho \int_{K_{a1}}^{K_{a2}} \frac{K_a\gamma_a[A]_m \mathrm{d}K_a}{1 + K_a\gamma_a[A]_m} \\ &= [Z_a]\left\{1 + \frac{1}{(K_{a2} - K_{a1})\gamma_a[A]_m} \ln\frac{1 + K_{a1}\gamma_a[A]_m}{1 + K_{a2}\gamma_a[A]_m}\right\} \end{aligned} \tag{11}$$

With increasing $[A]_m$ (8) tends to $[Z]_a$—the Langmuir sorption capacity of the polymer towards A.

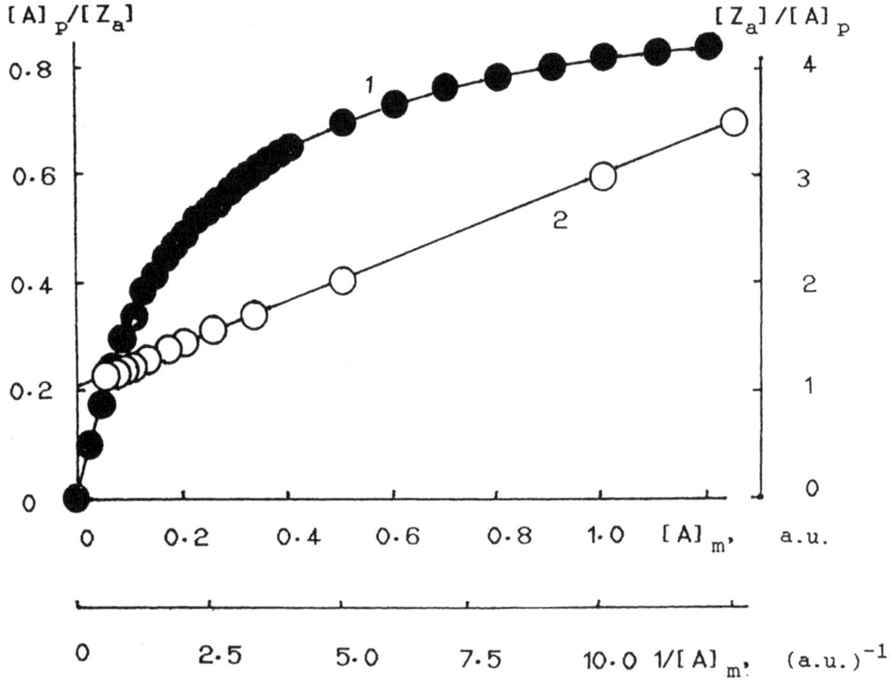

Figure 2 Dependence (11) in direct (1) and inverse (2) coordinates (calculated assuming $K_{2a}/K_{1a} = 10$).

As seen from Figure 2, in inverse coordinates ($1/[A]_m$ vs $1/[A]_p$) the dependence (11) transforms into the straight line, i.e. the isotherm (11) is virtually indistinguishable from Langmuir-type one (8)–(9).

The similar result follows from assumption that the equilibrium constants K_{ai} differ only in heat of sorption: $K_{ai} = \chi \exp(Q_i/RT)$ and the distribution of center concentration over the heat of sorption is symmetric about $(K_{a1}K_{a2})^{1/2}$.[3,7]

This similarity enables us to use the simple expression:

$$[A]_p = \frac{K_a[Z_a]\gamma_a[A]_m}{1 + K_a Y_a [A]_m} \tag{12}$$

instead of the complicated formula (8), in particular to solve the inverse task: to find the dependence of the concentration of mobile molecules $[A] = \gamma_a^{-1}[A]_m$ as function of $[A]_p$, $[Z_a]$ and certain average K_a:

$$[A] = \frac{[A]_p}{K_a([Z_a] - [A]_p)} \tag{13}$$

Apparently in the most cases we may divide the set of units of disorder and similarly the sorption centers according to any process into two groups: participating and non-participating, and sometimes into three groups always neglecting the differences inside each of them.

SOME REGULARITIES OF SORPTION OF LOW-MOLECULAR COMPOUNDS

At relatively small concentrations of low-molecular compounds their sorption from gas phase or liquids obeys the Langmuir law (4) with value of $[Z_a]$ independent of temperature, some-times in the range of about 180°C.[7] Thus the sorption isotherms of phenylbenzoate by isotactic polypropylene determined at various temperatures transformed into inverse coordinates (7) are the straight lines intersecting the ordinate axis in the same point $y = 1/[Z_a]$ (Figure 3). Analogously are sorbed low-molecular compounds from low-molecular liquids (Figure 4).[8]

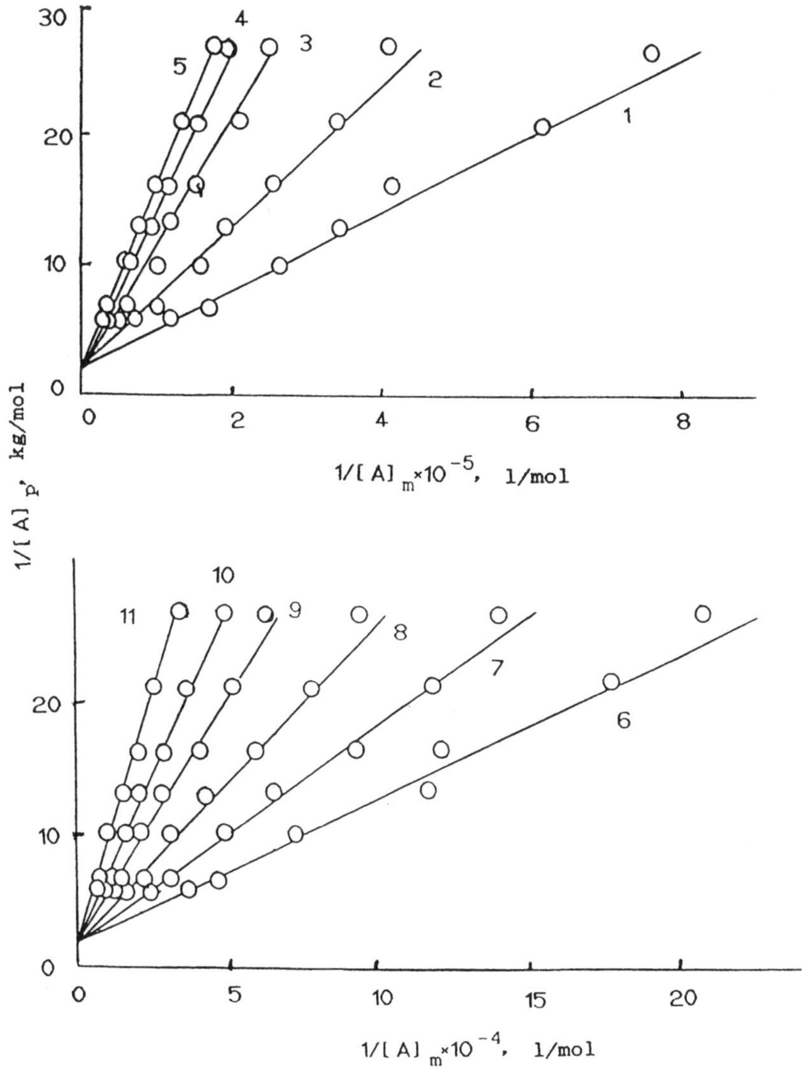

Figure 3 The sorption isotherms of phenylbenzoate by polyethylene from vapours. Temperatures: 80° (1), 90° (2), 100° (3), 110° (4), 120° (5), 130° (6), 140° (7), 150° (8), 160° (9), 170° (10), and 180° C (11).

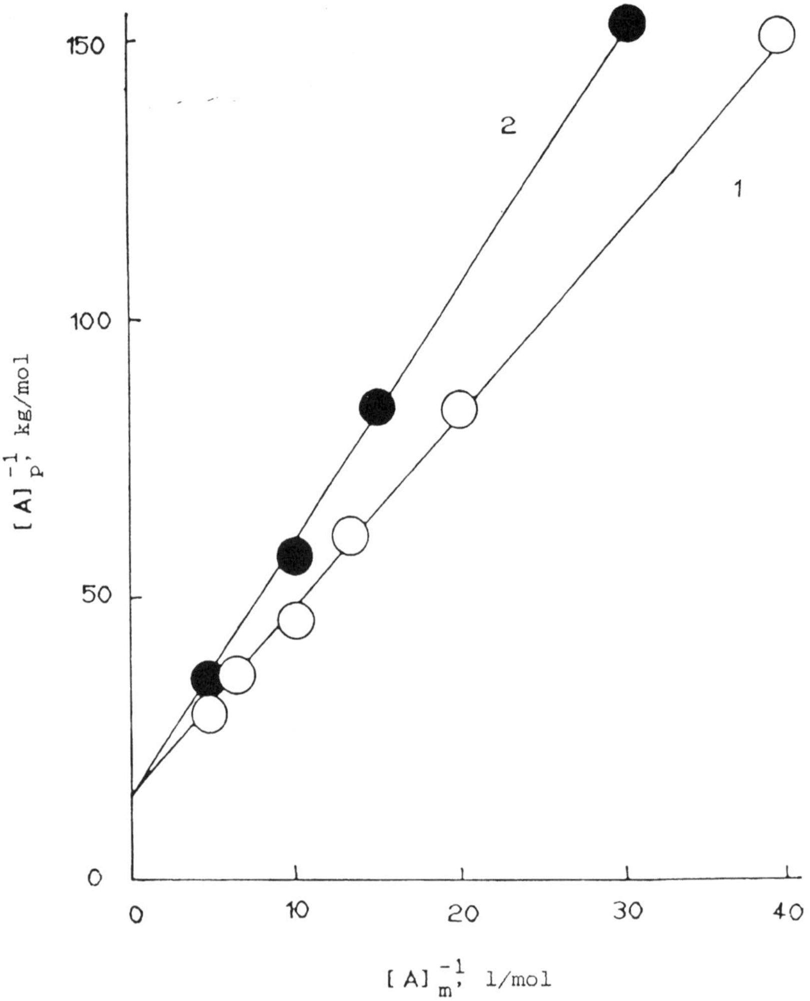

Figure 4 The sorption isotherms of phenylbenzoate (1) and diphenylamine (2) from hexane solutions, 50°C.[8]

On simultaneous sorption of two compounds A and B by the same polymer sample, the effects of mutual replacement of dissolved compounds are observed: at $[A]_m = \text{const.}$ with increasing $[B]_m$ the concentration of A in the polymer $[A]_p$ decreases because of substitution of A with B in some centers Z_{ab} (Figure 5):[8,9,10]

$$A{\cdot}Z_{ab} + B \Longleftrightarrow B{\cdot}Z_{ab} + A \qquad (14)$$

Occupying some centers capable of sorbing A and decreasing thus the value of $[Z]$ in denominator of (1), the second compound increases the ratio of mobile A molecules $[A]/[A]_p$.

On the sorption from low-molecular liquid, the molecules of solvent S can occupy some centers capable of sorption of A, as a result solubility of the same compound in

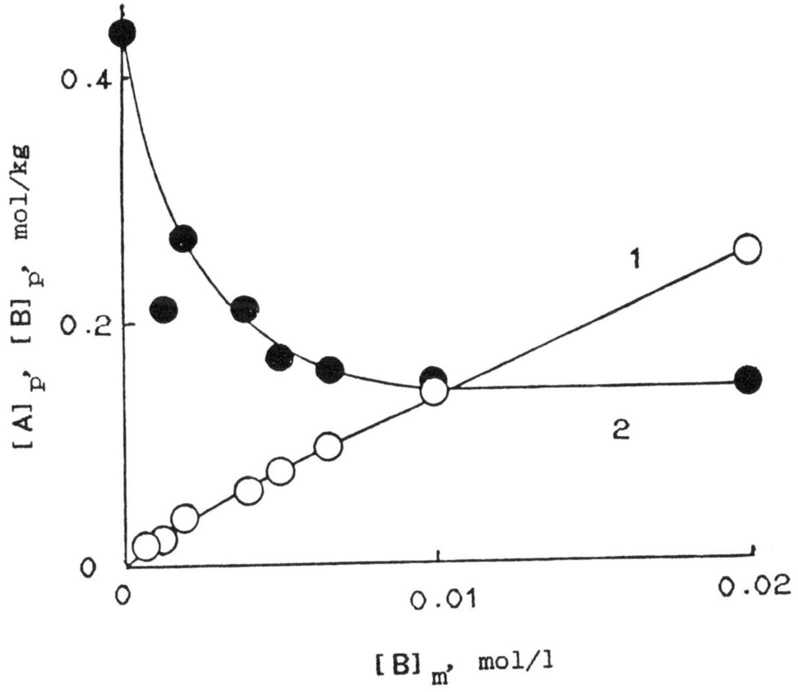

Figure 5 Dependence of concentration of α-naphthol $[A]_p$ and α-naphthylamine $[B]_p$ in high density polyethylene $[A]_p$ on α-naphthylamine concentration in hexane solution $[B]_m$ at $[A]_m = 0.02$ mol/kg = const. 50°C.[8]

the same polymer sample depends on the presence and nature of solvent into which it is immersed.

The more complex is UOD, the greater is the free volume it contains. We may find the relation between the volume of dissolved molecule v_a and the concentration of centers sorbing this molecules.

First we must postulate that in solution from which the polymer has been precipitated, the structures-precursors of the elements of topological disorder exist. These elements contain free volume occupied by the molecules of the solvent. The second assumption is: the energy of formation of these elements is proportional to their volumes $\varepsilon_i = v_i(q - q_s)$, where $q = \Delta\varepsilon_i/\Delta v_i$—the energy needed for formation of the unit of free volume in the absence of solvent and q_s—the decrease of this energy due to interaction of the polymer with the solvent. After precipitation the volume of the element decreases β times. Assuming that the volume of molecule dissolved in the polymer v_a is the same as in pure A, we find $v_a = M_a/\rho \mathrm{N_A}$, where M_a is molecular mass of A and $\mathrm{N_A}$ is the Avogadro number.

According to the Boltzmann law, the ratio of elements of formation needs an excess energy $\varepsilon \geq \varepsilon_a$ is $\exp(-\varepsilon_a/kT)$. Substituting ε_a with $\beta(q - q_s)M_a/\rho \mathrm{N_A}$ we find the meaning of the coefficient χ:[11]

$$\chi = \beta(q - q_s)(\rho \mathrm{N_A} k T_f)^{-1} \tag{15}$$

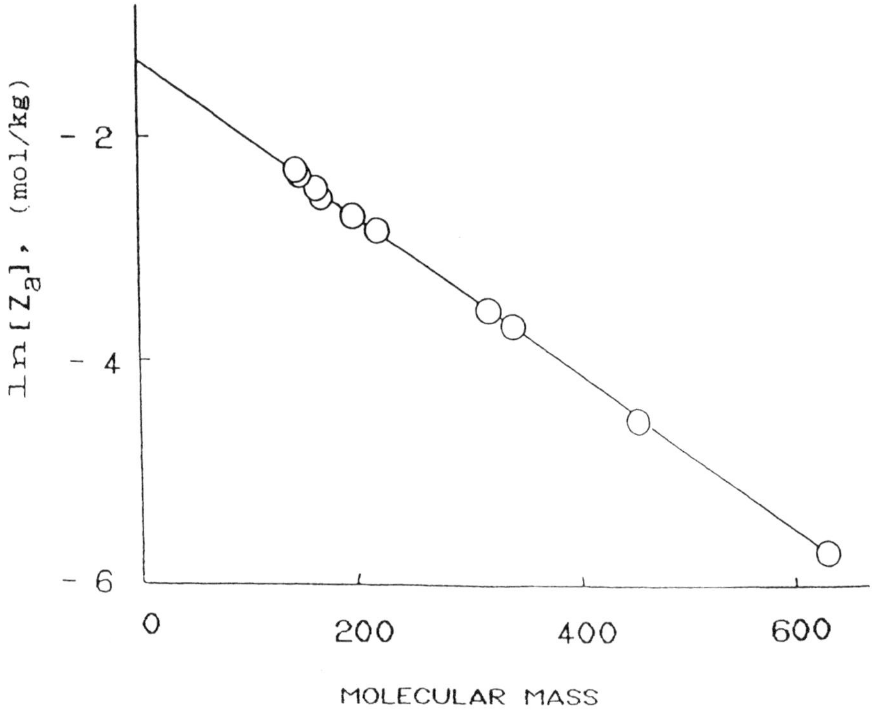

Figure 6 Logarithm of sorption centers concentration in high-density polyethylene as function of molecular mass of sorbed additive[12] (Formula (16)).

and finally:

$$[Z_a] = [Z]_0 \exp(-\chi M_a) \tag{16}$$

Formula (16) had been first found experimentally[12] for sorption of low-molecular compounds consisting of atoms C, N, O and H by polyethylene (Figure 6). The densities of these compounds were nearly the same ($\rho = 1.1 \pm 0.1$) which permitted to use of the same value of χ for all compounds studied.

The value of q_s for 'bad' solvent must be lower than for 'good' one, the values of χ are the opposite and must be greater for 'bad' and lower for 'good' one. The size-distribution of sorption centers can be varied also by variation of temperature of sedimentation and of polymer concentration in solution, all affecting $[Z]_0$.

Experiments have shown that, in accordance with (25) and (26) the parameters of sorption of antioxidant phenyl-β-naphthylamine by the same polypropylene precipitated from different solvents markedly differ (Figure 7):[13] the sorption capacity of the polypropylene precipitated from decane (PP-1) was $[Z_a] = 0.30$ mol/kg, the constant of sorption equilibrium $K_a = 3.5$ l/kg, for polypropylene precipitated from chlorobenzene (PP-2) $[Z_a] = 0.039$ mol/kg and $K_a = 3.0$ l/kg, all at 40°C, melting temperatures were, correspondingly, 158.5° and 160.0°C showing the difference in the structure.

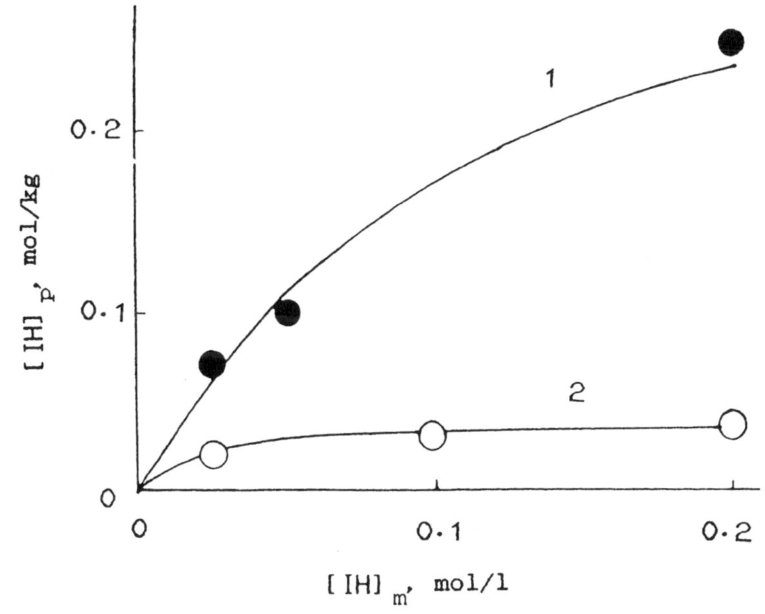

Figure 7 The sorption isotherms of phenyl-β-naphthylamine from its solutions in heptane at 40°C by polypropylene precipitated from n-decane (1) and chlorobenzene (2).

CONCENTRATION DEPENDENCE OF THE COEFFICIENT OF DIFFUSION IN POLYMER

Dividing the molecules of the low-molecular compound dissolved in a polymer into two groups: mobile and sorbed by centers Z_a results in dependence of diffusion coefficient on diffusant concentration.

If only mobile A molecules are moving in polymer and their coefficient of diffusion is D_0, so according to Ficks Law, the flow of A through the polymer in direction of x axis will be:

$$\Phi = -D_0 \frac{d[A]}{dx} \tag{17}$$

In the same time we register by the usual analytical methods, not the total A concentration $[A]_p$ and concentration of mobile A. To find the apparent diffusion coefficient we must apply the formula of derivative of function in respect to another function:

$$\Phi = -D_0 \frac{d[A]}{dx} = -D_0 \frac{d[A]}{d[A]_p} \cdot \frac{d[A]_p}{dx} = -\frac{D_0[Z_a]}{K_a([Z] - [A]_p)^2} \cdot \frac{d[A]_p}{dx} \tag{18}$$

or

$$D_a = \frac{D_0[Z_a]}{K_a([Z] - [A]_p)^2} \tag{19}$$

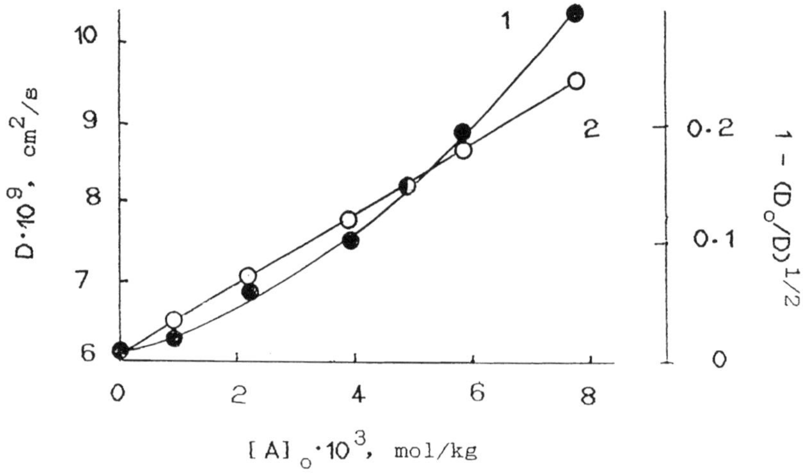

Figure 8 Coefficient of diffusion of 2,2′-methylene-bis(4-methyl-6-tert.butylphenol) in polyethylene as function of diffusant concentration (1, left axis), 2 (right axis)—transformation of this dependence in coordinates of formula (20) (right axis).[16]

Denoting $D_m[Z_a]/K_a = D(0)$ and $1/[Z_a] = \lambda$ we get the formula of Fujita:[14,15]

$$D_a = \frac{D_0}{(1 - \lambda[A]_p)^2} \tag{20}$$

According to (19) and (20) the apparent diffusion coefficient of the low-molecular compounds must increase with the diffusant concentration. The dependence of diffusion coefficient of antioxidant 2,2′-methylene-bis(4-methyl-6-tert.butylphenol) labelled with ^{14}C on the concentration of the same non-labelled compound is shown in Figure 8.[16] As seen from this figure, the experimental dependence may be transformed into the straight line in coordinates $1 - (D_0/D_a)^2$ vs $[A]_p$ following from (20).

SUBDIVIDING OF THE SORPTION CENTERS

For some purposes; it is convenient to divide the sorption centers of the same additive A into two groups: ones strongly binding the additive Z_{a1} (tight) and ones weakly binding (loose) Z_{a2}:$K_{a1} \gg K_{a2}$. Concentration of the first type centers, exactly fitting the A molecules, must be less then those of the second type $[Z_{a1}] \ll [Z_{a2}]$. The two equilibria will take place in the polymer:

$$A + Z_{a1} \overset{K_{a1}}{\rightleftharpoons} A{\cdot}Z_{a1} \tag{21}$$

and

$$A + Z_{a2} \overset{K_{a2}}{\rightleftharpoons} A{\cdot}Z_{a2} \tag{22}$$

To find relations between $[A]$, $[A{\cdot}Z_{a2}]$ and $[A]_p$ if the last two values are comparable with one another we must substitute the expression (6) with the sum:

$$[A]_p = \frac{K_{a1}[Z_{a1}][A]}{1+K_{a1}[A]} + K_{a2}[Z_{a2}][A] \tag{23}$$

Solving the equation (9) according to $[A]$ we get:

$$\begin{aligned} [A] &= \frac{K_{a1}[A]_p - K_{a1}[Z_{a1}] - K_{a2}[Z_{a2}]}{2K_{a1}K_{a2}[Z_{a2}]} \\ &= \frac{\sqrt{(K_{a1}[A]_p - K_{a1}[Z_{a1}] - K_{a2}[Z_{a2}])^2 + 4K_{a1}K_{a2}[Z_{a2}][A]_p}}{2K_{a1}K_{a2}[Z_{a2}]} \end{aligned} \tag{24}$$

The curves of relative concentration of mobile molecules $[A]/[A]_p$ as function of the ratio $[A]_p/[Z_{a1}]$ calculated using (13) and (24) are presented in the Figure 9. As seen from this figure, curve 1, if there is only one type of centers $[Z_{a1}]$ the ratio of mobile molecules rapidly increases when $[A]_p/[Z_{a1}]$ approaches to 1, i.e. $[A]_p$ is close to the concentration of centers strongly binding A, i.e. to $[Z_{a1}]$.

If two types of centers Z_{a1} and Z_{a2} exist, and $[Z_{a2}] \gg [Z_{a1}]$, the ratio of mobile $[A]$ calculated using formula (24), curve 2, though increases near $[A]_p/[A{\cdot}Z_{a1}] = 1$, but

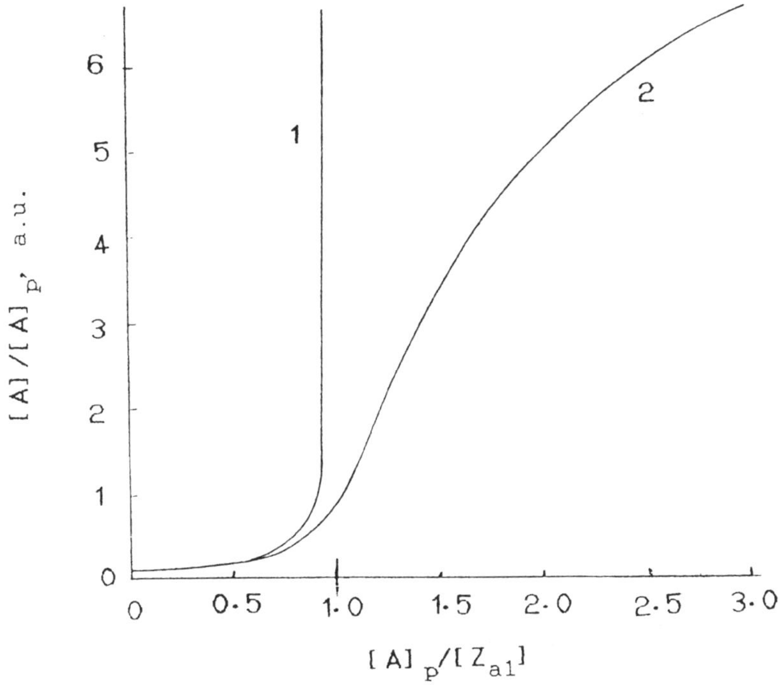

Figure 9 The ratio of mobile molecules of dissolved compound $[A]/[A]_p$ as function of its concentration (in the co-ordinates $[A]_p/[Z_a]$). 1—calculated from formula (10), 2—from formula (24).

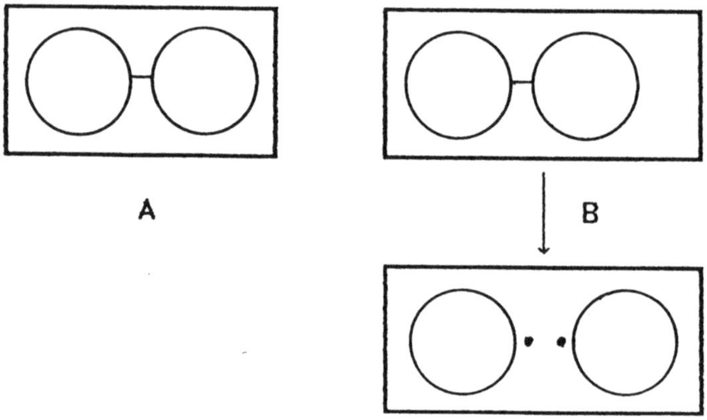

Figure 10 The scheme of monomolecular decomposition in "tight" sorption center (1) and in loose one (2).

does not tend to infinity and gradually bends to the right. The concentration of A molecules in the "loose" centers $[Z_{aw}]$ is directly proportional to $[A]([A \cdot Z_{a2}] = K_{a2}[Z_{a2}][A])$, thus the ratio of $[A \cdot Z_{aw}]$ to $[A]_p$ will have the same shape as the curve 2 in Figure 9.

The better the center Z_{a1} fits the A molecule, the more energy it needs to change its size or shape which is necessary for its transformation (Figure 10), thus we may wait that transition of A from Z_{a1} to Z_{a2} will result in increasing the rates of all reactions it participates. The similar effects are observed in behavior of many low-molecular compounds which are stable in crystalline state but decompose immediately after melting.

REARRANGEMENT OF THE SORPTION CENTERS

In many polymers, addition of low-molecular compounds results in marked changes of their physical properties, such as elasticity, these effects are known as plasticizing. In polyolefins the effects of low-molecular additives on their properties are not so pronounced.

Adding of low-molecular compound to the polymer melt we sometimes can introduce this compound into the polymer in concentrations several times exceeding not only its solubility,[9,17] but also the concentration of sorption centers $[Z_a]$ which normally sorb this compound.[18] After cooling of this polymer, a part of the additive evolves from the polymer sample (Figure 11), but residual concentration may also essentially exceed the equilibrium solubility.[18]

If the low-molecular compound A is extracted from the samples in which its concentration exceeded $[Z_a]$ by washing or evaporation at moderate temperature (for isotactic polypropylene at or below 60°C) and the sample is put into an atmosphere of saturated additive vapors, the concentration reaches the same value as before extraction:[19] the certain additional sorption centers $[Z_a^*]$ formed are stable enough, but above the certain temperature (80°C for polypropylene) they disappear.

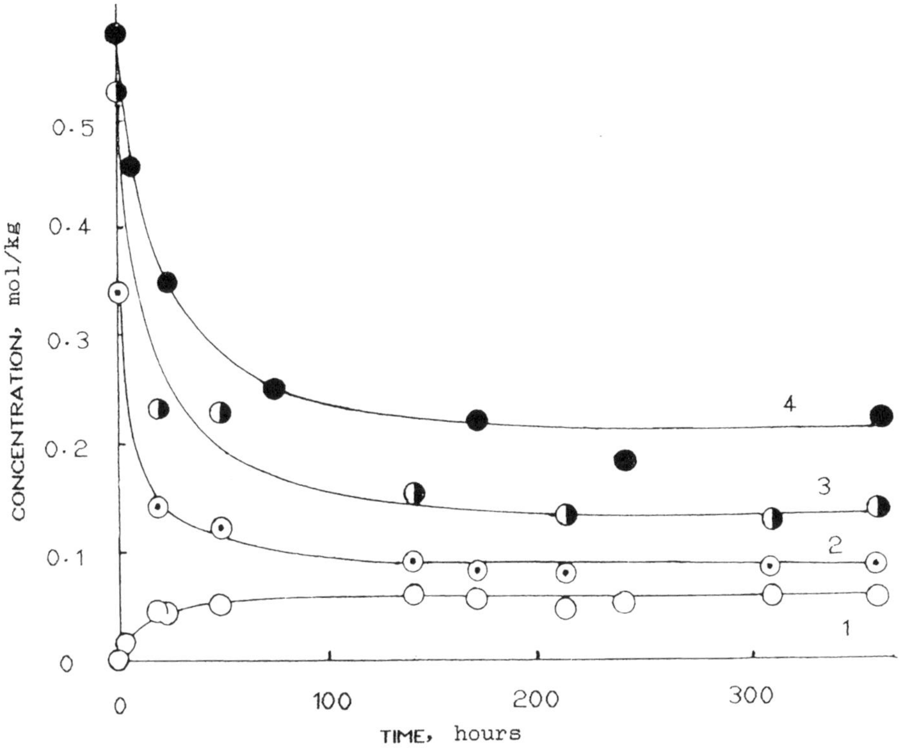

Figure 11 Variation of phenylbenzoate concentration in isotactic polypropylene samples prepared from the polymer melt without additives (1) and containing phenylbenzoate, 0.4 (2), 0.6 (3), and 0.8 mol/kg, 40°C.

To explain this phenomenon we assumed that some sorption centers are too small for compound A to be reversibly transformed into the centers of greater volume capable of sorbing this compound.

It follows from the assumption made above that the energy of the element of excess volume formation is proportional to its size: $\varepsilon_i = v_i(q - q_s)$, that if a compound A is occupying the volume $\Delta\varepsilon_i/\Delta v_i = q - q_a$ does not depend on both v_i and Δv_i values. Otherwise if the center Z_i already exists and its volume is less than that necessary for sorption of A molecules v_a, to increase the volume v_i to v_a, that is—to rearrange this center, the certain minimal (threshold) value of osmotic pressure of the additive $P_A = q - q_a$ is needed which does not depend on the size of v_i. In the polymer melt, when all volume of the polymer sample is accessible for the mobile part of the additive, this osmotic pressure P_A is connected with A concentration in the polymer $[A]_p$ by the expression:

$$P_a = [A]RT = \phi[A]_p RT \tag{25}$$

where $\phi = [A]/[A]_p$—the variable coefficient which may be calculated from expression (24). When $[A]_p \ll [Z_a]\phi = (K_a[Z_a])^{-1}$, but deviates from this when $[A]_p$ is comparable with $[Z]_a$. It follows from (25) that a certain minimal concentration of

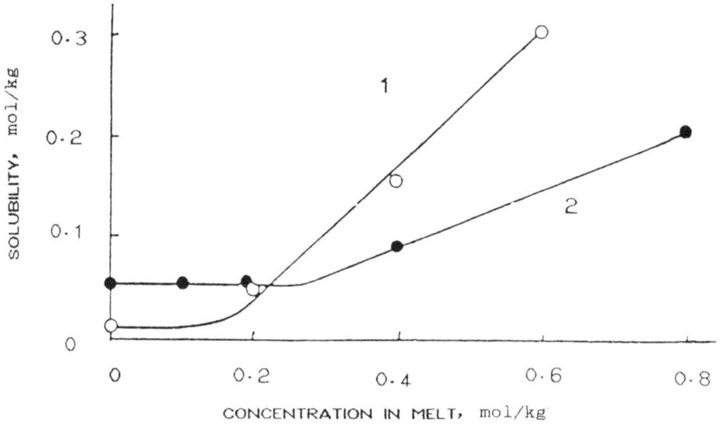

Figure 12 Solubility of phenyl-β-naphthylamine (1) and phenylbenzoate (2) in isotactic polypropylene at 40°C as function of their concenntrations in the polymer melt.[18]

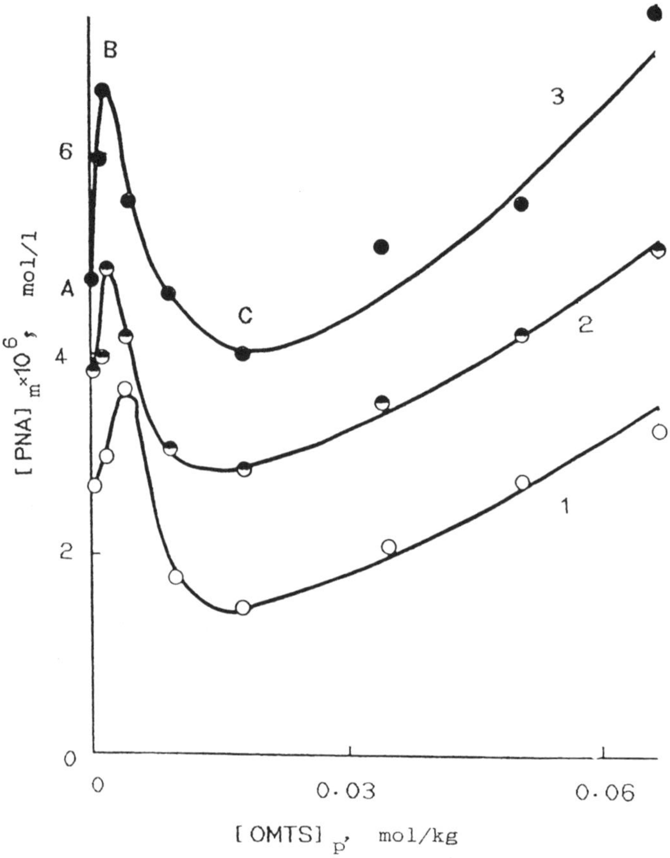

Figure 13 Concentration of phenyl-β-naphthylamine (PNA) in the gas phase above polyethylene as function of concentration of octamethylcyclotetrasiloxane (OMTS). $[PNA]_p = 8{\cdot}10^{-3}$ mol/kg, 180° (1), 190° (2), and 200° C (3).

low-molecular compound is needed above which the sorption centers will rearrange. Experiments support this conclusion: as seen from Figure 12, the certain concentration of compound added to the polymer melt is needed to change its solubility in the polymer.[18] If $q_a \geq q$ so $P_A \leq 0$ and the polymer will be swelling at any concentration of A.

Transformation of the element of disorder ζ_i into new sorption center Z^*_{ai} may be written as:

$$\zeta_i + A \longrightarrow Z^*_{ai}A \tag{26}$$

We now consider polymers with increased sorption centers concentrations.

The centers Z^*_{ai} disappear on heating of the polymer, but the topological structures on which they are based are preserve. This process is opposite to (26):

$$Z^*_{ai} \longrightarrow \zeta_i \tag{27}$$

Combination of substitution of one additive by another one along with rearrangement of sorption centers results in complicated but reproducible dependence of concentration of one additive in vapor (gas) phase on concentration of another one (Figure 13): In the section AB, the simple substitution of phenyl-B-naphthylamine (PNA) with octamethylcyclotetrasiloxane results in an increase of PNA concentration in the gas phase, then in the range BC the polymer structure is being broken and PNA concentration decreases, after the complete rearrangement of the structure substitution again results in increase of PNA concentration above the polymer.[19]

REACTIONS; GENERAL CONSIDERATION

Monomolecular transformation of a low-molecular mass compound A:

$$A \longrightarrow \text{product(s)} \tag{28}$$

proceeds with change of the size or (and) shape of the reacting molecule. For this reason the rate of such a reaction will depend on the shape or size of the element of free volume which contains the sorption center Z_i in which A is sorbed. As indicated above, the better the center fits for the A molecule the greater will be the equilibrium constant of its sorption K_{ai} and the less will be the rate of its transformation (Figure 10).

If we are studying the reaction of low-molecular compound A with a certain group G bound to the polymer chains which translational mobility is close to zero (these may be macroradicals formed at the polymer oxidation) two cases may take place: either reaction proceeds on nearly all encounters of mobile A with G, or the equilibrium exists:

$$G + A \underset{}{\overset{K_{ga}}{\rightleftharpoons}} G{\cdot}A \longrightarrow \text{products} \tag{29}$$

where $G{\cdot}A$ may be either complexes or simply a pair which can form and divide several times before the reaction will take place. In the first case, the reaction rate will be directly proportional to the concentration of the mobile molecules of A. In the second case the concentration of the complexes or pairs will be:

$$[G{\cdot}A] = K_{ga}[G][A] \tag{30}$$

i.e. also proportional to $[A]$—to the concentration of mobile molecules.

$$W_a = k_{a1}[A{\cdot}Z_{a2}] + k_{a2}[A{\cdot}Z_{a2}] = k_{a1}\left(1 + \frac{k_{a2}}{k_{a1}} \times \frac{[A{\cdot}Z_{a2}]}{[A]_p}\right)[A]_p \tag{31}$$

For $[A] = [AZ_{a2}](K_{a2}\,[Z_{a2}])^{-1}$ the rate constant of such reactions will also change with concentration as shown in Figure 9.

Bimolecular reactions between two low-molecular compounds A and B can follow one of three ways ($[Z_a] = [Z_{a1}] + [Z_{a2}]$ and $[Z_b] = [Z_{b1}] + [Z_{b2}]$):[20]

$$A + B{\cdot}Z_b \longrightarrow Z_b + \text{product(s)} \tag{32}$$

$$B + A{\cdot}Z_a \longrightarrow Z_a + \text{product(s)} \tag{33}$$

and through monomolecular transformation of triple complexes:

$$A{\cdot}B{\cdot}Z_{ab} \longrightarrow Z_{ab} + \text{product(s)} \tag{34}$$

The complexes $A{\cdot}Z_a$ and $B{\cdot}Z_b$ are immobile and can not react with one another, and direct interaction of two mobile molecules $(A + B)$ may be neglected because both concentrations $[A]$ and $[B]$ are too small. For the same reason we may assume $[A{\cdot}Z_a] \approx [A]_p$ and $[B{\cdot}Z_b] \approx [B]_p$.

The rates of reactions (32) and (33) are directly proportional to the product of reacting species, or $[A][B{\cdot}Z_b]$ and $[B][A{\cdot}Z_a]$.

The concentration of the triple complexes $A{\cdot}B{\cdot}Z_{ab}$ will be:

$$[A{\cdot}B{\cdot}Z_{ab}] = \frac{K_{ab}[A][B]}{1 + K_{ab}[A][B]} \tag{35}$$

Concentrations $[A]$ and $[B]$ rapidly increase with total concentration of both reagents, and the concentration of reacting complexes tends to the limit equal to $[Z_{ab}]$.

According to (35), the rate of reaction (34) will be:

$$W_{Zab} = K_{Zab}[A{\cdot}B{\cdot}Z_{ab}] = \frac{k_{Zab}K_{Zab}[A][B]}{1 + K_{ab}[A][B]} \longrightarrow k_{Zab}[Z_{ab}] = \text{const.} \tag{36}$$

and apparent rate constant of this reaction from a certain reagent concentrations will be $k_{Zab}[Z_{ab}]([A]_p[B]_p)^{-1}$, or const./$[A]_p[B]_p$.

SUBSTITUTIONAL CATALYSIS

As seen from Figure 9, curve 1, the rapid increase of the ratio $[A]/[A]_p$ or connected to it ratio $[A{\cdot}Z_{aw}]/[A]_p$ proceeds at $[A]_p \approx [Z_a]$ or, in the second case, at $[A]_p \approx [Z_{as}]$.

According to (10) we may decrease the concentration of centers participating in sorption of A by adding the second low-molecular compound B which will occupy these centers will exclude those from the processes connected with reactions of A. If compound B is sorbed by the same centers as A, substituting in denominator of (10) $[A]_p$ with the sum $([A]_p + [B]_p)$ we get:

$$[A] = k_{\text{eff}}[A]_p = \frac{[A]_p}{K_a([Z_a] - [A]_p - [B]_p)} \tag{37}$$

and, if $([A]_p + [B]_p) = \text{const.}$ denominator of (19) will remain constant, that is the effective (apparent) rate constant k_{eff} though dependent on initial A concentration in the course of separate reaction will remain constant.

EXPERIMENTAL DATA ON REACTIONS IN POLYMERS

First of all it must be noted that correct data on reaction kinetics in polymers can be obtained by only studying the processes in continuous samples (films, melt) and not in the polymer powder where we never know whether reaction proceeds in the polymer or in the separate phase between the polymer particles.

Reaction $A \longrightarrow$ product. An example of such reaction isomerization of dimethylbenzylsilylperoxide in polypropylene:[21]

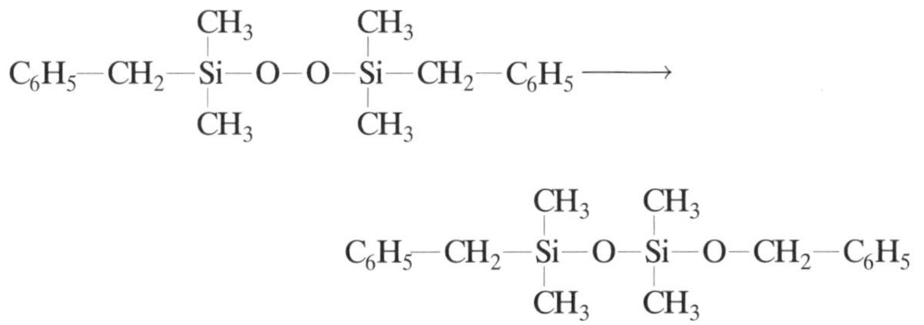

(38)

has been studied in films of isotactic polypropylene. As seen from Figure 14, in isotactic polypropylene and in polypropylene with an increased concentration of sorption centers, the rate constant increases with concentration according to curve 2 in Figure 9, but the curve for polypropylene with increased $[Z_a]$ lies below than that for usual polypropylene (Figure 14, curve 2). As seen from Figure 14, the addition of relatively “inert” compound—phenylbenzoate—increased the rate constant according to (20). Analogously depend on the initial concentration and on concentration of reaction products, the rate of benzoyl peroxide decomposition (Figure 16)[22] is observed to vary.

It has been shown that the yield of free radicals formed on decomposition of azo-bis-isobutyronitrile measured by method based on consumption of inhibitors varies with azo-bis-isobutyronitrile concentration according to Figure 9 (Figure 17).[23]

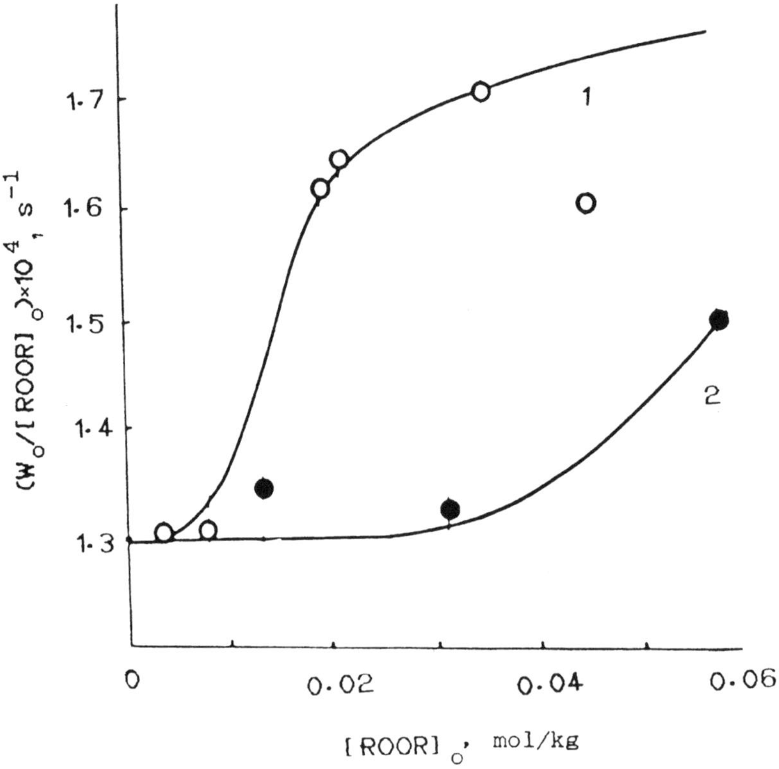

Figure 14 The rate constant of isomerization of dimethylbenzylsilylperoxide in usual isotactic polypropylene (1) and in polypropylene with increased sorption centers concentration (2) 100°C.

As an example of reaction $A + B \longrightarrow$ product, the reaction between benzoyl peroxide and dibenzylsulphide in atactic polypropylene and in polyisobutylene were studied:[20,24,25]

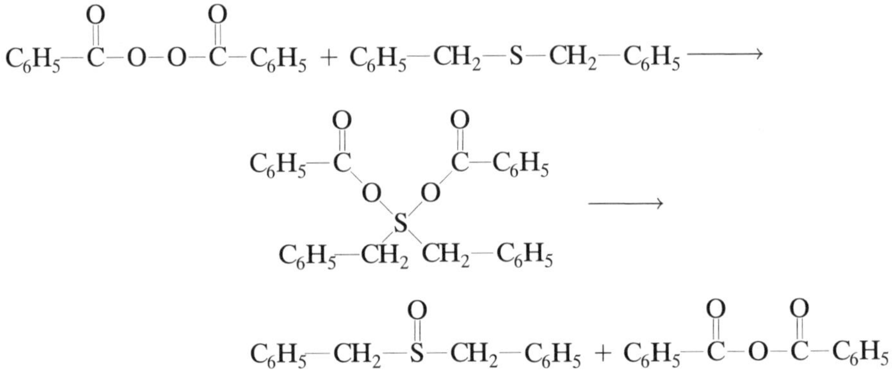

(39)

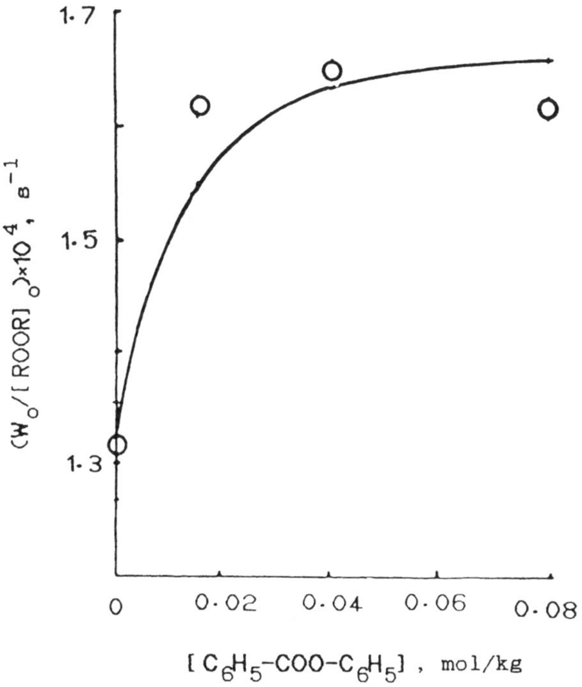

Figure 15 The rate constant of isomerization of dimethylbenzylsilylperoxide in polypropylene as function of phenylbenzoate concentration. 100°C, $[ROOR]_0 = 0.0085$ mol/kg.[20]

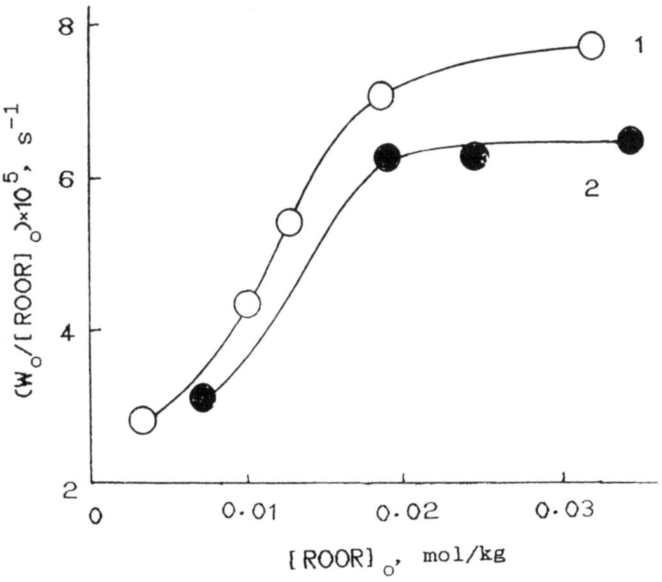

Figure 16 The rate constant of benzoyl peroxide decomposition in usual isotactic polypropylene (1) and in polypropylene with increased sorption centers concentration (2). 80°C.[19]

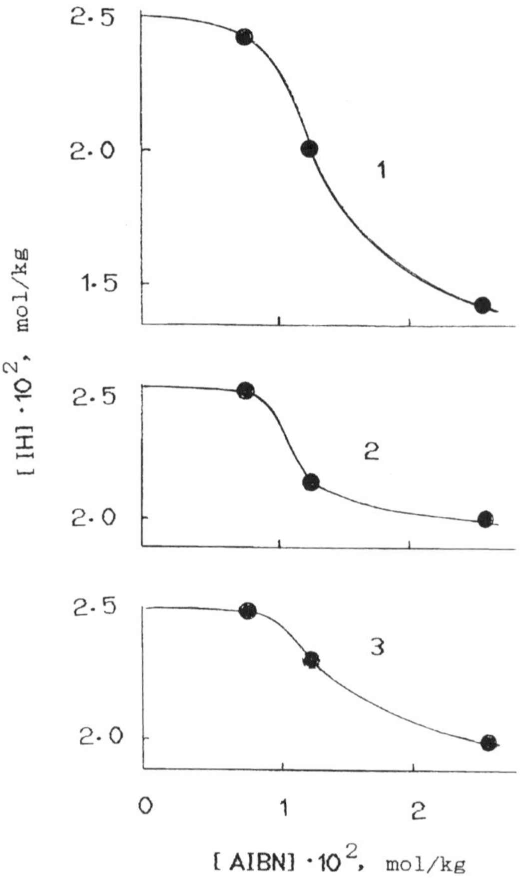

Figure 17 The change of inhibitor concentration during decomposition of azo-bis-isobutyronitrile in atactic polypropylene at heating during 6 hours at 80°C, inhibitors: benzoate of 2,2,4,4-tetramethylpiperidoleoxyl in absence of oxygen (1), 2,6-di-tert.butyl-4-phenylphenol (2), and phenyl-β-naphthylamine (3) in oxygen atmosphere, 150 mm Hg.

To achieve such a reaction two pieces of the polymer containing peroxide and sulphide were multiply folded and pressured together to obtain a sample with uniformly distributed reagents.

In separate experiments, these reactions follow the second kinetical order, but the dependencies of apparent rate constant $k_{\text{eff}} = W_{ab}([A]_p[B]_p)^{-1}$ on the initial reactant concentration have the intricate shape (Figure 18): the curves of k_{eff} as function of $[A]_p$ (and also of $[B]_p$) decreased, passed over minima and again increased. It is interesting that the rate of this reaction in the polymer may be greater than in low-molecular liquid.[19]

To explain the shapes of these dependencies it has been assumed that reaction follows all three ways (29), (30), and (31), the last process predominating at low and the two first—at high concentrations. To prove this, the effect of the third compound, which does not participate in the reaction, has been studied. Such a compound (C) phenylbenzoate, substituting either peroxide or sulphide in complexes

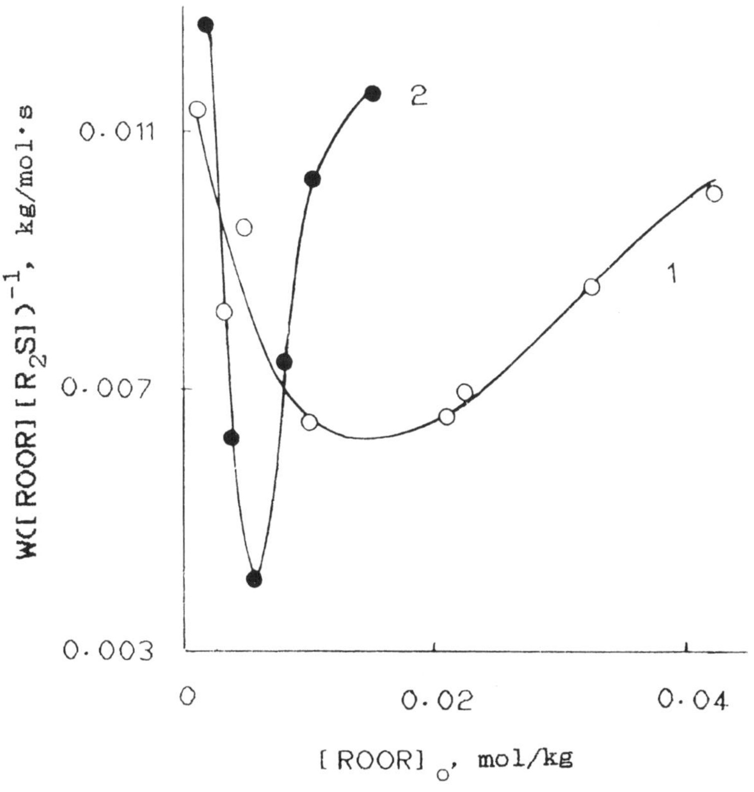

Figure 18 Dependence of apparent rate constant of reaction between benzoyl peroxide (ROOR) and dibenzylsulphide (R_2S). $k_a = W([ROOR][R_2S])^{-1}$ on benzoyl peroxide concentration at 50°C $[R_2S]_p = 0.01$ mol/kg: 1—in atactic polypropylene, and 2—in polyisobutylene.[24]

$A{\cdot}Z_a$ and $B{\cdot}Z_b$ increased the ratio of mobile reactant molecules and increased the rate at high concentrations, by turning the triple complexes $A{\cdot}B{\cdot}Z_{ab}$ into either $C{\cdot}B{\cdot}Z_{ab}$ or $A{\cdot}C{\cdot}Z_{ab}$, both enable the reaction, retarded at low concentrations.

The other type of reaction 2Q+ polymer, where Q was disubstituted *o*-quinone was studied in polyethylene, isotactic and atactic polypropylenes and in ethylene-propylene copolymers:[25,26,27]

$$\begin{array}{ll} O{=}C_6H_4{=}O & \sim CH_2{-}CH_2\sim \\ & + \\ O{=}C_6H_4{=}O & \sim CH_2{-}CH_2\sim \end{array} \longrightarrow \begin{array}{c} \sim CH_2{-}\underset{|}{C}H\sim \\ O{-}C_6H_4{-}\overset{}{O} \\ \sim CH_2{-}\overset{|}{C}H\sim \end{array} + HO{-}C_6H_4{-}OH \qquad (40)$$

Reaction is accompanied by crosslinking of the polymer. In accordance with (36) (substituting $[A][B] = [A]^2$), the reaction at relatively high concentrations follows the zero-order, i.e. its rate is independent of quinone concentration (Figure 19).

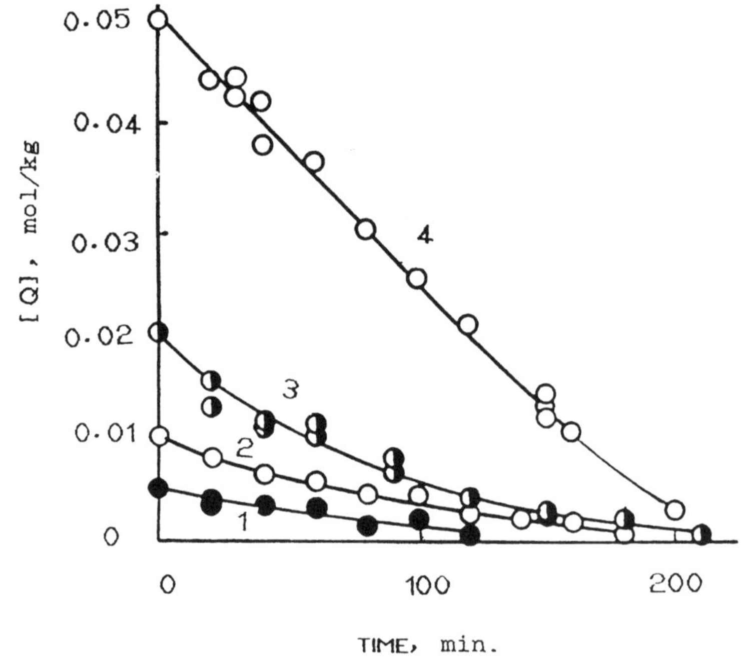

Figure 19 Consumption of 3,6-di-tert.butyl-1,2-benzoquinone in reaction with atactic polypropylene at 180°C and initial concentrations: 0.005 (1), 0.010 (2), 0.020 (3), and 0.050 mol/kg (4).[26]

SOME COMMENTS ON REACTIONS OF ANTIOXIDANTS

The main reaction of low-molecular antioxidants A = IH with macroradicals $RO_2^{\bullet}$ responsible for retardation of the oxidation processes is:[28]

$$RO_2^{\bullet} + IH \longrightarrow ROOH + I^{\bullet} \tag{41}$$

If the radicals $I^{\bullet}$ formed in this reaction disappear, at least partially, without formation of new active radicals $R^{\bullet}$ or $RO_2^{\bullet}$ this reaction leads to decrease of active radicals concentration and retards the oxidation.

No experiments were published in which the rate of this reaction in a polymer has been directly registered. For nondirect evaluation of this reaction rate, the method of critical antioxidant concentration[28,29] may be used.

In the oxidation reaction, formation of free radicals proceeds nearly completely through formation and decomposition of hydroperoxide groups:

$$RO_2^{\bullet} + RH \longrightarrow \boxed{ROOH + R^{\bullet} + nR_1H} \longrightarrow \begin{cases} \longrightarrow ROOH + RH + R_1^{\bullet} \\ \longrightarrow RO^{\bullet} + ROH + R_1H \end{cases} \tag{42}$$

Here the rectangle denotes the "cage" formed by surrounding monomeric units R_1H which can participate in intercage reactions. So-called "cage effect" decreases the yield of hydroperoxide groups α from about $\alpha \approx 1$ (100%) in low-molecular liquids to $\alpha = 0.05$–0.4 in low-mobile polymers.

Formation of additional radicals on decomposition of the hydroperoxide groups proceeds through formation of a caged radical pair, which participate in polymer recombine:

$$\mathrm{ROOH} + \mathrm{RH} \longrightarrow \boxed{\mathrm{RO^\bullet} + \mathrm{R^\bullet} + \mathrm{R_1H}} + \mathrm{H_2O} \longrightarrow \begin{cases} \longrightarrow \mathrm{ROH} + \mathrm{R^\bullet} + \mathrm{R^\bullet} \\ \longrightarrow \mathrm{ROR} + \mathrm{R_1H} \end{cases} \qquad (43)$$

The average yield of free radicals in reaction (43) is $\sigma \ll 1$ and depends on the oxygen concentration because of the reaction $\mathrm{R^\bullet} + \mathrm{O_2} \longrightarrow \mathrm{RO_2^\bullet}$ preventing recombination $\mathrm{RO^\bullet} + \mathrm{R^\bullet}$.

At high-temperature, polymer oxidation (above 250°C) of polymers containing side methyl-groups (—CH_3) provides another way of kinetic chain branching: formation of easy-oxidizing aldehyde groups:[31]

$$\sim\mathrm{CH_3} \longrightarrow \sim\mathrm{CH_2^\bullet} \longrightarrow \sim\mathrm{CH_2{-}O{-}O^\bullet} \longrightarrow \sim\mathrm{CHO} + {}^\bullet\mathrm{OH} \qquad (44)$$

$$\sim\mathrm{CHO} + \mathrm{O_2} \longrightarrow \sim\dot{\mathrm{C}}\mathrm{O} + \mathrm{HO_2^\bullet} \qquad (45)$$

In the simplified theory of critical antioxidant concentration so-called degenerate chain branching, that is formation of additional free radicals in reactions of non-stable intermediates[14] is substituted with direct branching. In this case the balance equation of active centers X (i.e. the radicals $\mathrm{R^\bullet}$ and $\mathrm{RO_2^\bullet}$ in polymer oxidation) will be:

$$\frac{\mathrm{d}[X]}{\mathrm{d}t} = W_0 + f[X] - k_t[\mathrm{IH}][X] \qquad (46)$$

where W_0 is the rate of primary radicals formation, f—the factor of chain branching, i.e. the average number of additional active centers formed by one center during the time unit, and k_t—the rate constant of chain termination. As seen from (46), if the factor of self-acceleration $\varphi = (f - k_t[\mathrm{IH}])$ is positive the number of reaction centers will be increasing with time even if we keep [IH] constant, i.e. reaction rate will grow. If φ is negative the radical concentration will be a uniform function of W_0, f, k_t, and [IH]:

$$[X] = \frac{W_0}{k_t[\mathrm{IH}] - f} \qquad (47)$$

The value of the antioxidant concentration dividing both regions of different reaction regimes is called "critical anti oxidant concentration" $[\mathrm{IH}]_{\mathrm{cr}} = f/k_t$. The critical concentration may be relatively easy determined as the concentration below which antioxidant occurs only slightly, but above which it—effectively retards the oxidation reaction.[29,30] Beginning from the critical concentration value, the induction period of the polymer oxidation rapidly increases. Consideration of the degenerate character of chain branching which proceeds through formation and decomposition of hydroperoxide groups changes only the nonessential details, especially at high temperatures (180° C and greater) when the lifetime of hydroperoxide groups vary from hours till fractions of seconds.

The reaction of polymer oxidation proceeds mainly in the zones of polymeric substance in which the oxygen dissolved in the polymer is present and mobility of its segments permits the changes of the valence angle necessary for reaction $RO_2^{\bullet} + RH$.[32] Some of these zones are the sorption centers not only for oxygen but also for antioxidants.

In reactions with virtually immobile macroradicals only two types of antioxidant molecules participate: mobile antioxidant molecules A and those sorbed by the same center. If $[A] \ll \sum[Z]_i$ only a small part of the zones of oxidation will contain antioxidant molecule, and the main role in the chain termination will be played by the reactions of mobile molecules.

As indicated above, we may change the ratio $[A]/[A]_p$ changing the level of topological disorder in the same polymer. The method of such variation had been precipitation of the same polypropylene from different solvents: the 'good' one *n*-decane (PP-1) and 'bad' chlorobenzene (PP-2).

Figure 20 shows that the values of critical concentration of antioxidant phenyl-β-naphthylamine at 180°C and oxygen pressure 300 mmHg were: at PP-1 $[IH]_{cr}$ =

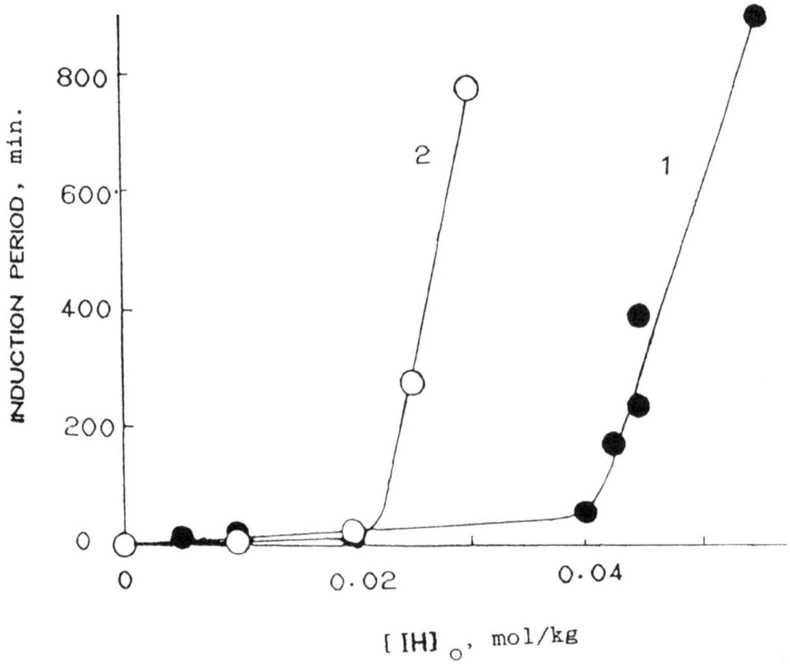

Figure 20 Induction period of isotactic polypropylene oxidation as function of initial antioxidant concentration. 180°C, oxygen, 300 mmHg, antioxidant phenyl-β-naphthylamine, polypropylene has been precipitated from *n*-decane (1) and chlorobenzene (2).

0.04 mol/kg, and at PP-2 $[IH]_{cr} = 0.021$ mol/kg.[33] Thus the difference between differently precipitated polypropylene samples is preserved even not only in the "solid" polymer (see Figure 7), but also in the polymer melt.

Though antioxidants are introduced into polymer for retardation of its oxidation, during the induction period the most part is consumed in side reactions, the main of which are direct oxidation by molecular oxygen and interaction with free radicals formed on the oxidation of antioxidant.[29] For this reason above critical concentration antioxidants are consumed in accordance with first kinetic order in the antioxidant concentration:

$$\frac{d[IH]}{dt} = k_{eff}[IH] \tag{48}$$

where the apparent rate constant k_{eff}, depends on the oxygen pressure above the polymer. When the antioxidant concentration [IH] becomes equal to $[IH]_{cr}$ the reaction rate rapidly increases and after a short period τ_{cr} the induction period ends. Integrating (48) from $[IH]_0$ at $t = O$ till $[IH]_{cr}$ at $t = \tau - \tau_{cr}$ we get a formula describing the induction period (τ) as a function of the initial antioxidant concentration $[IH]_0$:[29,30]

$$\tau = \tau_{cr} + \frac{1}{k_{eff}} \ln \frac{[IH]_0}{[IH]_{cr}} \tag{49}$$

It follows from (49) that the rate constant for the antioxidant consumption is: $k_{eff} = \Delta \ln[IH]_0/\Delta\tau$. Calculated values were $k_{eff} = 6.0\cdot10^{-6}\,s^{-1}$ in PP-1 and $k_{eff} = 7.6\cdot10^{-6}\,s^{-1}$ in PP-2,[33] i.e. differ in agreement with general theory (24).

In our experiments after melting of polypropylene with antioxidant tri-tert. butylphenol, 0.6 mol/kg, extracted from cooled samples with alcohol, the concentration of sorption centers increased from $[Z_a] = 0.14$ mol/kg to $[Z_a] = 0.52$ mol/kg. As shown in [33], the induction periods of oxidation of isotactic polypropylene in the presence of various concentrations of this antioxidant at 80°C markedly differs for treated and nontreated samples (Figure 21). The rate constants of antioxidant consumption calculated from these data were $4.2\cdot10^{-7}\,s^{-1}$ in non-treated and $1.6\cdot10^{-7}\,s^{-1}$ in treated. The differences in rate constants of the same reactions may be due to the same difficulties of reaction complex formation in the 'tight' centers formed around the same molecules of antioxidant as discussed above (Figure 10).

According to (37) we may increase the ratio of mobile molecules by adding the third compound to the polymer.

As seen from Figure 22, in the presence of phenylbenzoate, 0.1 mol/kg, the critical concentration of antioxidant, the ester of pentaerythrol and 3,5-di-tert.butyl-4-hydroxyphenyl-propionic acid at 200°C and oxygen pressure 300 mmHg decreased from $1.5\cdot10^{-2}$ mol/kg to $6\cdot10^{-3}$ mol/kg.[35] At the same time the rate constant of antioxidant consumption increased from $7.7\cdot10^{-6}\,s^{-1}$ to $1.4\cdot10^{-5}\,s^{-1}$ because the third compound occupied some centers which mostly fit to antioxidant molecules. As discussed above, such centers restricting mobility of molecules and retard all reactions they participate in. In some cases, relatively "inert" compounds thus increase the effectivity of antioxidant that in the curves "induction period vs mixture of antioxidant—inert compound composition" appear as distinct maxima (Figure 23).[35]

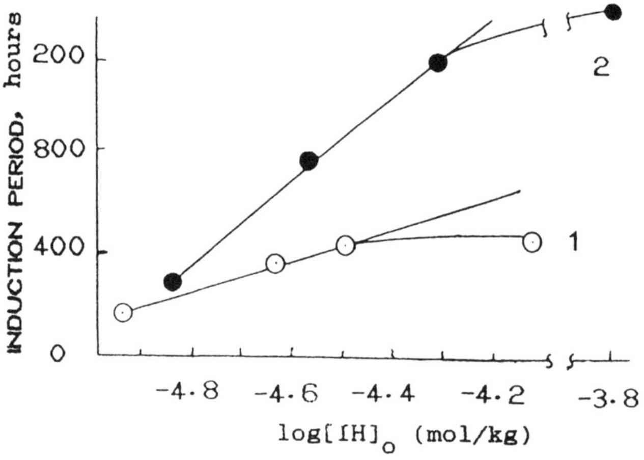

Figure 21 Induction period of oxidation of usual isotactic polypropylene (1) and of polypropylene treated with 2,4,6-tri-tret.butylphenol, 0.6 mol/kg in melt state as function of logarithm of initial concentration of the same additive. 80°C, oxygen, 500 mmHg.

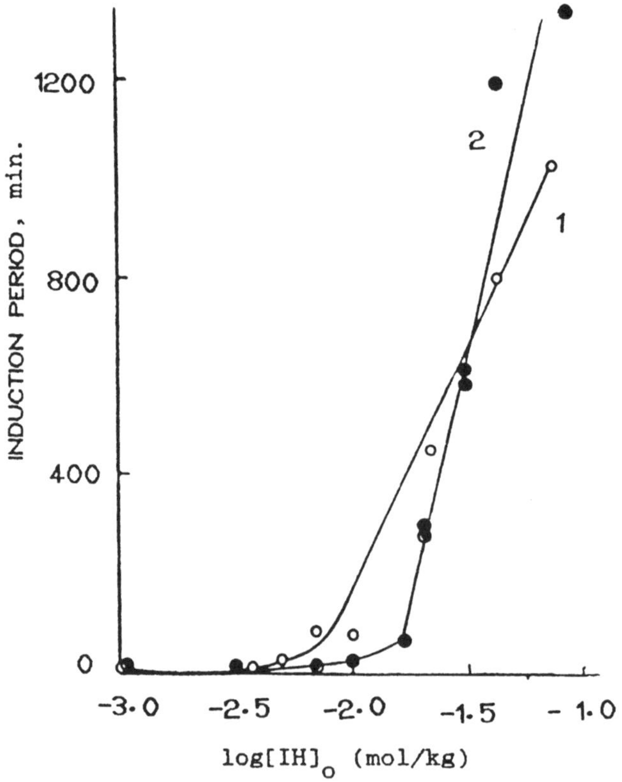

Figure 22 Induction period of isotactic polypropylene oxidation as function of initial antioxidant concentration in the absence (1) and in the presence of phenylbenzoate, 0.1 mol/kg. 200°C, oxygen, 300 mmHg, antioxidant—the ester of pentaerythrol and 3,5-di-tert.butyl4-hydroxyphenylpropionic acid.

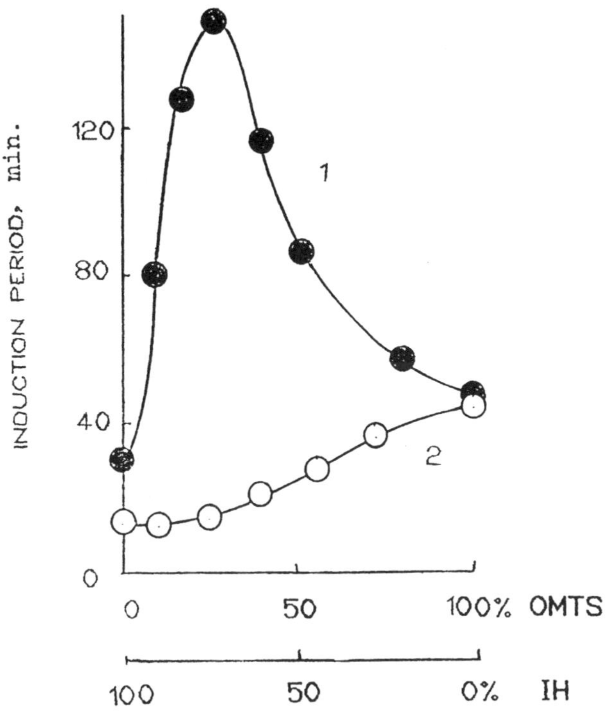

Figure 23 Induction period of oxidation of polyamide-12 as function of composition of mixture of 2,2′-methylenebis (4-methyl-6-tert.butylphenol) (IH) and octamethylcyclotetrasiloxane (OMTS) at 170° (1) and 190°C (2). Oxygen, 300 mmHg, [IH] + [OMTS] = 0.02 mol/kg.[35]

Increase in molecular mass of antioxidant, decreases the diffusion coefficient of its mobile molecules. On the other side it decreases the concentration of centers capable of the antioxidant sorption. The interesting phenomenon may be foreseen: when the concentration of centers strongly binding antioxidant molecules which changes with molecular mass of antioxidant according to (15).

Figure 24 shows the variation of the concentration of sorption centers with molecular mass of sorbed additive: of strongly binding ones (line 1) and of weakly binding (line 2). Varying the molecular mass at constant antioxidant concentration (line 3) we first intersect line 1 (point A). Beginning from this point only a part of the antioxidant molecules can be strongly bound and the amount of weakly bound increases till after intersection of the line 2 in the point B amount of antioxidant becomes greater than sorption center concentration. After passing point B, the solubility of the antioxidant becomes lower than the sorption center concentration and excess either remains undissolved, or breaks the polymer structure as described above (Figures 11–13). As a result the effectivity of antioxidants with relatively high molecular masses can become sufficient. But when the total concentration of sorption centers becomes smaller than antioxidant concentration (line 2), the solubility of antioxidant and its concentration in the polymer rapidly decreases. The example of such an antioxidant is the ester of pentaerythrol and 3,5-di-tert.butyl-4-hydroxyphenylpropionic acid known as Irganox 1010.

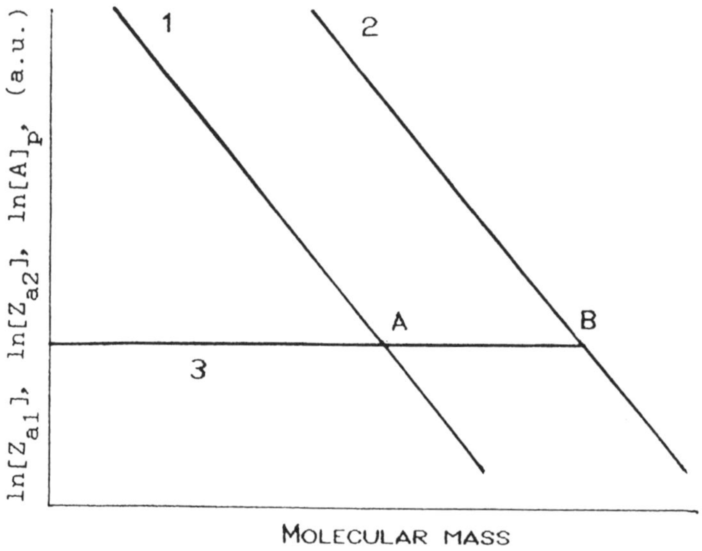

Figure 24 Concentration of sorption centers: 1—strongly binding antioxidant, and 2—weakly binding, 3—antioxidant concentration. To the left side from A apparently all antioxidant is strongly bound, in the range AB the increasing part remains weakly bound, and after point B the concentration becomes greater than solubility.

Thus taking into account the topological structure of polymer we may help understanding of many phenomena existing only in polymers or showing various regularities in polymers and their low-molecular analogous.

REFERENCES

1. Yu.A. Shlyapnikov, *Doklady Akademii Nauk SSSR* (Rus.), 1972, **202**, p. 1377.
2. Yu.A. Shlyapnikov, *Europhysics Conference Abstract*, 1981, **51**, p. 311.
3. Yu.A. Shlyapnikov, *Soviet Journ. Chem. Phys.*, 1993, **11**, p. 1898.
4. J.M. Braun and J.E. Guillet, *J. Polym. Sci., Polym. Chem.* Ed., 1975, **12**, p. 1119.
5. A.S. Michaels, W.R. Vieth and J.A. Barrie, *J. Appl. Phys.*, 1963, **34**, p. 13.
6. Yu.A. Shlyapnikov and A.P. Mar'in, *Acta Chimica Hungarica*, 1987, **124**(4) p. 531.
7. Yu.A. Shlyapnikov and A.P. Mar'in, *Europ. Polym. J.*, 1987, **23**, p. 623.
8. G.B. Giedraytite, *Regularities of Dissolution of Low-Molecular Compounds in Polymers*, Candidate of Science (PhD), 1989, Thesis, Vilnius, Liethuania.
9. A.P. Mar'in and Yu.A. Shlyapnikov, *Doklady Akademii Nauk SSSR*, 1974, **219**, p. 1409.
10. J. Sataite, A.P. Mar'in, S. Juskeviciute and Yu.A. Shlyapnikov, *Vysokomolek. soedin. B*, 1985, **27**, p. 215.
11. Yu.A. Shlyapnikov, *Polymer*, 1994, **35**, p. 1031.
12. G.B. Gedraitite, A.P. Mar'in and Yu.A. Shlyapnikov, *Eur. Polym. J.*, 1989, **25**, p. 39.
13. Yu.A. Shlyapnikov, T.V. Monakhova and T.A. Bogaevskaya, *Polym. Degrad. Stability*. 1994, **46**, p. 247.
14. A.P. Mar'in and Yu.A. Shlyapnikov, *Vysokomolek. soedin. B*, 1981, **23**, p. 825.
15. H. Fujita, *J. Phys. Soc. Japan*, 1953, **8**, p. 271.
16. V.A. Bagdonayte and S.S. Juskeviciute, *Vysokomolek. soedin. B*, 1981, **23**, p. 229.
17. T.A. Bogaevskaya and Yu.A. Shlyapnikov, *Doklady Akademii Nauk SSSR* (Rus.), 1973, **210**, p. 1362.
18. Yu.A. Shlyapnikov and N.N. Kolesnikova, *Int. J. Polym. Materials*, 1996, **32**, p. 75.
19. A.P. Mar'in, E.A. Sviridova and Yu.A. Shlyapnikov, *Polym. Degrad. Stability*, 1995, **47**, p. 349.

20. Yu.A. Shlyapnikov and N.N. Kolesnikova, *Europ. Polym. J.*, 1987, **23**, p. 633.
21. A.P. Mar'in and V.A. Yablokov, A.N. Sunin and Yu.A. Shlyapnikov, *Izvestiya Akad. Nauk SSSR*, 1975, p. 2251.
22. A.P. Mar'in and Yu.A. Shlyapnikov, *Doklady Akademii Nauk SSSR*, 1974, **215**, p. 1160.
23. Yu.A. Shlyapnikov, T.V. Monakhova and I.S. Gaponova, *Vysokomolek. soedin., A*, 1979, **21**, p. 875.
24. N.N. Kolesnikova and Yu.A. Shlyapnikov, *Vysokomolek. soedin. A*, 1976, **18**, p. 2401.
25. N.N. Kolesnikova and Yu.A. Shlyapnikov, *Vysokomolek. soedin. B*, 1977, **19**, p. 184.
26. E.S. Torsueva and Yu.A. Shlyapnikov, *Vysokomolek. soedin. B*, 1977, **19**, p. 377.
27. E.S. Torsueva and Yu.A. Shlyapnikov, *Vysokomolek. soedin. B*, 1978, **20**, p. 446.
28. I.G. Latyshkaeva, T.A. Bogaevskaya, G.P. Belov and Yu.A. Shlyapnikov, *Vysokomolek. soedin. B*, 1977, **19**, p. 531.
29. Yu.A. Shlyapnikov, S.G. Kiryushkin and A.P. Mar'in, *Antioxidative Stabilization of Polymers*. 1996, Taylor & Francis, London.
30. Yu.A. Shlyapnikov, *Pure & Appl. Chem.*, 1980, **32**, p. 337.
31. Yu.A. Shlyapnikov, I.A. Serenkova, *Polym. Degrad. Stability*, 1992, **35**, p. 67.
32. Yu.A. Shlyapnikov, *Kinetika i kataliz*, 1978, **19**, p. 504.
33. Yu.A. Shlyapnikov, T.V. Monakhova and T.A. Bogaevskaya, *Polym. Degrad. Stability*, 1994, **46**, p. 247.
34. A.P. Mar'in and Yu.A. Shlyapnikov, *Vysokomolek. soedin. B*, 1975, **17**, p. 582.
35. Yu.A. Shlyapnikov and A.P. Mar'in, *Polym. Degrad. Stability*, 1993, **40**, p. 337.

Biodegradable Polymeric Microparticles in Biomedical Applications

K.Z. GUMARGALIEVA, DANIEL HORAK* and G.E. ZAIKOV

Institute of Chemical Physics Academy of Sciences of Russia ul. Kosygina, 4, 117334, Moscow

INTRODUCTION

A wide range of polymeric materials are available for biomedical applications. The number of materials that are approved for human use, however, is small. Much attention has recently been paid to materials used in controlled drug delivery over a prolonged period of time, targeting drugs to specific sites in cancer chemotherapy[1] and intracellular parasitic diseases.[2] If drug delivery devices are resistant to biodegradation, upon repeated treatment they accumulate in the liver of the patient which could eventually result in adverse effects. As a consequence, many hydrophilic addition polymers have been banned from medicinal use. Therefore, the use of biodegradable polymers is required in these systems.[3] Degradable systems have the advantage of obviating the need of surgical removal of the drug-depleted device which can always be the source of infection.[4] Potentially, degradable matrix systems also have a number of other advantages such as simplicity of design and predictability of release, if the release is controlled solely by matrix degradation.[5]

For many medical applications it is desirable to have a biodegradable polymer in the form of spherical microparticles[6] with diameters ranging from below 1 μm to over 100 μm and nanoparticles[7] with a size less than 1000 nm. The spherical sample geometry offers distinct advantages relative to the more conventional film and fiber gometries, since microspheres cannot only control delivery of the incorporated agent, but also protect the agent, such as proteins and peptides, from proteolytic degradation. Moreover, their application is easier than that of other forms: they can be subcutaneously, intravenously and intramuscularly injected. Nanoparticles can have a matrix-type structure or can be nanocapsules with a reservoir-like structure, consisting of a solid shell and an inner liquid core. Various other particulate systems have been described, including emulsions,[8,9] phospholipid vesicles,[10,11] microcapsules[12,13] and microspheres prepared from a variety of materials, such as polysaccharides,[14–16] alkylcyanoacrylates,[17,18] lactic acid and related polymers[19,20] and proteins.[21–23]

*Institute of Macromolecular Chemistry Academy of Sciences of the Czech. Republic, 16206, Prague, 6 Czech. Repulic.

The drug release from biodegradable microparticles is governed by various properties of the polymer, drug and carrier system.[24] Polymer dependent factors include the molecular weight and molecular weight distribution, the co-polymer ratio and distribution, and the crystallinity. Effective ways to increase the drug release from microspheres are to increase the drug loading or to decrease molecular weight of polymer or to prefer amorphous to crystalline polymer. Important drug dependent parameters are the solubility of the drug in dissolution or biological fluids, the molecular weight and possible polymer-drug interactions. These can be influenced through pH changes. Carrier system dependent factors comprise the type of microparticle (microsphere vs. microcapsule), the drug loading, the physical state of the drug in the polymer matrix (dissolved vs. dispersed), the particle size and particle size distribution, and the porosity and internal structure of the microparticles.[25] An increase in matrix porosity enhances the drug release because of the easier accessibility of the drug by dissolution fluids. Porous microspheres are also essential to deliver high molecular weight substances which cannot diffuse out of a nonporous matrix and to deliver substances which have high affinity for polymer and are not released unless the matrix is eroding.

BIODEGRADATION

Polymeric implant materials designed to safely degrade in the body are usually referred to as degradable, biodegradable, resorbable or absorbable polymers.[26] Some general review articles on biodegradation of polymers[27] and biodegradable polymers for medical applications have been written.[28,29] For clinical applications, it is often important to distinguish clearly between "biodegradable polymers" and "bioabsorbable polymers".[30] Biodegradable polymers are polymers which are decomposed in the living body but whose degradation products remain for a long-term in tissue. On the other hand, bioabsorbable polymers can be defined as polymers which degrade after implantation into nontoxic products which are then eliminated from the body or metabolized therein.[30] Polymers that are decomposed by enzyme-specific reactions are called "enzymatically degradable polymers" while polymers that are decomposed by contact with water or serum are "non-enzymatically degradable polymers".[31] Technically, only enzymatically degradable polymers should be considered as truly "biodegradable". However, in this review, nonenzymatically degradable polymers will also be included. In nonenzymatically degradable polymers, a relatively fast degradation rate is found for synthetic polymers consisting of easily hydrolyzable chemical bonds, such as amides, enamines, esters, orthoesters, acetals, urea, urethane, glycosides and related groups and carbonate linkages.[30]

A few critical requirements for the design of biodegradable/bioerodible polymers must be considered. First, they should hydrolyze at an appropriate, well-defined, rate to suit a specific application.[26] Second, their degradation products must be nontoxic and preferably should be a normal constituent of a human biochemical metabolic pathway. Besides these two factors, the other important quality is biological compatibility.[32] Finally, the mechanical and chemical properties of the polymer must be able to satisfy the requirements of the device, e.g. stiffness, permeability, elasticity or blood compatibility, depending on the nature of the device.[26] If the degradation occurs at the surface of the particles and approaches the center, surface erosion is achieved. In contrast, bulk erosion is characterized by degradation that occurs simultaneously through the particle.[33] Five important factors control the type of erosion taking place: (1) bond stability, (2) hydrophobicity, (3) crystallinity, (4) dissolution of the degradation products, and (5) porosity. In any degradation process the first step is the penetration of water into the polymer, followed by the hydrolysis of the chemical bond and dissolution of the degradation products. If water penetration is slower than hydrolysis and dissolution, surface erosion will take place. However, if water penetration is faster than the dissolution rate, bulk erosion will dominate. Ideal polymers for surface erosion would have a hydrophobic backbone but very labile linkages connecting monomers.[33] Since the degradation rate is proportional to the surface area of microspheres, the degradation rate increases with decreasing microsphere size (increasing surface area).[33] Porous materials degrade at higher rate than the nonporous ones.[33] Degradation also depends on drug loading: microspheres with higher drug loading degrade faster than those with low drug loading.[33] Crystalline regions will erode more slowly than amorphous regions.[33]

Natural polymers such as polypeptides, polysaccharides, polynucleotides, and bacterial polyesters are generally degraded in biological systems by hydrolysis followed by oxidation. Most of these biopolymers are enzymatically biodegradable,[30] except for highly crystalline celluloses and "hard" proteins like keratin and silk fibroin. On the other hand, most nonenzymatically degradable polymers are synthetic polymers, including aliphatic polyesters and polycarbonates prepared from fatty acids and diols. These polymers are hydrolyzed into low molecular weight oligomers and then to monomers by water or serum. For this reason, degradation rates for nonenzymatically degradable polymers are almost the same *in vivo* compared with *in vitro*.[30] From the standpoint of the degradation mechanism, biodegradable polymers may be divided into three general classes: (1) polymers whose main chain bonds are hydrolyzed to produce oligomers and monomers; (2) polymers which are converted to soluble polymers by hydrolysis of side groups; and (3) cross-linked polymers which are solubilized by a dissociation of their cross-links. In the latter two cases, the molecular weight of the resulting soluble polymers should be low enough so that they can be excreted by kidney dialysis.[34]

ENZYMATICALLY DEGRADABLE BIOPOLYMER MICROPARTICLES

All naturally occuring polymers such as starch, cellulose, proteins, nucleic acids and lignin are biodegradable, since they have existed on earth for a sufficient length of time for enzymes and microorganisms to evolve that can degrade or utilize these materials as food. Unfortunatelly, all of these materials which evolved through on aqueous medium contain very polar groups, mostly either peptide (—CONH—) or ester (—COO—) in their main chain, and therefore decompose upon heating before they melt.[35] It might seem that natural polymers would be well suited for use as biomedical materials because of their structural similarity to components in host tissues. However, there are some significant disadvantages to natural polymers. These include: (1) strong physiological activities and the potential for rejection; (2) a difficulty in evaluating degradation rates *in vivo* because of differences in enzyme concentrations in different parts of living tissues; and (3) the mechanical strength of natural polymers is generally insufficient. For these reasons, their application as biomedical materials has been limited to only a few specific areas.

Polysaccharides

The polysaccharides[30] occupy a central position among the natural polymers and are ubiquitous throughout nature. Modified cellulose, starch, various dextrans, alginic acid, hyaluronic acid, chitin and chitosan are polysaccharides that may serve as potential biomaterials.

Cellulose and its Acetate

Cellulose (β-1,4-polyanhydroglucose) (Figure 1) is the major naturally occurring storage and structural polymer in the vegetable kingdom.[30] Although native cellulose is poorly digestible in living tissue, it can be made biodegradable through modifications that disturb its higher ordered structure. One of such modifications include the reaction of acetic anhydride with cotton linters of wood pulp, resulting in cellulose acetate.[36] Cellulose esters can also be produced from recycled paper and sugar cane.[37] Commercially available cellulose acetate has a degree of substitution between 1.7 and 3.0. Cellulose acetate is biodegradable,[38] if its degree of substitution is less than 2.5. Rates of biodegradation decrease as the degree of substitution increases.

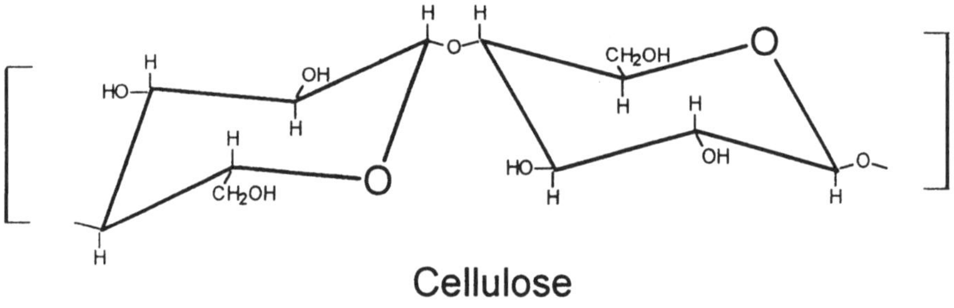

Figure 1

Starch

Starch[30] (Figure 2) consists of glucopyranose residues in an α-*D*-(1,4)-linkage that yield *D*-glucose upon hydrolysis. Starch is produced in plants and contains the polysaccharides amylose [α-(1,4)-linked glucose] and amylopectin [α-(1,4)-linked glucose main chains with α-(1,6)-linked branches of α-(1,4)-linked glucose].[36] Corn is the primary source of starch, although potato, wheat and rice starch also have markets in Europe, the Orient and USA.[39] Starch is a potentially useful polymer for thermoplastic biodegradable materials because of its low cost, availability and pro-

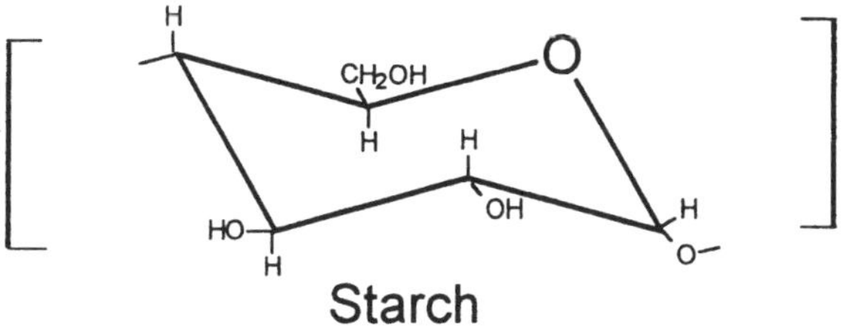

Figure 2

duction from annually renewable resources. The degradation rate and extent to which the starch gel could be degraded by α-amylase are dependent on the degree of modification of starch chains during the crosslinking reaction.[40]

Dextran

Dextrans[30] consist of α-*D*-glucose units joined predominantly by 1-6 glycosidic bonds (Figure 3). They are cleaved by dextranases which are not present in blood, but are present in the liver, spleen, intestinal mucosa, and colon.[41]

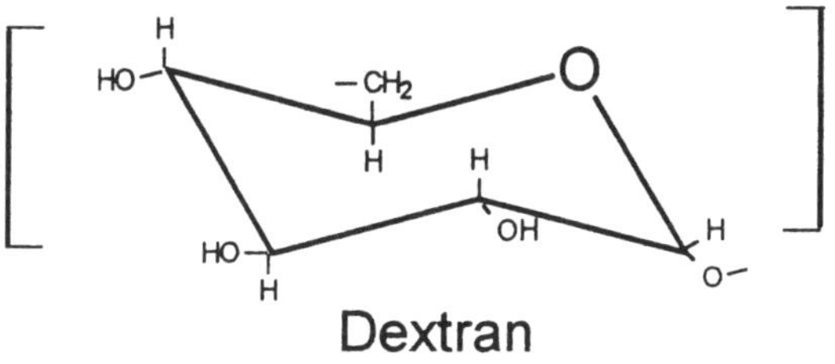

Figure 3

Alginic and Hyaluronic acid

Sodium alginate is a linear polymer of β-(1-4)-*D*-mannuronic acid and α-(1-4)-*L*-glucuronic acid residues[30] (Figure 4). Alginic acid forms water-soluble salts with monovalent cations, low molecular weight amines, and quaternary ammonium compounds. Upon introduction of polyvalent cations such as Ca^{2+}, Be^{2+}, Cu^{2+}, Co^{2+}, Al^{3+} and Fe^{3+} it becomes water-insoluble and forms gels. The degree of crosslinking is dependent on various factors such as pH, ionic strength, type of counterion, and the functional charge density of these polymers.[42] The polymeric anionic character of alginate renders the polymer suitable for enteric coating of oral delivery systems.[43] Similarly alginates, also gellan which is of microbial origin, is capable of gelation in the presence of mono- and divalent ions.[44] Gellan beads show a slightly slower release than obtained with alginate beads.[44]

Hyaluronic acid is a naturally occurring nonsulfated glycosaminoglycan consisting of a linear sequence of *D*-glucuronic acid and *N*-acetyl-*D*-glucosamine (Figure 5). It is present in connective tissue, in the synovial fluid of articular joints, and in the

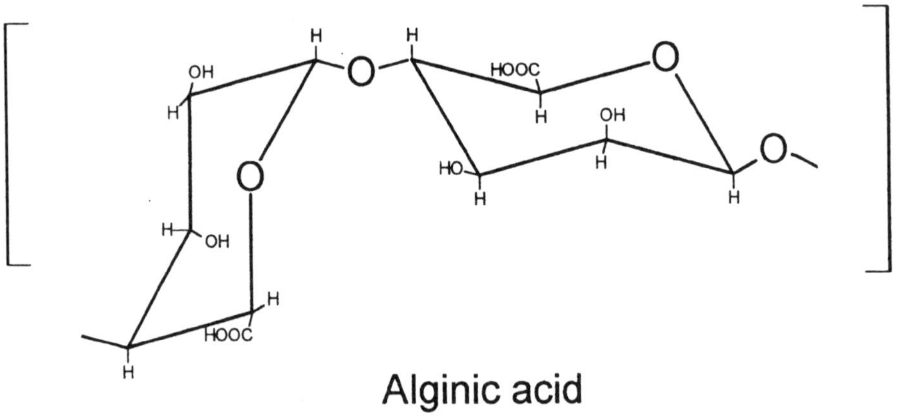

Figure 4

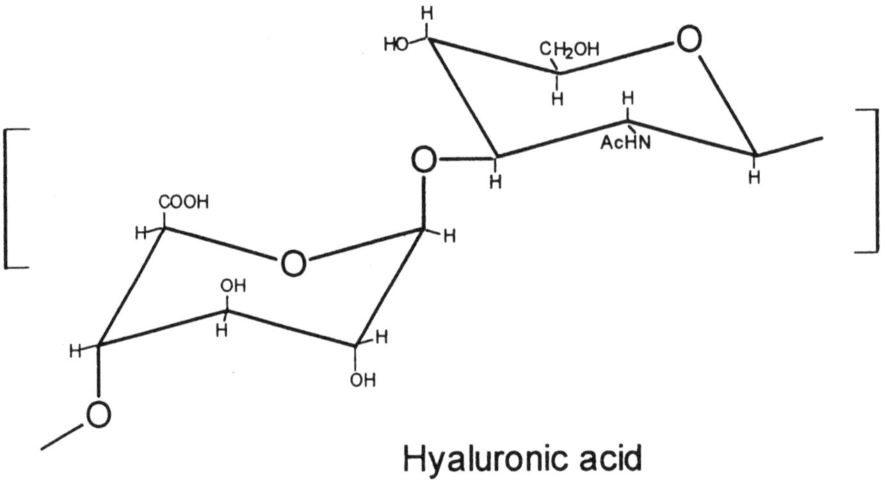

Figure 5

vitreous humor of the eye. In dilute solutions under physiological conditions, hyaluronate molecules exist as random coils with their own solvent shells.[30]

Chitin and Chitosan

Chitosan is deacetylated chitin and a linear polymer of 2-amino-2-deoxy-β-*D*-glucan (Figure 6). It is abundant in nature as a major hexose of the crustacean skeleton, insects, etc. It contains primary and secondary alcoholic groups and its amine group renders the polymer soluble in dilute organic acids. Chitin (Figure 7) can be degraded by chitinase. Its immunogenicity is exceptionally low in spite of the presence of nitrogen atoms. The polymeric cationic character along with its potentially reactive functional groups has given it unique properties for utilization in controlled

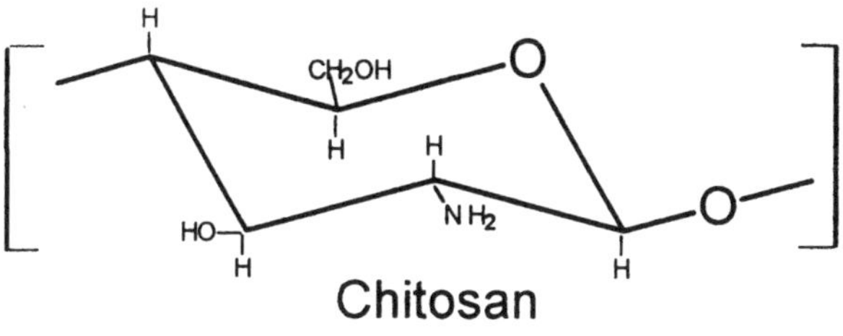

Figure 6

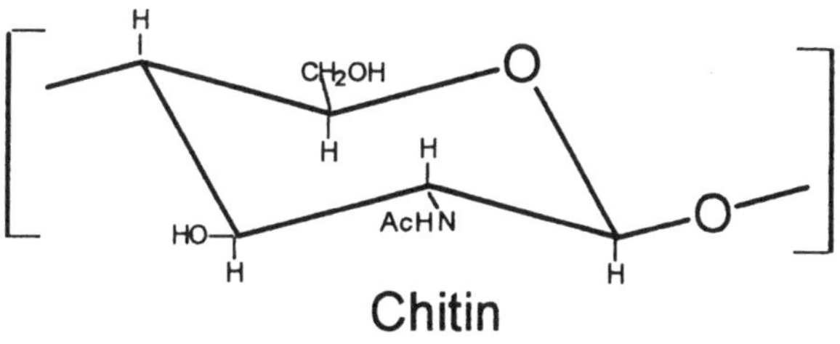

Figure 7

release systems.[45] Chitosan has ability of gelling by controlling inter and intramolecular interaction of its positively charged amino groups with the tripolyphosphate counterion.[46]

Proteins

Albumin and Heparin

Serum albumin is a blood plasma protein that is soluble in water half saturated with a salt such as ammonim sulfate. Albumin (molecular weight 68 000) has a single free sulfhydryl (-SH) group, which on oxidation forms a disulfide bond with the sulfhydryl group of another serum albumin molecule thus forming a dimer. The resulting albumin-cross-linked networks are susceptible to proteolytic degradation. Degradation of albumin microspheres depends on concentration of glutaraldehyde used in preparation of protein microspheres. Iodine labelling, drug loading and scaling up batch sizes has no effect.[47] Heparin is a well known anticoagulant and widely used for the prevention and treatment of thrombotic diseases.[48]

Collagen and Gelatin

Collagen is the major component of all mammalian tissues, including skin, bone, cartilage, tendons, and ligaments.[30] Different types of collagenous material are known, from collagen type I to X. Among them, the most abundant and widely investigated material is collagen type I. It contains high content of glycine and the imino acids proline and hydroxyproline, hydroxylysine and small amount of aromatic and sulfur containing amino acids.

Gelatin[30] is a variant of collagen, that is, a denaturated collagen. Since a heat denaturation method cannot be applied to the microsphere preparation of gelatin, microspheres or hydrogels of gelatin require stabilization by chemical cross-linking.

Other Poly(amino acid)s

The polymers synthesized from α-amino acids present a unique opportunity and distinct advantage over other polymeric systems because of the wide choice of amino acids with different side-group functionalities.[49] These side groups can be manipulated to afford tailor-made systems for specific applications. However, the antigenicity of polypeptides containing three or more amino acids excludes their use in biomedical applications.[50] Due to these difficulties, only a few synthetic polypeptides have been investigated as implant materials.[51] Their greatest potential lies in the area of drug-delivery systems, where research has concentrated mainly on homopolymers and copolymers derived from *L*-glutamic acid (*L*-Glu) and *L*-aspartic acid (*L*-Asp). This is mainly because of the side-chain carboxyl groups, which enable attachment of other functional groups including drug molecules (polyagents). Other systems are based on a sequential polydepsipeptide containing a tripeptide sequence *L*-alanyl-*L*-alanyl-*g*-ethyl *L*-glutamyl and an α-hydroxy acid *L*-lactic acid, such as poly [Ala-Ala-Glu(OEt)-Lac]. In $[\text{Glu(Ome)}]_m(\text{Sar})_n$ and $[\text{Lys(z)}]_m$ polysarcosine segment in polypeptide $(\text{Sar})_n$ synthesized by N-carboxyanhydride method is soluble either in water or in organic solvents which enables the preparation of microcapsules by a solvent evaporation technique.[52] The membrane permeability of these polypeptide microcapsules is pH-sensitive.[53]

Polyesters

Poly(β-hydroxyalkanoates)

Poly(β-hydroxyalkanoates), PHA, such as poly(β-hydroxyvalerate), PHV, and their copolymers, are naturally occuring bacterial polyesters synthesized by microbial fermentation.[36] They accumulate as energy storage reserves within the cells of many bacteria and fungi under growth-limiting conditions[54] in the same way that animals use fat. For example, *Alcaligenes eutrophus NCIB 11599* can accumulate 80% of total cell dry weight as PHA,[55] and the species is used in the commercialized production of poly(hydroxybutyrate-*co*-valerate). Polyhydroxybutyrate, PHB, random copolymers of butyrate and valerate, PHBV, long-side-chain PHAs,[56] novel functionalized side chains,[57] and copolymers containing 4-hydroxybutyrate, 4-HB,[58] or 3-hydroxybutyrate, 3-HB,[59] are biosynthesized depending on the carbon source, the organism and the growth conditions.[60] Biosynthesis of PHB with inexpensive carbon sources such as methanol or hydrogen gas and carbon dioxide,[61] and by halophilic microorganisms, *Haloferax mediterranei*, with glucose[62] or starch[63] as the carbon source, have also been demonstrated. The biodegradability of PHB, PHBV (with various valeric acid contents), longer side chains and 4-PHB has been well documented.[64] In addition, some of the esterase enzymes involved in the initial hydrolytic depolymerization step have been identified and characterized.[65] However, the degradation rates *in vivo* appear to be extremely slow.

Poly(caprolactone)

Poly(ε-caprolactone), PCL, is an aliphatic polyester synthesized by the ring-opening polymerization of ε-caprolactone with a catalyst like stannous octanoate in the presence of an initiator that contains an active hydrogen atom.[36] Molecular weight vary from 2000 to 80 000 Da.[66] PCL can be degraded by microorganisms (enzymes, lipases) and also by a hydrolytic mechanism under physiological conditions.[67] Also, low-molecular-weight fragments of PCL are reportedly taken up by microphages and degraded intracellularly.[68] As the molecular weight of PCL increases the rates of biodegradation decrease.[69] PCL degrades at a much slower pace than PLA and can therefore be used for the design of long-term, implantable drug delivery systems that remain active for more than one year. Interest in slowly degrading polymers has, however, decreased.

NONENZYMATICALLY DEGRADABLE SYNTHETIC MICROPARTICLES

By contrast to naturally occuring polymers, synthetic polymers have not, in general, been in existence long enough to have enzymes or microorganisms evolve that can utilize them as food. Degradable synthetic polymers offer several advantages over enzymatically degradable natural polymers. Generally, the nonenzymatically degradable synthetic polymers are less immunogenic and more biocompatible than many natural polymers. Synthetic polymers can be prepared reproducibly under carefully controlled conditions and can be made available, if needed, in almost unlimited quantities. The mechanical properties of some synthetic polymer materials are maintained even in harsh biological environments, and are easily modified by chemical and physical modifications. Thus, degradable synthetic polymers have been considered to be more useful as biomedical materials than the natural polymers.

Poly(α-hydroxy esters)

Poly(α-hydroxy esters) such as poly(glycolic acid), PGA, or poly(lactic acid), PLA, are crystalline polymers with relatively high melting point. They are obtained by ring-opening polymerization of cyclic glycolides and lactides or the direct condensation of lactic and glycolic acids and depending on the method of synthesis, the molecular weight can be varied. Poly(glycolic acid) often called poly(glycolide) (Figure 8), is the simplest linear, aliphatic polyester.[30] Poly(lactic acid) also called poly(lactide), is more hydrophobic than PGA, due to the presence of an extra methyl group. It has been studied since the 1960s as degradable polymer.[70] Since lactic acid is a chiral molecule, it exists in two stereoisomeric forms (enantiomers) which give rise to four morphologically distinct polymers. They degrade more slowly than a *DL* mixture.[71] The *L*-form is highly crystalline and the melt transition temperature decreases with lower molecular weight.[72] *D,L*-Lactide is the racemic polymer significantly more amorphous, with a correspondingly lower melting point. The release rate of drugs molecularly dispersed in poly(lactide) microspheres is governed by glass temperature of the polymer matrix.[73] Rates of hydrolysis and thus the drug release rate

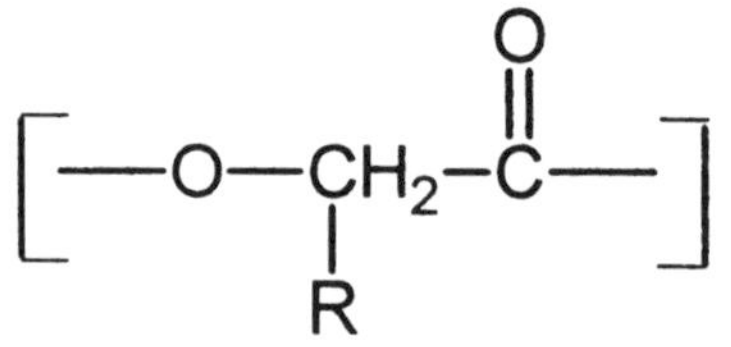

Polyglycolide (R = H), polylactide (R = CH_3)

Figure 8

increase in polymers with lower glass temperature, i.e. as molecular weight decrease. Variations in the molecular weight of polymer, however, usually alter not only glass temperature but also the particle size and surface area of prepared microspheres. These factors also affect the drug release rate of the microspheres. Adjusting the glass temperature of microspheres without altering other physical properties may be achieved by γ-irradiation of the particles after preparation.[74] Introduction of poly(ethylene glycol) within poly(*DL*-lactide) increases the degradation rate.[75] The role of enzymatic versus chemical hydrolysis is, to date, not clear.[76] Certain hydrolytic enzymes, such as pronase, proteinase K and bromelain, accelerate the rate of PLA degradation, other enzymes such as liver esterase do not.[77] Nevertheless it is supposed that in aqueous environments, such as body fluids, PGA and PLA degrade by simple hydrolysis of the ester backbone. The polymer breaks down to lactic or glycolic acid, a normal product of carbohydrate metabolism. Furthermore, the degradation products are ultimately metabolized to carbon dioxide and water or are excreted via the kidneys.[30] Poly(glycolic acid) exhibits a more rapid rate of bioabsorption than poly(lactic acid). Poly(lactic acid-*co*-glycolid acid) (PLGA) materials can be prepared so that their degradation rates range between PLA and PGA extremes. Especially low molecular weight PLGA microspheres are known to be able to incorporate high peptide load.[78]

If formulated as nanoparticles, the major problem is their rapid clearance from the bloodstream, which is non-specific and characteristic for all colloidal drug carriers. Therefore surfactants containing poly(ethyleneoxide) have been explored to alter surface properties such as surface charge and hydrophobicity of poly(lactide) nanoparticles. *In vivo* studies with rats confirmed that the circulation half-life of these particles was significantly higher than the half-life of the degradable part alone.[79]

Poly(ortho esters)

Poly(*ortho* esters), POE, are a family of synthetic degradable hydrophobic polymers that can undergo an erosion process confined to the polymer-water interface under certain conditions. The properties of POEs can be controlled to a large extent by the choice of the diols used in the synthesis. The *ortho*-ester linkage is far more stable in base than in acid. Upon hydrolysis, these POEs release acidic by-products that autocatalyze the degradation process, resulting in degradation rates that increase with time.

Polyanhydrides

Polyanhydrides, such as poly(sebacic anhydride), SA, hydrolyze more quickly (*in vivo* after 72 days) than poly(lactic acid).[80] By varying the ratio of the aliphatic to the aromatic monomers during the copolymerization of sebacic acid and 1,3-bis-(carboxyphenoxypropane), CPP, the type of erosion taking place could be controlled. Polymers with high SA content erode more quickly than those with a high CPP content, causing increased rates of protein release. It is theoretically possible to deliver drugs for periods ranging from hours to years just by changing the ratio of SA to CPP in the polymer.[81] The hydrophobicity and crystallinity of the polyanhydrides are two of the most important factors controlling the type of erosion.[82] Polymers made of aromatic monomers degrade much more quickly than polymers of aliphatic monomers. Poly(adipic anhydride) prepared by ring-opening polymerization of oxepan-2,7-dione initiated with triethyl amine[82] displays surface erosion which completely releases entrapped drug after 7 h at 37°C. Characteristic for the surface-eroding polyanhydrides is the approximately constant release rate.[82] On the contrary, bulk-eroding polyesters, such as poly(lactic-*co*-glycolic acid), reveal an S-shaped release profile at low loadings.

Poly(alkylcyanoacrylates)

Previously, polymers based up on alkylcyanoacrylates received considerable attention, however, the interest in these systems has declined because of concerns over toxicity. Formaldehyde is produced during degradation of the polymers *in* vivo. Poly(isobutyl 2-cyanoacrylate) (Figure 9) degrades in two enzyme-free media at pH 7 and pH 12 in the presence of rat-liver microsomes.[83] The formaldehyde-producing degradation route is less efficient, and the ester hydrolysis is catalyzed by enzymes. The degradation of poly(ethylcyanoacrylate), PECA, microspheres which are produced by dispersion polymerization occurres mainly by surface erosion.[84] Higher degradation rates are observed with the PECA microspheres produced with higher poly(ethylene oxide-*co*-propylene oxide) stabilizer and lower hydrochloric acid concentrations.

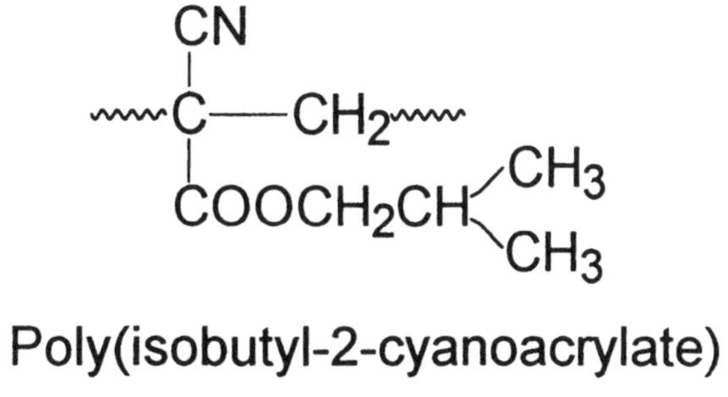

Figure 9

Polyphosphazenes

Polyphosphazenes with hydrolytically labile substituents also have a potential for biodegradable applications. With proper choice of substituents, polymers can be prepared which can degrade into harmless products.[30] Certain side-group structures impart hydrolytic sensitivity to polyphosphazenes, examples being those with amino acid ester or imidazolyl side groups.[85] For example, the ethyl glycinato derivative[36] hydrolyzes slowly in aqueous media to yield ethanol, glycine, phosphate, and ammonia. Polyphosphazenes are suitable for a production of microparticles that range in size from 5 to 200 μ or small 100–200 nm.

PREPARATION METHODS

A great number of techniques are available for the preparation of biodegradable microspheres. They include solvent evaporation after aqueous microemulsification, organic phase separation, often referred as coacervation, dispersion polymerization, spray-drying, hot melt encapsulation,[33] supercritical fluid technology,[86] etc. The last two techniques are potentially suitable for the encapsulation of peptide and protein drugs. Hot melt encapsulation has, however, the disadvantage that the drug must be exposed to higher temperature. The most popular methods for the preparation of biodegradable microparticles are therefore solvent evaporation and phase separation techniques since they can readily be performed in the laboratory without specialized equipment. The choice of one particular method is primarily determined by the solubility characteristics of the drug and of the polymer. If the core material is water insoluble, either of the methods can be considered. For water-soluble core materials, only the organic phase separation procedure is suitable.[87] Organic phase separation method results in the formation of microcapsules (core-shell structure) vs. microspheres (matrix structure) formed by the solvent evaporation method. The disadvantage of both these manufacturing processes stems from the fact that commonly used sovents for polymers are harmful compounds like halogenated hydrocarbons, cyclic ethers, nitrides or amides.

Organic Phase Separation Method

In the organic phase separation method, the wall-forming polymer is precipitated around a dispersed drug phase. This can be induced by the addition of nonsolvents to the polymer, addition of a second polymer incompatible with the wall-forming polymer, and change in temperature.[88] As an example of a nonsolvent (coacervating agent) added to a polymer solution containing an active compound, silicon oil can be named.[89] The dispersion is then transferred into a hardening agent, where solid microspheres are formed.

Temperature can be used as another means to induce phase separation. Phase separation induced by temperature change is used for the preparation of gelatin microspheres crosslinked with glutaraldehyde[90] or uncrosslinked.[8] It takes advantage of the fact that gelatin is soluble in a hot aqueous solution but insoluble on cooling to room temperature. The extent of crosslinking is an effective parameter in the control of the size of the microspheres. When the amount of crosslinker is increased, the size of the microspheres decreases and this occurrence may be explained by increased crosslinking density resulting in the formation of densely packed structure like helical formation causing a shrinkage of the particles. Increasing crosslinking results in slower rate of water evaporation and leads to the formation of microspheres with a smooth surface. Another insolubilization process may involve spraying of warm aqueous gelatin solution through a capillary into cold water containing glutaraldehyde forming a Schiff base.[91] Narrow particle size distribution results. The particle size is about 1 mm and smaller, depending on the concentration of the crosslinker, the conditions of spraying and the temperature of the medium.[90] Drug-loaded gelatin microspheres can also be prepared by ultrasonically emulsifying an aqueous drug/gelatin solution in excess sesame seed oil.[92] In these systems environmentally undesirable solvents such as diethyl ether or chloroform are required to remove the oil phase of the emulsion and the resulting microspheres often contain residual surfactants used as emulsifiers.

Solvent Evaporation Method

In the solvent extraction/evaporation method, an aqueous solution of the drug (e.g., peptide, aclarubicin,[93] adriamycin[94]) is dispersed or emulsified into an organic polymer solution (typically polyanhydride,[95] poly(lactide-*co*-glycolide), poly(lactide-*co*-glycolide) and poly(ethylene glycol), poly(d,l-lactide),[93] or poly(D,L-lactide-*co*-ethylene glycol)[75] in dichloromethane), to form a primary water in organic emulsion (w/o), which is then emulsified by sonication into an external aqueous or oil (e.g., linseed or peanut oil) continuous phase[96] to form a w/o/w or w/o/o emulsion. The organic solvent diffuses from the emulsion droplets into the external aqueous (or oil) phase and evaporates. Inner oil phase gives a solid dispersion. Resulting microspheres are usually collected by centrifugation, washed with water and lyophilised.[97] Advantage of w/o/o double emulsion technique, when compared with more conventional protein encapsulation using water-in oil-in water (w/o/w) methods, include much higher protein entrapment, a marked reduction of burst effect and more uniform and controllable release characteristics.[98] Typical size is 75–150 μm or even in tens of micrometers. A reduction in particle size of polylactide and poly(lactide-*co*-glycolide) microspheres to a submicron size range can be achieved by introduction of water-miscible organic solvent to the organic phase of the emulsification solvent evaporation protocol. This modification was named "spontaneous emulsification solvent evaporation method".[99] Further reduction in the particle size to sub-200 nm range can be reached applying a preparation method based on precipitation of the polymer from its solution by the addition of miscible nonsolvent.[100]

In most cases, a surfactant is required to stabilise the dispersed phase. Poly(vinyl alcohol), poly(vinylpyrrolidone), or methyl cellulose are the most frequently used polymeric surfactants,[101] however, bovin serum albumin emulsifies poly(α-hydroxy acids) as well.[102] Mean particle size of the microspheres is inversely related to the stirring speed and the emulsifier (surfactant) counterion. Sorbitan monooleate (Span 80) as an emulsifier and *n*-hexanol as a cosurfactant are used in preparation of porous chitosan beads with typical diameter 70 or even 250 μm in toluene continuous phase. Hydroxypropyl chitosan hollow microbeads are manufactured from w/o (toluene) emulsion stabilized with sorbitan monooleate by crosslinking hydroxyl groups with epichlorohydrin under alkaline condition.[103] Using an oil-in-oil solvent removal technique, poly(adipic anhydride) microspheres with an average size 40 μm are prepared by adding methylene chloride solution of polymer to sesame oil containing Span 80 under vigorous stirring.[82] Using the same technique[104] poly(glycolic-*co*-lactic acid) is dissolved in dimethyl formamide containing cisplatin and the solution was added dropwise to liquid paraffin containing Span 80 resulting in 5 to 40 μm microspheres. Solvent extraction/evaporation method involves intrinsic variables, such as solvent-polymer interaction parameters, molecular weight of polymer, and extrinsic variables, such as dispersed phase/continuous phase ratio, temperature, dispersed phase composition. These variables control the particle size. Higher viscosities of the organic phase caused by higher molecular weights or by increasing solvent/polymer ratio result in larger particles.[75]

Dispersion Polymerization

The term of dispersion polymerization usually covers the polymerization of apolar monomers by using the dispersion media in which all ingredients, including monomer, are completely soluble initially. The nucleation occurs when the polymer chains reach to a certain molecular weight at which they become insoluble in the dispersion medium. Thermal initiation is usually selected and macromolecular stabilizers are used to prevent the aggregation of microspheres in the medium. Under optimum conditions in the system with fast particle nucleation in the initial period of the polymerization, followed with a continuous size increase of growing particles, and accompanied with an efficient stabilization, monosize microspheres in the micron-size range can be obtained.[105] In the dispersion polymerization of ethylcyanoacrylate the polymerization occurs via an anionic mechanism involving initiation by nucleophilic attack on the β-carbon of ethylcyanoacrylate.[106] This polymerization is performed by using a stabilizer system containing a poly(ethylene oxide-*co*-propylene oxide) and dextran in the aqueous hydrochloric solution as a dispersion medium. Phosphoric acid is then used as a catalyst. The average size in the range 0.5–2.5 μm and the size distribution (monodispersity) of poly(ethylcyanoacrylate) microspheres does not change significantly with the phosphoric acid concentration and molecular weight and concentration of dextran. The microsphere size significantly decreases with increasing poly(ethyleneoxide-*co*-propyleneoxide) and hydrochloric acid concentration.[84]

Poly(*D*,*L*-lactide), poly(*L*,*L*-lactide) and poly(ε-caprolactone) particles smaller than 5 μm can be prepared in heptane-1,4-dioxane mixed solvent by the dispersion ring-opening polymerization initiated with tin(II) 2-ethylhexanoate in the presence of poly(dodecyl acrylate)-*g*-poly(ε-caprolactone) stabilizer.[107]

Other Techniques

Various other techniques for preparation of biodegradable particles are described. For example, microspheres with size of 150 μm are prepared from 2-vinyl-4,4′-

dimethyl-2-oxazolin-5-one derivatized starch through interfacial crosslinking with dipropyleneglycol diacrylate by a water-in-oil polymerization using Pluronic F68 emulsifier.[108] An interesting technique to prepare thermo-sensitive poly(γ-benzyl *L*-glutamate-*b*-N-isopropylacrylamide) core/shell nanoparticles 70–360 nm in size consists in dialysing the block copolymer dissolved in N,N-dimethylformamide.[109] Nanoparticle size depends on the nature of the solvent, temperature and dialysis speed. Such particles release a higher content of drug (indomethacin) at 28°C than 34° and if the content of hydrophobic glutamate blocks is lower.

Thermal denaturation at an elevated temperature (95–170°C) or chemical crosslinking in vegetable oil or organic solvent emulsions are two basic methods for the production of albumin microspheres. In the latter case, an aqueous protein is prepared by dissolving a lyophilised quantity of human serum albumin in a phosphate buffer, saline and drug (e.g., doxorubicin or daunorubicin). Solution of human serum albumin is added to an oil phase consisting of petroleum ether and cotton seed oil containing Span 80 and the mixture homogenised. The droplets are stabilised by cross-linking effect of varying amount of glutaraldehyde. The diameter of albumin microspheres prepared by these methods ranges from 0.2 μm to 100 μm.

Thermal condensation of oligoamino acids synthesized by oligomerization of amino acid N-carboxyanhydrides, such as *L*-aspartic and *L*-glutamic acids, *L*-phenylalanine and *L*-tyrosine under benzylamine[110] or *L*-tyrosine methyl ester[111] initiation produces proteinoids. The driving force for microspheres formation might be related to a combination of hydrogen-bonding, hydrophobic interaction, and charge transfer interaction. The capability of an amino acid oligomer to form microspheres is strongly affected by its composition, which is selected to balance the hydrophilicity and hydrophobicity. The stability of microspheres the diameter of which varies from 0.5 to 20 μm, has been found to be pH dependent. They appear at low pH's (< 4) and spontaneously disassemble under neutral pH conditions.

BIOMEDICAL APPLICATIONS

Drug Delivery

Particulate drug delivery systems, often also termed as micro (or nano)sphere-based controlled release systems, are utilised in various areas of modern medicine as a means of improving therapeutic efficiency of bioactive materials such as proteins and peptides, antigens and other drugs.[112] Much attention has focused especially on poly(lactic acid), poly(glycolic acid) and poly(*D,L*-lactide-*co*-glycolide) particles[113] in which a branched peptide immunogen (200 M), representing a portion of the principal neutralizing determinant of HIV-1, indomethacin,[114] progesterone,[115] aclarubicin HCl, somatostatin acetate,[116] thyrotropin releasing hormone,[117] a somatostatin antagonist,[118] several LH-RH analogues,[119] porcine somatotropin,[120] interleukin-2,[121] norgesterol, bone morphogenic protein[122] have been encapsulated. Alginate microspheres have also been used to encapsulate various vaccines, antigens, microorganisms and cells.[30,123] Ideally, the controlled release device enables the agent to be delivered over prolonged time periods. Its advantages include the use of lower amounts of drug and hence, reduction in costs and toxic side effects, and improved patient compliance. Recent advances in delivery systems are focusing on drug targeting. Drug targeting is especially useful for cancer treatment whereby the cancer drug is selectively delivered into the malignant tumor cells. Decreasing the particle polymer molecular weight is believed to result in a faster drug release rate due to the faster degradation of the polymer matrix.[124] Once encapsulated, the active agent can exist in several different physical states: crystalline, molecularly dispersed in the polymer matrix, or existing as a metastable dispersion with the carrier matrix. This can also greatly influence the drug release rate and storage stability of the microspheres.[125] The level of drug loading in the microspheres significantly affects the initial burst phase. To prevent the loss of encapsulated materials and to reduce the burst effect, the microcapsules can be coated with another polymer that forms a membrane at the bead surface. This membrane acts as a rate controlling barrier to drug release and thereby prolongs release of drug when compared to uncoated microspheres. The most well-known and promising system is the encapsulation of alginate beads with poly(*L*-lysine)[126] or with a polyelectrolyte complex of sodium alginate, an anionic polysaccharide, and a derivative of chitosan, a cationic polysaccharide.[127] The release rate of drug from such microcapsules may depend mainly on two factors. One is the thickness, and the other is the compactness of the membrane that forms the outer shell of the microcapsule. This can be controlled by the pH where the capsules are formed and the kind of groups in the chitosan.[127]

Particulate drug delivery systems are gaining attention for use in oral, systemic and parenteral drug delivery routes.[128]

Oral Drug Administration

Oral drug administration is the most popular, convenient, and traditionally preferred mode of delivery of therapeutic agents. Conventionally, therapeutic drug levels are achieved by taking multiple and regularly spaced daily doses of medicine.[129] The need to remember to take the pills or tablets frequently is obviated by using colloidal particulate carriers such as microspheres as an oral delivery system. They are ideal in providing a constant therapeutic and nontoxic level of the drug. Many small drug molecules are chemically and structurally stable and remain unchanged by oral delivery. However, macromolecular drugs such as heparin, insulin and human growth hormone are very sensitive to the components of the gastrointestinal tract. Specific digestive processes, especially hydrolysis, can efficiently transform these agents into molecular fragments that are pharmacologically ineffective since their activity is directly dependent on specific molecular structures.[110] One primary approach to protect the incorporated drug in the system as well as the system itself from degradation in the gastric juice is to coat (encapsulate) the drug system with biocompatible, nontoxic polymers, such as alginate, that are insoluble at acidic pH of the stomach but dissolve in the alkaline pH of the intestine and release the drug. On the other hand, different pH sensitivity is obtained at chitosan coats on gelatin microspheres containing the anticancer drug methotrexate.[129] Chitosan, which is soluble at acidic pH but insoluble at alkaline pH, prolonged the release of methotrexate in intestinal fluid. It is possible to control release rate of methotrexate by selecting appropriate concentrations of the coating polymers or by varying the size of the gelatin microspheres.[129] Chitosan/gelatin hybrid polymer network microspheres loaded with cimetidine are suggested for treatment of gastric ulceration.[130]

In some cases, oral administration of protein and polar macromolecular drugs results in extremely low to no bioavailability due to their poor membrane permeability from the gastrointestinal tract. Therefore proteinoid microspheres are being developed aimed at delivering therapeutics such as polysaccharides and proteins, e.g. insulin and heparin, which are being presently administred *via* injection. To encapsulate a drug, the proteinoid material is dissolved in an aqueous solution at pH 7. This solution is added to a therapeutically desirable drug solution at low pH and vigorously shaken. Under these acidic conditions,[131] the proteinoids form stable microspheres with encapsulated drugs ranging in size from 5 to 10 μm. The size is usually dependent on the proteinoid used and the agitation, i.e., smaller spheres are formed by ultrasonic agitation (0.5 μm) compared to hand agitation (10–15 μm). In this manner, the proteinoid microspheres are able to protect a therapeutic agent, such as standard and low-molecular weight heparin, heparinoids, calcitonin, human growth hormone, vaccines, monoclonal antibody IgG2a, polar compounds such as sodium cromolyn and desferoxamine, from gastric acids and enzymes in the stomach and then release it into the intestinal adsorption area.[48] By using proteinoid microsphere oral delivery system, high plasma levels and higher bioavailability are obtainable.[48] In essence, proteinoids have a dual function: in the microsphere phase, proteinoids have the ability to protect drug cargoes from acids and enzymes; and as soluble materials, the proteinoids facilitate the absorption of a therapeutic agent from the intestine into the blood stream.[48]

Other oral biodegradable carriers include poly(lactide) and poly(lactide-co-glycolide) particles and poly(alkylcyanoacrylate) nanoparticles with physically entrapped or adsorbed drugs. Oral immunization via targeting to Peyers patches by antigen encapsulated in poly(lactide-co-glycolide) microparticles has been studied and its many advantages compared to parenteral administration of vaccines have been shown.[132] Target diseases include influenza, polio, measles, pertunis, cholera, tetanus and so on. Nanoparticles of ~100 nm diameter containing covalently bound peptide prepared by copolymerization of lutenizing hormone releasing hormone-vinylacetate with n-butylcyanoacrylate are also described.[133]

Parenteral Drug Administration

Micro- and nanoparticles, such as those based on chitosan, human albumin or poly(caprolactone-β-(*d,l*)lactide), are a promising vehicle for parenteral delivery of the protein and polar macromolecular drugs, genes, antigens and vaccines,[48] which are currently administred via injection into the muscle to provide enhanced immune response. To avoid difficulty during injection, particles with high degree of sphericity and monodispersity and with much smaller size than those administered orally are required. By gellation of chitosan in the presence of poly(ethylene oxide) and poly(ethylene oxide-*b*-propylene oxide) pH-sensitive nanoparticles are formed, the size of which increases with the increasing concentration and molecular weight of both stabilizers.[46] Temperature-sensitive nanoparticles for parenteral administration are developed from poly(γ-benzyl L-glutamate-b-N-isopropylacrylamide).[109] The uptake of micron-size monosized polymeric particles by white blood cells and macrophages is higher than that of polymeric particles in the submicron size range.[134] Injectable poly(lactide) microspheres containing antimetabolic agent adriamycin are suggested as a therapeutic agent for glaucoma filtering surgery.[94] Poly(glycolic-*co*-L-lactic acid) particles containing cisplatin are promising to enhance the antitumor effect of the drug and to reduce its systemic toxicity.[104] They enable to increase drug dose to the level 5-times higher than its LD_{50} value. A sustained release of cisplatin can be achieved over 20 days without a large initial burst. About 70% of the incorporated drug is released within the initial 7 days and the microspheres are completely digested after about 8 months. Cisplatin loaded poly(lactic-*co*-glycolic acids) microspheres ranging from 180 to 250 μm were suggested for direct injection into brain tumors.[124] Release of cisplatin, approximately 80% of which took place within over 30 days, is a combination of diffusion and erosion processes.

Intra-arterial Applications

Popular drug carrier used in intra-arterial applications are albumin microspheres with entrapped adriamycin. In order to overcome problems connected with low adriamycin payloads and with a large burst effect usually observed (80–90% of the drug is released within 30 min. in any aqueous medium), highly negatively charged albumin-heparin conjugate microspheres having thus ion-exchange properties are developed.[135] Pendent amino groups of the lysine residues of the albumin are used to crosslink the material in order to obtain stable microspheres. The anionic groups of the heparin (such as sulfamate groups and carboxylic acid groups) allow ionic interaction with the adriamycin, thus enabling high payloads (up to 34%) and ion-controlled drug release. Other biodegradable microspheres, which behave as an ion-exchanger and which can be loaded with adriamycin up to a payload of 60%, are based on sulfamated polylysine stabilized using glutaraldehyde or oxidized dextran as a crosslinking agent.[136]

Another microspherical particles of about 58 μm diameter are produced from polydepsipeptide (poly(Ala-Ala-Glu(OEt)-Lac)) containing β-estradiol. If implanted into the animal, the effective pharmacological level of the drug is kept during the first 12-week period. This is followed by an incomplete supplying of drug until the implant is perfectly degraded in the 25th week from the start of implantation.[137]

Chemoembolization

Classical cytostatic agents widely used for the treatment of cancer have, in general, a narrow therapeutic window. Due to the high systemic levels of the drug needed to achieve sufficiently high drug levels at the tumor site, severe side effects such as cardiomyopathy can occur.[138] A reduction of the side effects can be achieved if the drug is targeted to the site of action using microspheres which is known as chemoembolization.[139] Chemoembolization refers to transcatheteral administration of drug-loaded particles of the requisite size (15–60 μm), to cause tumor infarction by occlusion or to induce transient ischemia within the tumor vasculature, whereupon the entrapped drug (e.g. 5-fluorouracyl, mitomycin) can be released locally.[140] The great advantage of this procedure consists in that toxicity of the microsphere-formulated drug decreases as compared with the free drug, thus improving the therapeutic index.[141] An essential aspect of chemoembolization as a targeting technique is the biodegradation of the system.[83] Therefore microspheres and microcapsules from ethylcellulose,[13] starch,[14] casein,[22] human serum albumin,[142,143] poly(*D*,*L*-lactide),[19,144] hyaluronic acid[145] (sympo Berlin 1992) and poly(isobutyl 2-cyanoacrylate)[83] have been utilised for targeting as (chemo) embolic agents in the treatment of vascular and tumoral lesions. Particles greater than 7 μm in diameter become embolized in the first capillary bed encountered after intravenous administration.[6] Then larger and larger particles follow, obturating blood vessels from periphery to proximal region of the tumor.

Other Applications

Other applications include the use of the particles in designing supports for cell growth and the design of cyanoacrylic nanoparticles as a lysosometric and biodegradable drug carrier.[146] Cyanoacrylic nanoparticles have been also used in applications such as occular drug carriers to enhance the corneal penetration of polar drugs and as carriers with monoclonal antibodies for targeting cytotoxic agents to tumor cells.[147] Likewise polyanhydride microspheres with incorporated trimolal maleate seem to be promising in ophthalmology.[82] Starch particles are suggested as a model of the human ocyte during its transport through the oviduct (Fallopian tube). These biocompatible ocyte surrogates could thus provide the information about functional disorders of tubal transport, unavailable yet by classical diagnostic methods, in female patients who were indicated for tubal potency examination because of long-term unexplained infertility.[40]

REFERENCES

1. P.K. Gupta, Drug targeting in cancer chemotherapy: A clinical perspective, *J. Pharm. Sci.*, 1990, **79**, pp. 1–14.
2. T. Laakso, P. Stjarnkvist and I. Sjoholm, Biodegradable microspheres VI: Lysosomal release of covalently bound antiparasitic drugs from starch microparticles, *J. Pharm. Sci.*, 1987, **76**, pp. 134–140.
3. G.E. Visscher, R.L. Robison, H.V. Maulding, J.W. Fong, J.E. Pearson and G.J. Argentieri, Biodegradation of and tissue reaction to 50:50 poly(DL-lactide-co-glycolide) microcapsules, *J. Biomed. Mater. Res.*, 1985, **19**, pp. 349–365.
4. R.S. Langer and N.A. Peppas, Present and future applications of biomaterials in controlled drug delivery systems, *Biomaterials*, 1981, **2**, pp. 201–214.
5. R. Langer and N.A. Peppas, Chemical and physical structure of polymers as carriers for controlled release of bioactive agents: A review, *Rev. Macromol. Chem. Phys.*, 1983, **C23**, pp. 61–126.
6. L. Illum and S.S. Davis, The targeting of drugs parenterally be use of microspheres, *J. Parenter. Sci. Technol.*, 1982, **36**, pp. 242–247.
7. R. Gurny, N.A. Peppas, D.D. Harrington and G.S. Banker, Development of biodegradable and injectable latices for controlled release of potent drugs, *Drug Dev. Ind. Pharm.*, 1981, **7**, pp. 1–25.

8. M. Hashida, S. Muranishi, H. Sezaki, N. Tanigawa, K. Satomura and Y. Hikasa, Increased lymphatic delivery of bleomycin by microsphere in oil emulsion and its effect on lymph node metastasis, *Int. J. Pharm.*, 1979, **2**, pp. 245–256.
9. D.M. Lidgate, R.C. Fu, N.E. Byars, L.C. Foster and J.S. Fleitman, Formulation of vaccine adjuvant muramylpeptides. 3. Processing optimisation, characterisation and bioactivity of an emulsion vehicle, *Pharm. Res.*, 1989, **6**, pp. 748–752.
10. F.H. Roerding, T. Daemen, I.A.J.M. Baker-Woundenburg, G. Storm, D.J.A. Crommelin and G.L. Scherphof, *Drug Delivery Systems: Foundamentals and Techniques*, Ellis Horwood, Chichester, 1987, pp. 66–80.
11. A.T. Florence and A.J. Baillie, Non-ionic surfactant vesicles—alternatives to liposomes in drug delivery, in: *Novel Drug Delivery and Its Therapeutic Application*, (L.F. Prescott and W.S. Nimmo, eds), John Wiley, New York, 1989, pp. 281–296.
12. T. Kato, R. Nemoto, H. Mori, M. Takahashi and M. Harada, Arterial Chemoembolization with mitomycin C microcapsules in the treatment of primary or secondary carcinoma of the kidney, liver, bone and intrapelvic organs, *Cancer*, 1981, **48**, pp. 674–680.
13. D.J. Kerr, J. Goldberg, C.S. McArdle and T. Whateley, Intrahepatic arterial administration of mitomycin C microcapsules, *Br. J. Cancer*, 1990, **62**, pp. 527–533.
14. R.F. Tuma, The use of degradable starch microspheres for transient occlusion of blood flow and for drug targeting to selected tissues, in: *Microspheres and Drug Therapy. Pharmaceutical, Immunological and Medical Aspects*, (S.S. Davis, L. Illum, J.G. McVie and E. Tomlinson, eds), Elsevier, Amsterdam, 1984, pp. 189–203.
15. P. Artursson, E. Arro, P. Edman, J.L.E. Ericsson and I. Sjoholm, Biodegradable microspheres. V. Stimulation of macrophages with microparticles made of various polysaccharides, *J. Pharm. Sci.*, 1987, **76**, pp. 127–133.
16. T. Laakso, J. Andersson, P. Artursson, P. Edman and I. Sjoholm, Acrylic microspherees in vivo. X. Elimination of circulating cells by active targeting using specific monoclonal antibodies bound to microparticles, *Life Sci.*, 1986, **38**, pp. 183–190.
17. J. Kreuter and H.R. Hartmann, Comparative study on the cytostatic effects and the tissue distribution of 5-flurouracil in a free form and bound to polybutylcyanoacrylate nanoparticles in sarcoma 180-bearing mice, *Oncology*, 1983, **40**, pp. 363–366.
18. P.G. Wasser, U. Muller, J. Kreuter, S. Berger, K. Munz, E. Kaiser and B. Pfluger, Localization of colloidal particles (liposomes, hexylcyanoacrylate nanoparticles and albumin nanoparticles) by histology and autoradiography in mice, *Int. J. Pharm.*, 1987, **39**, pp. 312–327.
19. P. Flandroy, C. Grandfils, J. Collignon, A. Thibaut, N. Nihard, S. Barbette, R. Jérome and P. Teyssie, (D,L)-Polylactide microspheres as embolic agent. A preliminary study, *Neuroradiology*, 1990, **32**, pp. 311–315.
20. R. Verrijk, I.J.H. Smoders, N. Bosnie and A.C. Begg, Reduction of systemic exposure and toxicity of cisplatin by encapsulation in polylactide-co-glycolide, *Cancer Res.*, 1992, **52**, pp. 6653–6656.
21. S. Miyazaki, N. Hashiguchi, C. Yokouchi, M. Takada and W.-M. Hou, Antitumour effect of fibrinogen microspheres containing doxorubicin on Ehrlich ascites carcinoma, *J. Pharm. Pharmacol.*, 1986, **38**, pp. 618–620.
22. Y. Chen, N. Willmott, J. Anderson and A.T. Florence, Comparison of albumin and casein microspheres as a carrier for doxorubicin, *J. Pharm. Pharmacol.*, 1987, **39**, pp. 978–985.
23. Y. Chen, N. Willmott, J. Anderson and A.T. Florence, Haemoglobin, transferrin and albumin/polyaspartic acid microspheres as carriers for the cytotoxic drug adriamycin. I. Ultrastructural appearance and drug content, *J. Control. Release*, 1988, **8**, pp. 93–101.
24. T. Kissel, Z. Brich, S. Bantle, I. Lancranjan, F. Nimmerfall and P. Vit, Parenteral depot-systems on the basis of biodegradable polyesters, *J. Control. Release*, 1991, **16**, pp. 27–42.
25. C. Washington, Drug release from monodisperse systems: A critical review, *Int. J. Pharm.*, 1990, **58**, pp. 1–12.
26. B.D. Ratner, Biomedical applications of synthetic polymers, in: *Comprehensive Polymer Science*, 1989, **7**, pp. 201–247. (G. Allen, J.C. Bevington, S.L. Aggarwal, eds), Pergamon Press, Oxford.
27. G.E. Zaikov, Quantitative aspects of polymer degradation in the living body, *J. Macromol. Sci., Rev. Macromol. Chem. Phys.*, 1985, **C25**, pp. 551–597.
28. T.H. Barrows, *Clin. Mater.*, 1986, **1**, p. 233.

29. M. Vert, P. Christel, F. Chabot and J. Lerry, in: *Macromolecular Biomaterials*, (G.W. Hastings and P. Duckeyne, eds), CRC Press, Boca Raton, 1984, p. 119.
30. T. Hayashi, Biodegradable polymers for biomedical uses, *Prog. Polym. Sci.*, 1994, **19**, pp. 663–702.
31. Y. Ikada, Kobunshi Shinsozai Binran (Japanese), Maruzen, Tokyo, 1989, p. 322.
32. J.A. Hubbell, Chemical modification of polymer surfaces to improve biocompatibility, *Trends Polym. Sci.*, 1994, **2**, pp. 20–25.
33. E. Mathiowitz and R. Langer, Polyanhydride microspheres as drug delivery systems, in *Microcapsules and Nanoparticles in Medicine and Pharmacy*, (J. Dunbrow ed.), CRC Press, Boca Raton, 1992, pp. 99–123.
34. Y. Kimura, in *Biomedical Applications of Polymeric Materials*, (T. Tsuruta ed.), CRC Press, Boca Raton, 1993, pp. 163–189.
35. W.J. Bailey, Ring-opening polymerization, in: *Comprehensive Polymer Science*, (G. Allen, J.C. Bevington, G.C. Eastmond, A. Ledwith, S. Russo and P. Sigwalt, eds), Pergamon Press, Oxford 1989, pp. 283–320.
36. J.M. Mayer and D.L. Kaplan, Biodegradable materials: Balancing degradability and performance, *Trends Polym. Sci.*, 1994, **2**, pp. 227–235.
37. G.R. Elion, *US Patent*, 5 244 945, 1993.
38. C.M. Buchanan, R.M. Gardner and R.J. Komarek, Aerobic biodegradation of cellulose acetate, *J. Appl. Polym. Sci.*, 1993, **47**, pp. 1709–1719.
39. O.B. Wurzburg, Modified starches: Properties and uses, CRC Press, Boca Raton, 1986.
40. F. Rypáček, S. Matějková and J. Uher, Biodegradable hydrogel microspheres for studies of oocyte transport in human salpinx, 36th Microsymposium High-Swelling Gels, Prague, 1995, **SL1**.
41. R. Ammon, The occurence of dextranase in human tissues, *Enzymologia*, 1963, **25**, pp. 245–251.
42. G. Pfister, M. Bahadir and F. Korte, Release characteristics of herbicides from Ca alginate gel formulations, *J. Control. Release*, 1986, **3**, pp. 229–233.
43. E.R. Edelman, F. Mathiowitz, R. Langer and M. Klagsbrun, Controlled and modulated release of basic fibroblast growth factor, *Biomaterials*, 1991, **12**, pp. 619–626.
44. E. Santucci, F. Alhaique, M. Carafa, T. Coviello, E. Murtas and F.M. Riccieri, Gellan for the formulation of sustained delivery beads, *J. Control. Release*, 1996, **42**, pp. 157–164.
45. T. Chandy and C.P. Sharma, Biodegradable chitosan matrix for the controlled release of steroids, *Biomater., Artif. Cells, Immobilization Biotechnol.*, 1991, **19**, pp. 745–760.
46. P. Calvo, C. Remuñán-López, J.L. Vila-Jato and M.J. Alonso, Novel hydrophilic chitosan-polyethylene oxide nanoparticles as protein carriers, *J. Appl. Polym. Sci.*, 1997, **63**, pp. 125–132.
47. G.A. Magee, G.W. Halbert and N. Vilmott, Effect of process variables on the in vitro degradation of protein microspheres, *J. Control. Release*, 1995, **37**, pp. 11–19.
48. R.M. Ottenbrite, R. Zhao and S. Milstein, A new oral microsphere drug delivery system, *Macromol. Symp.*, 1996, **101**, pp. 379–387.
49. K.E. Gonsalves and P. Mungara, Synthesis and properties of degradable polyamides and related polymers, *Trends Polym. Sci.*, 1996, **4**, pp. 25–33.
50. J.M. Anderson, K.L. Spilizewski and A. Hiltner, in Biocompatibility of Tissue Analogs, (D.F. Williams, ed.), CRC Press, Boca Raton, 1985, **1**, p. 67.
51. F. Lescure, R. Gurny, E. Doelker, M.L. Pelaprat, D. Bichon and J.M. Anderson, Acute histopathological response to a new biodegradable polypeptidic polymer for implantable drug delivery system, *J. Biomed. Mater. Res.*, 1989, **23**, pp. 1299–1313.
52. T. Kidchob, S. Kimura and Y. Imanishi, Preparation, structure and release profile of polypeptide microcapsules, *J. Control. Release*, 1996, **40**, pp. 285–291.
53. T. Kidchob, S. Kimura and Y. Imanishi, pH-Responsive release from polypeptide microcapsules, *J. Appl. Polym. Sci*, 1997, **63**, pp. 453–458.
54. A. Steinbuechel, Biodegradable plastics, *Curr. Opin. Biotechnol.*, 1992, **3**, pp. 291–297.
55. P.A. Holmes, S.H. Collins and L.F. Wright, *US Patent*, 4 477 654, 1984.
56. R.A. Gross, C. DeMello, R.W. Lenz, H. Brandl and R.C. Fuller, Biosynthesis and characterization of poly(β-hydroxyalkanoate)s produced by pseudomonas oleovorans, *Macromolecules*, 1989, **22**, pp. 1106–1115.
57. B. Hazer, R.W. Lenz and R.C. Fuller, Biosynthesis of nethyl-branched poly(β-hydroxyalkanoate)s produced by pseudomonas oleovorans, *Macromolecules*, 1994, **27**, pp. 45–49.

58. S. Nakamura, Y. Doi and M. Scandola, Microbial synthesis and characterization of poly(3-hydroxybutyrate-co-4-hydroxybutyrate), *Macromolecules*, 1992, **25**, pp. 4237–4241.
59. S. Nakamura, M. Kunioka and Y. Doi, Biosynthesis and characterization of bacterial poly(3-hydroxybutyrate-co-3-hydroxypropionate), *Macromol. Rep.*, 1991, **A28**, pp. 15–24.
60. W.J. Page and O. Knosp, Hyperproduction of poly-β-hydroxybutyrate during exponential growth of azobacter vinelandii UWD, *Appl. Environ. Microbiol.*, 1989, **55**, pp. 1334–1339.
61. S.H. Collins, Choice of substrate in polyhydroxybutyrate synthesis, *Spec. Publ. Soc. Gen. Microbiol.*, 1987, **21**, pp. 161–168.
62. J. Anton, I. Meseguer and F. Rodriguez-Valera, Production of an extracellular polysaccharide by Haloferax mediterranei, *Appl. Environ. Microbiol.*, 1988, **54**, pp. 2381–2386.
63. A.L. Allen and D.H. Ball, Continuous cultivation of haloferx mediterranei for the production of polyhydroxyalkanoates, *Proc. Am. Chem. Soc., Div. Polym. Mater.: Sci. Eng.*, 1992, **67**, pp. 132–133.
64. Y. Doi, Y. Kanesawa, M. Kunioka and T. Saito, Biodegradation of microbial copolyesters: Poly(3-hydroxybutyrate-co-hydroxyvalerate) and poly(3-hydroxybutyrate-co-4-hydroxybutyrate), *Macromolecules*, 1990, **23**, pp. 26–31.
65. A. Schimmer, D. Jendrossek and H.G. Schlegel, *Appl. Environ. Microbiol.*, 1993, **59**, p. 1222.
66. C.V. Benedict, J.A. Cameron and S.J. Huang, Polycaprolactone degradation by mixed and pure cultures of bacteria and yeast, *J. Appl. Polym. Sci.*, 1983, **28**, pp. 335–342.
67. C.G. Pitt, F.I. Chasalow, Y.M. Hibionada, D.M. Klimas and A. Schindler, Aliphatic polyesters. I. The degradation of poly(ε-caprolactone) in vivo, *J. Appl. Polym. Sci.*, 1981, **26**, pp. 3779–3787.
68. S.C. Woodward, P.S. Brewer, F. Moatamed, A. Schindler and C.G. Pitt, The intracellular degradation of poly(ε-caprolactone), *J. Biomed. Mater. Res.*, 1985, **19**, pp. 437–444.
69. R.D. Fields, F. Rodriguez and R.K. Finn, Microbial degradation of polyesters: Polycaprolactone degraded by P. pullulans, *J. Appl. Polym. Sci.*, 1974, **18**, pp. 3571–3579.
70. R.K. Kulkarni, K.C. Pani, C. Neuman and F. Leonard, Poly(lactic acid) for surgical implants, *Arch. Surg.*, Chicago, 1966, **93**, pp. 839–854.
71. R.K. Kulkarni, E.G. Moore, A.F. Heggyeli and F. Leonard, Biodegradable poly(lactic acid) polymers, *J. Biomed. Mater. Res.*, 1971, **5**, pp. 169–181.
72. K. Jamshidi, S.-H. Hyon and Y. Ikada, Thermal characterization of polylactides, *Polymer*, 1988, **29**, pp. 2229–2234.
73. Y. Aso, S. Yoshioka, A. Li Wan Po and T. Terao, Effect of temperature on mechanism of drug release and matrix degradation of poly(*D,L*-lactide) microspheres, *J. Control. Release*, 1994, **31**, pp. 33–39.
74. S. Yoshioka, Y. Aso and S. Kojima, Drug release poly(*dl*-lactide) microspheres controlled by γ-irradiation, *J. Control. Release*, 1995, **37**, pp. 263–267.
75. E. Celikkaya, E.B. Denbas and E. Piskin, Poly(DL-lactide)/poly(ethylene glycol) copolymer particles. I. Preparation and characterization, *J. Appl. Polym. Sci.*, 1996, **61**, pp. 1439–1446.
76. M. Vert, S.M. Li, G. Spenlehauer and P. Guerin, Bioresorbability and biocompatibility of aliphatic polyesters, *J. Mater. Sci.: Mater. Med.*, 1992, **3**, pp. 432–446.
77. D.F. Williams, *Eng. Med.*, 1981, **10**, p. 5.
78. R.C. Mehta, B.C. Thanoo and P.P. DeLuca, Peptide containing microspheres from low molecular weight and hydrophilic poly(*d,l*-lactide-co-glycolide), *J. Control. Release*, 1996, **41**, pp. 249–257.
79. D. Bazile, C. Prud'Homme, M.-T. Bassoullet, M. Marland, G. Splenlehauer, M. Veillard and M. Stealth, PEG-PLA nanoparticles avoid uptake by the mononuclear phagocytes system, *J. Pharm. Sci.*, 1994, **84**, pp. 493–498.
80. K.J. Pekarek, M.J. Dyrud, K. Ferrer, Y.S. Jong and E. Mathiowitz, *In vitro* and *in vivo* degradation of double-walled polymer microspheres, *J. Control. Release*, 1996, **40**, pp. 169–178.
81. K.W. Leong, B.C. Brott and R. Langer, Bioerodible polyanhydrides as drug-carrier matrices. I. Characterization, degradation and release characteristics, *J. Biomed. Mater. Res.*, 1985, **19**, pp. 941–955.
82. A.-Ch. Albertsson, J. Carlfors and C. Sturesson, Preparation and characterization of poly(adipic anhydride) microspheres for ocular drug delivery, *J. Appl. Polym. Sci.*, 1996, **62**, pp. 695–705.
83. S.J. Huang, Biodegradable Polymers, in *Encycl. Polym. Sci. and Eng.*, (H.F. Mark, N.M. Bikales, Ch.G. Overberger and G. Menges eds), John Wiley, New York, 1985, **2**, pp. 220–243.
84. A. Tuncel, H. Cicek, M. Hayaran and E. Piskin, Monosize poly(ethylcyanoacrylate) microspheres: Preparation and degradation properties, *J. Biomed. Mater. Res.*, 1995, **29**, pp. 721–728.

85. R. Alkock, *Polyphosphazenes, in Encyclopedia of Polymer Science and Engineering*, (H.F. Mark, N.M. Bikales, Ch.G. Overberger and G. Menges, eds), John Wiley, New York, 1988, pp. 31–41.
86. J. Bleich, B.W. Müller and W. Waßmus, Aeorosol solvent extraction system: A new microparticle production technique, *Int. J. Pharm.*, 1993, **97**, pp. 111–117.
87. R. Alex and R. Bodmeier, Encapsulation of water-soluble drugs by a modified solvent evaporation method. I. Effect of process and formulation variables on drug entrapment, *J. Microencapsulation*, 1990, **7**, pp. 347–355.
88. J.M. Ruiz and J.P. Benoit, *In vitro* peptide release from poly(*D,L*-lactic acid-co-glycolic acid copolymer) 50/50 microspheres, *J. Control. Release*, 1991, **16**, pp. 177–186.
89. C. Thomasin, P. Johansen, R. Alder, R. Bemsel, G. Hottinger, H. Altorfer, A.D. Wright, G. Wehrli, H.P. Merkle and B. Gander, A contribution to overcoming the problem of residual solvents in biodegradable microspheres prepared by coacervation, *Eur. J. Pharm. Biopharm.*, 1996, **42**, pp. 16–24.
90. H. Akin and N. Hasirci, Preparation and characterization of crosslinked gelatin microspheres, *J. Appl. Polym. Sci.*, 1995, **58**, pp. 95–100.
91. P.R. Chatterji, Gelatin with hydrophilic/hydrophobic grafts and glutaraldehyde crosslinks, *J. Appl. Polym. Sci.*, 1989, **37**, pp. 2203–2212.
92. T. Yoshioka, M. Hashida, S. Muranishi and H. Sezaki, *Chem. Pharmacol. Bull.*, 1980, **28**, p. 1009.
93. R. Wada, S.-H. Hyon, Y. Ikada, Y. Nakao, H. Yoshikawa and S. Muranishi, Lactic acid oligomer microspheres containing an anticancer agent for selective lymphatic delivery: I. *In vitro* studies, *J. Bioactive Compat. Polym.*, 1988, **3**, pp. 126–136.
94. S.-H. Hyon, Ophthalmic drug delivery systems using biodegradable polymers, *Polym. Preprints*, 1996, **37**(2), pp. 125–126.
95. M. Chiba, J. Hanes and R. Langer, Controlled protein delivery from biodegradable tyrosine-containing poly(anhydride-co-imide) microspheres, *Biomaterials*, 1997, **18**, pp. 893–901.
96. H.T. Wang, E. Schmitt, D.R. Flanagan and R.J. Linhardt, Influence of formulation methods on the *in vitro* controlled release of protein from poly(ester) microspheres, *J. Control. Release*, 1991, **17**, pp. 23–32.
97. R. Wada, S.-H. Hyon and Y. Ikada, Kinetics of diffusion-mediated drug release enhanced by matrix degradation, *J. Control. Release*, 1995, **37**, pp. 151–160.
98. M.K. Yek, P.G. Jenkins, S.S. Davis and A.G.A. Coombes, Improving the delivery capacity of microparticle system using (resorbable) blends of poly(*DL*-lactide-co-glycolide) and poly(ethylene glycol), *J. Control. Release*, 1995, **37**, pp. 1–9.
99. T. Niwa, H. Takeuchi, T. Hino, N. Kunou and Y. Kawashima, *In vitro* drug release behaviour of D,L-lactide/glycolide copolymer (PLGA) nanospheres with naferelin acetate prepared by a novel spontaneous emulsification solvent evaporation method, *J. Pharm. Sci.*, 1994, **83**, pp. 727–732.
100. F. Fawaz, F. Bonini, M. Guyot, A.M. Lagueny, H. Fessi and J.P. Devissaguet, Disposition and protective effect against irritation after intravenous and rectal administration of indomethacin loaded nanocapsules to rabbits, *Int. J. Pharm.*, 1996, **133**, pp. 107–115.
101. J.W. Fong, *French Patent*, No. FRA 81 11694, 1981.
102. F. Boury, H. Marchais, J.P. Benoit and J.E. Proust, Surface characterization of poly(α-hydroxy acid) microspheres prepared by a solvent evaporation/extraction process, *Biomaterials*, 1997, **18**, pp. 125–136.
103. B.-J. Ha, O.-S. Lee and Y.-S. Lee, Novel hollow microbeads based on hydroxypropyl chitosan by w/o emulsion cross-linking method, *Macromol. Reports*, 1996, **A33**, pp. 297–308.
104. K. Itoi, C.-Y. Tabata, O. Ike, Y. Shimizu, M. Kuwabara, M. Kyo, S.-H. Hyon and Y. Ikada, *In vivo* suppressive effect of copoly(glycolic/L-lactic acid) microspheres containing CDDP on murine tumor cells, *J. Control. Release*, 1996, **42**, pp. 175–184.
105. S. Shen, E.D. Sudol and M.S. El-Aasser, Control of particle size in dispersion polymerization of methyl methacrylate, *J. Polym. Sci.*, Part A, 1993, **31**, pp. 1393–1402.
106. S.J. Douglas, L. Illum, S.S. Davis and J. Kreuter, Particle size and size distribution of poly(butyl-2-cyanoacrylate) nanoparticles, *J. Colloid Interface Sci.*, 1984, **101**, pp. 149–158.
107. S. Sosnowski, M. Gadzinowski and S. Slomkowski, Poly(*L,L*-lactide) microspheres by ring-opening polymerization, *Macromolecules*, 1996, **29**, pp. 4556–4564.
108. M.G. Duarte, D. Brunnel, M.H. Gil and E. Schacht, Microcapsules prepared from starch derivatives, *J. Mater. Sci.: Mater. Med.*, 1997, **8**, pp. 321–323.

109. Ch.-S. Cho, J.-B. Cheon, Y.-I. Jeong, I.-S. Kim, S.-H. Kim and T. Akaike, Novel core-shell type thermo-sensitive nanoparticles composed of poly(γ-benzyl L-glutamate) as the core and poly(N-isopropylacrylamide) as the shell, *Macromol. Rapid Commun.*, 1997, **18**, pp. 361–369.
110. J.-Z. Yang, S. Antoun and R.M. Ottenbrite, Amino acid oligomer microspheres as drug delivery systems. I. Synthesis of oligo(amino acids) via NCAs and their microsphere formation, *J. Bioactive Compat. Polym.*, 1996, **11**, pp. 219–235.
111. J.-Z. Yang, M. Wang and R.M. Ottenbrite, Amino acid oligomer microspheres as drug delivery systems. II. Oligomerization of NCAs initiated with L-tyrosine methyl ester, *J. Bioactive Compat. Polym.*, 1996, **11**, pp. 236–247.
112. C.G. Pitt, The controlled parenteral delivery of polypeptides and proteins, *Int. J. Pharm.*, 1990, **59**, pp. 173–196.
113. H. Jeffery, S.S. Davis and D.T. O'Hagan, The preparation and characterization of poly(lactide-co-glycolide) microparticles II.: The entrapment of a model protein using a (water-in-oil)-in-water emulsion solvent evaporation techniques, *Pharm. Res.*, 1993, **10**, pp. 362–368.
114. T. Richey and F.W. Harris, Preparation and characterization of indomethacin-loaded microspheres, *Polym. Preprints*, 1995, **36**(2), pp. 255–256.
115. A. Carrio, G. Schwach, J. Coudane and M. Vert, Preparation and degradation of surfactant-free PLAGA microspheres, *J. Control. Release*, 1995, **37**, pp. 113–121.
116. J. Herrmann and R. Bodmeier, The effect of particle microstructure on the somatostatin release from poly(lactide) microspheres prepared by a W/O/W solvent evaporation method, *J. Control. Release*, 1995, **36**, pp. 63–71.
117. T. Heya, H. Okada, Y. Tanigawara, Y. Ogawa and H. Toguchi, Effects of counteranion of TRH and loading amount on control of TRH release from copoly(*dl*-lactic/glycolic acid) microspheres prepared by an in-water drying method, *Int. J. Pharm.*, 1991, **69**, pp. 69–75.
118. M. Mason-Garcia, M. Vaccarella, J. Horvath, T.W. Redding, K. Groot, P. Orsolini and A.V. Schally, Radioimmunoassay for octapeptide analogs of somatostatin: Measurement of serum levels after administration of long-acting microcapsule formulations, *Proc. Natl. Acad. Sci.*, USA, 1985, **85**, pp. 5688–5692.
119. J.M. Ruis and J.P. Benoit, *In vivo* peptide release from poly(D,L-lactic acid-co-glycolic acid) copolymer 50/50 microspheres, *J. Control. Release*, 1991, **16**, pp. 177–186.
120. J.W. Wyse, Y. Takahashi and P.P. DeLuca, Instability of porcine somatotropin in polyglycolic acid microspheres, *Proc. Int. Symp. Control. Rel. Bioact. Mater.*, 1989, **16**, pp. 334–360.
121. M.S. Hora, R.K. Rana, T.A. Taforo, J.H. Nunbeerg, R.R. Tice, R.M. Gilley and M.E. Hudson, Development of a controlled release microspheres formulation of interleukin-2, *Proc. Int. Symp. Control. Rel. Bioact. Mater.*, 1989, **16**, pp. 509–510.
122. S.C. Lee, M.Shea, M.A. Battle, K. Kozitza, E. Ron, T. Turek, R.G. Schaub and W.C. Hayes, Healing of large segmental defects in rat femurus is aided by RhBMP-2 in PLGA matrix, *J. Biomed. Mater. Res.*, 1994, **28**, pp. 1149–1156.
123. T.L. Bowersock, H. HogenEsch, M. Suckow, R.E. Porter, R. Jackson, H. Park and K. Park, Oral vaccination with alginate microsphere systems, *J. Control. Release*, 1996, **39**, pp. 209–220.
124. L. Garcí-Contreras, K. Abu-Izza and D.R. Lu, Biodegradable cisplatin microspheres for direct brain injection: Preparation and characterization, *Pharm. Develop. Technol.*, 1997, **2**, pp. 53–65.
125. J.P. Benoit, F. Courteille and C. Thies, A physicochemical study of the morphology of progesterone-loaded poly(D,L-lactice) microspheres, *Int. J. Pharm.*, 1986, **29**, pp. 95–102.
126. P. De Vos, B. De Haan and R. Van Schilfgaarde, Effect of the alginate composition on the biocompatibility of alginate-polylysine microcapsules, *Biomaterials*, 1997, **18**, pp. 273–278.
127. K.Y. Lee, W.H. Park and W.S. Ha, Polyelectrolyte complexes of sodium alginate with chitosan or its derivatives for microcapsules, *J. Appl. Polym. Sci.*, 1997, **63**, pp. 425–432.
128. M. Donbrow, in Microcapsules and Nanoparticles in Medicine and Pharmacy, (M. Donbrow, ed.), CRC Press, Boca Raton, 1992, pp. 1–14.
129. R. Narayani and K.P. Rao, pH-Responsive gelatin microspheres for oral delivery of anticancer drug methotrexate, *J. Appl. Polym. Sci.*, 1995, **58**, pp. 1761–1769.
130. K.D. Yao, M.X. Xu, Y.J. Yin, J.Y. Zhao and X.L. Chen, pH-Sensitive chitosan/gelatin hybrid polymer network microspheres for delivery of cimetidine, *Polymer Int.*, 1996, **39**, pp. 333–337.
131. N. Santiago, S. Milstein, T. Rivera, E. Garcia, T. Zaidi, H. Hong and D. Buck, Oral immunization in rats with microspheren encapsulating influenza virus, *Pharm. Res.*, 1993, **10**, pp. 1243–1247.

132. S.S. Davis, L. Illum and S. Stolnik, Polymers in drug delivery, *Curr. Opin. Colloid Interface Sci.*, 1996, **1**, pp. 660–666.
133. A.M. Hillery, I. Toth, A.J. Shaw and A.T. Florence, Co-polymerised peptide particles (CPP) I: Synthesis, characterisation and *in vitro* studies on a novel oral nanoparticulate delivery system, *J. Control. Release*, 1996, **41**, pp. 271–281.
134. Y. Tabata and Y. Ikada, Macrophage phagocytosis of biodegradable microspheres composed of L-lactic acid/glycolic acid homo and copolymers, *J. Biomed. Mater. Res.*, 1988, **22**, pp. 837–858.
135. H.F.M. Cremers, K. Lam, R.F.E. Wolf, E.H. Blaauw, J.M. Schakenraad, R. Verrijk, G.S. Kwon, Y.H. Bae, S.W. Kim and J. Feijen, Degradation and intrahepatic compatibility of albumin-heparin conjugate microspheres, *Biomaterials*, 1994, **15**, pp. 577–585.
136. H.F.M. Cremers, J.P. Lens, L. Seymour and J. Feijen, Biodegradable ion-exchange microspheres based on modified polylysines, *J. Control. Release*, 1995, **36**, pp. 167–179.
137. M. Yoshida, M. Asano, M. Kumakura, R. Katazaki, T. Mashimo, H. Yuasa, K. Imai and H. Yamanaka, A new bidegradable polydepsipeptide microsphere for application in drug delivery systems, *Colloid Polym. Sci.*, 1990, **268**, pp. 726–730.
138. J.H. Doroshow, Doxorubicin-induced cardiac toxicity, *New Engl. J. Med.*, 1991, **324**, pp. 843–845.
139. S.S. Davis and L. Illum, Polymeric microspheres as drug carriers, *Biomaterials*, 1988, **9**, pp. 111–115.
140. H.P.J.M. Noteborn and J.G. McVie, Chemoembolization in regional chemotherapy, in: Drug Delivery in Cancer Treatment, *ESO Monographs*, (L. Domellöf, ed.), Springer Verlag, Berlin-New York, 1989, pp. 55–78.
141. J.P. Codde, M. Burton, D.K. Kelleher, S.G. Archer and B.N. Gray, Reduced toxicity of adriamycin by incorporation into ion exchange microspheres: A therapeutic study using a rat liver tumor model, *Anticancer Res.*, 1990, **10**, pp. 1715–1718.
142. J.A. Goldberg, N.S. Willmott, J.H. Anderson, G. McCurrach, R.G. Bessent, J.H. McKillop and C.S. McArdle, The biodegradation of albumin microspheres used for regional chemotherapy in patients with colorectal liver methastases, *Nucl. Med. Commun.*, 1991, **12**, pp. 57–63.
143. C.S. McArdle, H. Lewi, D. Hansell, D.J. Kerr, J.H. McKillop and N.S. Willmott, Cytotoxic-loaded albumin microspheres: A novel approach to regional chemotherapy, *Br. J. Surg.*, 1988, **75**, pp. 132–134.
144. C. Grandfils, P. Flandroy and R. Jérome, Control of the biodegradation rate of poly(D,L-lactide) microparticles intended as chemoembolization materials, *J. Control. Release*, 1996, **38**, pp. 109–122.
145. N.E. Larsen, S.T. Pollak, K. Hers, E.A. Leshchiner and E.A. Balaers, Use of Hylan gel composition for embolization of cerebral vessel in a rabbits, 4th World Biomaterial Symp., Berlin, 1992, p. 576.
146. P. Courvreur, B. Kante, M. Roland, P. Guiot, P. Bauduin and P. Speiser, Polyalkylcyanoacrylate nanocapsules as potential lysosomotropic carriers: Preparation, morphological and sorptive properties, *J. Pharm. Pharmacol.*, 1979, **31**, pp. 331–332.
147. L. Manil, L.R. Trupel and P. Couvreur, Isobutylcyanoacrylate nanoparticles as a solid phase for an efficient immunoradiometric assay, *Biomaterials*, 1986, **7**, pp. 212–216.

Ecological Aspects of Polymer Flame Retardation

G.E. ZAIKOV and S.M. LOMAKIN

Institute of the Biochemical Physics of Russian Academy of Sciences, Kosygin 4, 117334, Russia

INTRODUCTION

Plastics have played an important role in shaping our history. After the invention of the celluloid billiard ball in 1860's, plastics demonstrated their endless possibilities. Since then, plastics have become an integral part of our everyday life.

The interest in flame retarding plastics goes back to the mid nineteenth century with the discovery of highly flammable cellulose nitrate and celluloid. More recently the conventional large volume of plastics such as phenolics, rigid PVC and melamine resins possess adequate flame retardancy. By the 1970s, the major flame retardant polymers were the thermosets, namely, unsaturated polyesters and epoxy resins which utilized reactive halogen compounds and alumina hydrate as an additive. There was also a large market for phosphate esters in plasticized PVC, cellulose acetate film, unsaturated polyesters and modified polyphenylene oxide. Alumina trihydrate (ATH) was the largest volume flame retardant into unsaturated plastics. Consumption of halogen-containing flame retardant additives in 70s was much less than the other additives. The halogenated flame retardant additives were Dechlorane Plus, a chlorinated alicyclic (for polyolefins), tris-(dibromopropyl) phosphate, brominated aromatics, pentabromochlorocyclohexane and hexabromocyclododecane (for polystyrene). The next five years was to see a number of new brominated additives on the market. There were produced a number of chlorinated flame retardant products under the Dechlorane trade name. The products included of two moles of hexachlorocyclopentadiene and contained 78% chlorine, Dechlorane Plus, a Diels-Alder reaction product of cyclooctaliene and hexachlorocyclopentadiene with 65% chlorine, a Diels-Alder product with furan and a product containing both bromine and chlorine with 77% halogen developed for the polystyrene and ABS materials.

In 1985–86, a German study detected brominated dioxins and furans from pyrolysis of a brominated diphenyl oxide in the laboratory at 510–630°C. The relevance of these pyrolysis studies to the real hazard presented by these flame retardants under actual use conditions has been questioned. Germany and Holland have considered a ban or curtailed use of brominated diphenyl oxide flame retardants because of the potential formation of highly toxic and potentially carcinogenic brominated furans and dioxins during combustion. The issue spread to other parts of

Europe where regulations were proposed to restrict their use. Nevertheless, demand for brominated flame retardants including decabromo- and pentabromodiphenyl oxides continues to be strong and growing.

Halogenated Diphenyl Ethers, Dioxins

Chlorinated dibenzo-*p*-dioxins and related compounds (commonly known simply as dioxins) are contaminants present in a variety of environmental media. This class of compounds has caused great concern in the general public as well as intense interest in the scientific community. Laboratory studies suggest the probability that exposure to dioxin-like compounds may be associated with other serious health effects including cancer. Recent laboratory studies have provided new insights into the mechanisms involved in the impact of dioxins on various cells and tissues and ultimately, on toxicity. Dioxins have been demonstrated to be potent modulators of cellular growth and differentiation, particularly in epithelial tissues. These data, together with the collective body of information from animal and human studies, when coupled with assumptions and inferences regarding extrapolation from experimental animals to humans and from high does to low doses, allow a characterization of dioxin hazards.

Polychlorinated dibenzodioxins (PCDDs), polychlorinated dibenzofurans (PCDFs), and polychlorinated biphenyls (PCBs) are chemically classified as halogenated aromatic hydrocarbons. The chlorinated and brominated dibenzodioxins and dibenzofurans are tricyclic aromatic compounds with similar physical and chemical properties, and both classes are similar structurally. Certain of the PCBs (the so-called coplanar or mono-ortho coplanar congeners) are also structurally and conformationally similar. The most widely studied of these compounds is 2,3,7,8-tetrachlorodibenzo-*p*-dioxin (TCDD). This compound, often called simply dioxin, represents the reference compound for this class of compounds. The structure of TCDD and several related compounds is shown in Figure 1.

These compounds are assigned individual toxicity equivalence factor (TEF) values as defined by international convention (U.S. EPA, 1989). Results of *in vitro* and *in vivo* laboratory studies contribute to the assignment of a relative toxicity value. TEFs are estimates of the toxicity of dioxin-like compounds relative to the toxicity of TCDD, which is assigned a TEF of 1.0. All chlorinated dibenzodioxins (CDDs) and chlorinated dibenzofurans (CDFs) with chlorines substituted in the 2, 3, 7, and 8 positions are assigned TEF values. Additionally, the analogous brominated dioxins and furans (BDDs and BDFs) and certain polychlorinated biphenyls have recently been identified as having dioxin-like toxicity and thus are also included in the definition of dioxin-like compounds. Generally accepted TEF values for chlorinated dibenzodioxins and dibenzofurans are shown in Table 1.

A recent World Health Organization/International Program on Chemical Safety meeting held in The Netherlands in December 1993 considered the need to derive internationally acceptable interim TEFs for the dioxin-like PCBs. Recommendations arising from that meeting of experts[1] suggest that in general only a few of the dioxin-like PCBs are likely to be significant contributors to general population exposures to dioxin-like compounds. Dioxin-like PCBs may be responsible for approximately one-

2,3,7,8-Tetrachlorodibenzo-*p*-dioxin

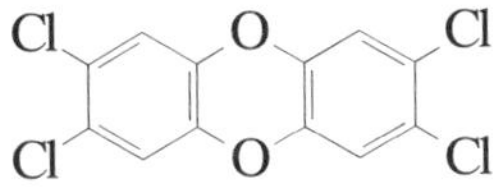

1,2,3,7,8-Pentachlorodibenzo-*p*-dioxin

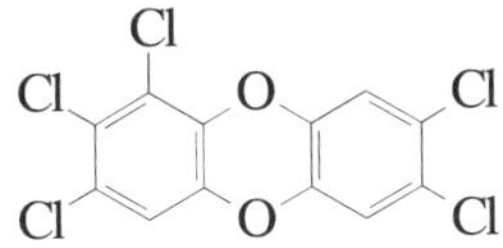

2,3,7,8-Tetrachlorodibenzofuran

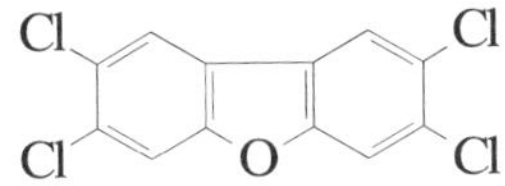

2,3,4,7,8-Pentachlorodibenzofuran

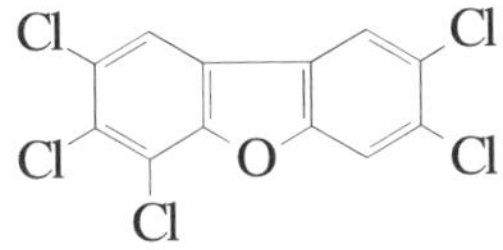

3,3′,4,4′,5,5′-Hexachlorobiphenyl

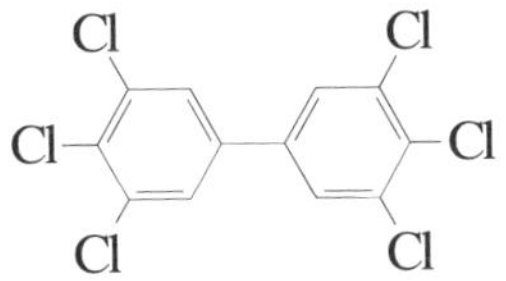

3,3′,4,4′,5,′-Pentachlorobiphenyl

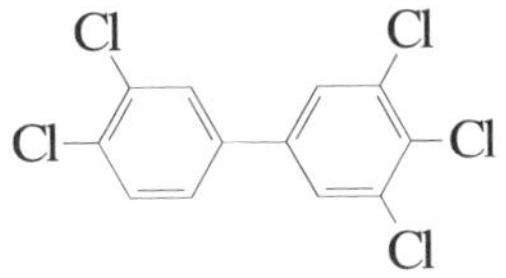

Figure 1 The structures of dioxin and similar compounds.

fourth to one-half of the total toxicity equivalence associated with general population environmental exposures to this class of related compounds.

There are 75 individual compounds comprising the CDDs, depending on the positioning of the chlorine(s), and 135 different CDFs. These are called individual congeners. Likewise, there are 75 different positional congeners of BDDs and 135 different congeners of BDFs. Only 7 of the 75 congeners of CDDs or of BDDs are thought to have dioxin-like toxicity; these are ones with chlorine/bromine substitutions in, at least, the 2, 3, 7, and 8 positions. Only 10 of the 135 possible congeners of CDFs or of BDFs are thought to have dioxin-like toxicity; these also are ones with substitutions in the 2, 3, 7, and 8 positions. While this suggests 34 individual CDDs, CDFs, BDDs, or BDFs with dioxin-like toxicity, inclusion of the mixed chloro/bromo congeners substantially increases the number of possible congeners with dioxin-like activity. There are 209 PCB congeners. Only 13 of the 209 congeners are thought to have dioxin-like toxicity; these are PCBs with 4 or more chlorines with just 1 or no substitution in the ortho position. These compounds are sometimes referred to as coplanar, meaning that they can assume a flat configuration with rings in the same plane. Similarly configured polybrominated biphenyls are likely to have similar

TABLE 1
Toxicity Equivalency Factors (TEF) for CDDs and CDFs.

Compound	Toxicity Equivalency Factors, TEF
Mono-, Di-, and Tri-CDDs	0
2,3,7,8-TCDD	1
Other TCDDs	0
2,3,7,8-PeCDD	0.5
Other PeCDDs	0
2,3,7,8-HxCDD	0.1
Other HxCDDs	0
2,3,7,8-HpCDD	0.01
Other HpCDDs	0
Mono-, Di-, and Tri-CDFs	0
2,3,7,8-TCDF	0.1
Other TCDFs	0
1,2,3,7,8-PeCDF	0.05
2,3,4,7,8-PeCDF	0.5
Other PeCDFs	0
2,3,7,8-HxCDF	0.1
Other HxCDFs	0
2,3,7,8-HpCDF	0.01
Other HpCDFs	0
OCDF	0.001

properties; however, the data base on these compounds with regard to dioxin-like activity has been less extensively evaluated. Mixed chlorinated and brominated congeners also exist, increasing the number of compounds considered dioxin-like. The physical/chemical properties of each congener vary according to the degree and position of chlorine and/or bromine substitution. Very little is known about the occurrence and toxicity of the mixed (chlorinated and brominated) dioxin, furan, and biphenyl congeners.

In general, these compounds have very low water solubility, high octanol-water partition coefficients, and low vapor pressure and tend to bioaccumulate.

Although these compounds are released from a variety of sources, the congener profiles of CDDs and CDFs found in sediments have been linked to combustion sources.[3]

The Hazards Substance Ordinance in Germany specifies the maximum level of chlorinated dibenzodioxins and furans that can be present in materials marketed in Germany. This has been extended to the brominated compounds. The two largest volume flame retardants decabromodiphenyl oxide and tetrabromo bis-phenol A are said to meet these requirements.[1,2]

The International Program for Chemical Safety (IPCS) of the World Health Organization has made several recommendations. Polybrominated diphenyls production (France) and use should be limited because of the concern over high persistency, bioaccumulation and potential adverse effects at low levels. There is limited toxicity data on deca- and octabromodiphenyls. Commercial use should cease unless safety is demonstrated. For the polybrominated diphenyl oxides, a Task Group felt that polybrominated dibenzo furans, and to a lesser extent the dioxins, may be formed. For decabromodiphenyl oxide, apropriate industrial hygiene measures need to be taken and environmental exposure minimized by effluent and emission control. Controlled incineration procedures should be instituted. For octabromodiphenyl oxide, the hexa and lower isomers should be minimized. There is considerable concern over persistance in the environment and the accumulation in organisms, especially, for pentabromodiphenyl oxide.

There are no regulations proposed or in effect anywhere around the world banning the use of brominated flame retardants. The proposed EU Directive on the brominated diphenyl oxides is withdrawn. Deca and tetrabromo bis-phenol A as well as other brominated flame retardants meet the requirements of the German Ordinance regulating dioxin and furan content of products sold in Germany.

The European search for a replacement for decabromodiphenyl oxide in HIPS has led to consideration of other bromoaromatics such as Saytex 8010 from Albemarle and a heat-stable chlorinated paraffin from ATOCHEM. The former product is more costly, and the latter, if sufficiently heat stable, lowers the heat distortion under load (HDUL) significantly. Neither approach has been fully accepted.

In September 1994, the US Environmental Protection Agency (EPA) released a final draft of exposure and risk assessment of dioxins and like compounds.[3,4] This reassessment finds the risks greater than previously thought. Based on this reassessment, a picture emerges that tetrachlorodiphenyl dioxins and related compounds are potent toxicants in animals with the potential to produce a spectrum of effects. Some of these effects may be occurring in humans at very low levels and some may be resulting in adverse impacts on human health. The EPA also concluded that dioxin should remain classified as a probable human carcinogen. The American Industrial Health Council disagrees with EPA's declaration that dioxin is definitely linked to lung cancer and soft-tissue sarcoma.[5] Polymer producers have been seeking non-halogen flame retardants and the search has been successful in several polymer systems. Non-halogen flame retardant polycarbonate/ABS blends are now commercial. They contain triphenyl phosphate or resorcinol diphosphate (RI)P as the flame retardant. Modified polyphenylene oxide (GE's Noryl) has used phosphate esters as the flame relardant for the past 15–20 years and the industry recently switched from the alkylated triphenyl phosphate to RDP. Red phosphorus is used with glass-reinforced nylon 6/6 in Europe and melamine cyanurate is used in unfilled nylon. Magnesium hydroxide is being used commercially in polyethylene wire and cable. The non-halogen solutions present other problems such as poor properties (plasticizers lower heat distortion temperature), difficult processing (high loadings of ATH and magnesium hydroxide), corrosion (red phosphorus) and handling problems (red phosphorus). In this paper we have tried to look at some new trends in the search of the new ecologically-friendly flame retardants.

MODE OF ACTION OF FLAME RETARDANTS

The main flame retardant systems for polymers currently in use are based on halogenated, phosphorous, nitrogen, and inorganic compounds (Scheme 1). All of these flame retardant system basically inhibit or even suppress the combustion process by chemical or physical action in the gas or condensed phase. The main process are:

POLYMER FLAME RETARDANTS

HALOGENATED FR

PHOSPHOROUS FR
PHOSPHATE ESTERS

ANTIMONY OXIDE

Mg HYDROXIDE, ALUMINA TRIHYDRATE,
BORON FR, AMMONIUM POLYPHOSPHATE,
MELAMINES, MOLYBDENUM FR

- -

Ecologically-friendly FR

POLYMER-ORGANIC CHAR FORMERS:
PVA, STARCH, GLUCOSE DERIVATIVES,
POLYFUNCTIONAL ALCOHOLS

LOW-MELTING GLASSES AND GLASS-CERAMICS:
$K_2CO_3-SiO_2$, $K_2SO_4-Na_2SO_4-ZnSO_4$

INTERCALATION STRUCTURES, GRAPHITE

POLYMER MORPHOLOGY MODIFICATION,
POLYPROPYLENE–POLYETHYLENE COMPOSITIONS

Scheme 1

1. Physical process acting by cooling (endothermic process), or by dilution. (Aluminium and magnesium hydroxides, melamines)
2. Chemical process taking place in the Gas Phase are based on radical chain mechanisms supported by high-energy H and OH radicals. These radicals can be removed by chemical species like halogen halides, metal halides and P-containing fragments (flame poisoning).
   (Halogenated flame retardants and antimony trioxide)
3. In the Condensed Phase the flame retardants can cause carbonization of polymer material, which protect the "native" polymer against heat and oxygen attack. (Phosphorous compounds and another intumescent systems)

The empirical approach to fire retardance can no longer meet alone the present requirements either in terms of effectiveness or hazard. The above mentioned, commercially the most effective flame retardants so far are halogen, phosphorous, antimony and heavy metal based compounds which however have the most environmental impact either while they perform their action or when burned in incineration of waste containing fire retardant polymeric materials.

The search for new ecologically-friendly flame retardants requires cooperation between industrial and academic research. Much remains to be solved in complete replacement of ecologically harmful flame retardants. This has been a problem for many years. It is not our goal today to try to complete that approach, but it's our aim to point out only some new trends in this field. The first example of ecologically-friendly flame retardant system is polymer-organic char former.

POLYMER-ORGANIC CHAR FORMER

Our recent study[7,8] has been directed at finding ways to increase the tendency of plastics to char when they are burned. There is a strong correlation between char yield and fire resistance. This follows because char is formed at the expense of combustible gases and because the presence of a char inhibits further flame spread by acting as a thermal barrier around the unburned material. It has been studied polymeric additives (polyvinyl alcohol systems) which promote the formation of char in polyvinyl alcohol-nylon 6,6 system.[7] These polymeric additives usually produce a highly conjugated system—aromatic structures which char during thermal degradation and/or transform into cross-linking agents at high temperatures.

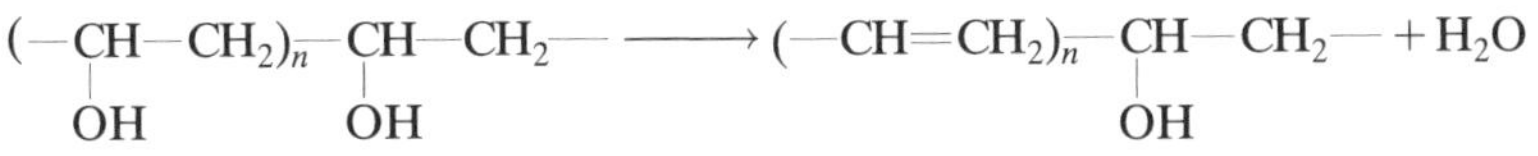

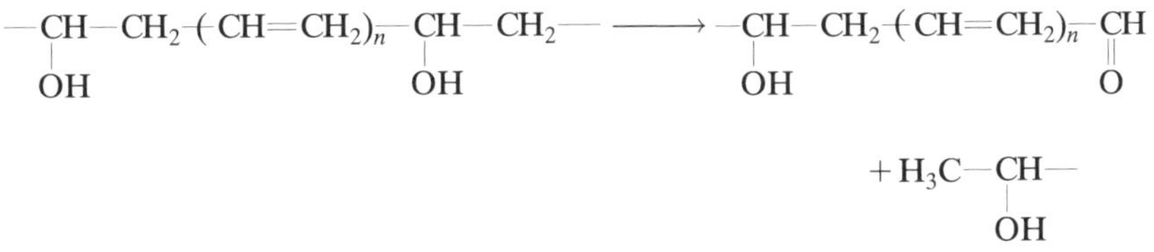

Scission of several carbon-carbon bonds leads to the formation of carbonyl ends. For example, aldehyde ends arise from the reaction.

The identification of a low concentration of benzene among the volatile products of PVA has been taken to indicate the onset of a crosslinking reaction proceeding by a Diels-Alder addition mechanism.[7] Clearly benzenoid structures are ultimately formed in the solid residue, and the IR spectrum of the residue also indicated the development of aromatic structures.

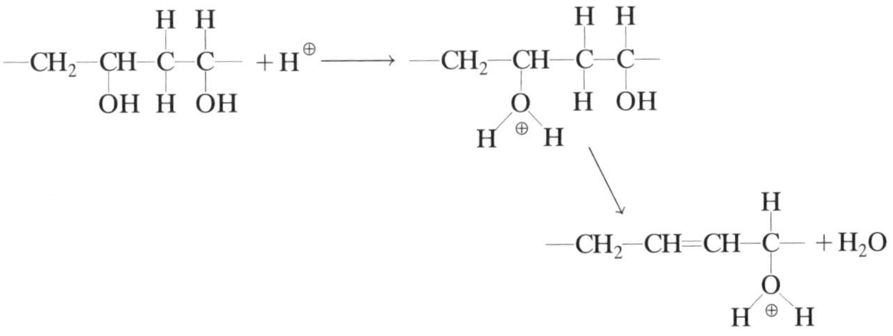

Acid-catalyzed dehydration promotes the formation of conjugated sequences of double bonds (a) and Diels-Alder addition of conjugated and isolated double bonds in different chains may result in intermolecular crosslinking producing structures which form graphite or carbonization (b):

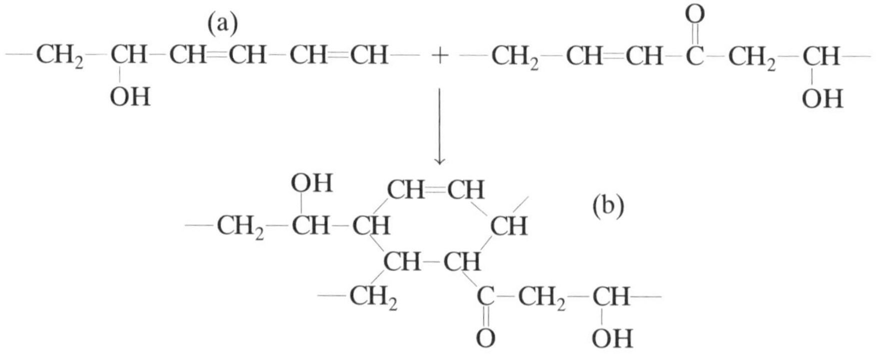

In contrast to PVA, nylon 6,6 which was subjected to temperatures above 300°C in an inert atmosphere it completely decomposed. The wide range of degradation products, which included several simple hydrocarbons, cyclopentanone, water, CO, CO_2 and NH_3 suggested that the degradation mechanism must have been highly complex. Further research has led to a generally accepted degradation mechanism for aliphatic polyamides.[7]

The idea of introducing PVA into nylon 6,6 composition is based on the possibility of high temperature acid-catalized dehydration.

This reaction can be provided by the acid products of nylon 6,6 degradation hydrolysis which would promote the formation of intermolecular crosslinking and

TABLE 1
Cone Calorimeter Data of nylon 6,6—PVA.

Material, Heat flux, kW/m^2	Initial wt., g	Char yield, % wt.	Ignition time, sec.	Peak R.H.R., kW/m^2	Total Heat Release, MJ/m^2
PVA, 20	27.6	8.8	39	255.5	159.6
PVA, 35	28.3	3.9	52	540.3	111.3
PVA, 50	29.2	2.4	41	777.9	115.7
PVA-ox $KMnO_4$, 20	27.9	30.8	1127	127.6	36.9
PVA-ox $KMnO_4$, 35	30.5	12.7	774	194.0	103.4
PVA-ox $KMnO_4$, 50	29.6	9.1	18	305.3	119.8
Nylon 6,6, 50	29.1	1.4	97	1124.6	216.5
Nylon 6,6 + PVA(8:2), 50	26.4	8.7	94	476.7	138.4
Nylon 6,6 + PVA-ox(8:2) $KMnO_4$, 50	29.1	8.9	89	399.5	197.5

char. Such a system we have called "synergetic carbonization" because the char yield and flame suppression parameters of the polymer blend of poly(vinyl alcohol) and nylon 6,6 are significantly better than pure poly(vinyl alcohol) and nylon 6,6 polymers.

The next step in our plan to improve the flame resistant properties of poly(vinyl alcohol)—nylon 6,6 system was the substitution of pure poly(vinyl alcohol) by poly(vinyl alcohol) oxidized by potassium permanganate (PVA-ox). This approach was based on the fire behavior of the (PVA-ox) itself. It was shown experimentally (Cone Calorimeter) the dramatic decrease of the rate of the heat release and significant increase in ignition time for the oxidized PVA in comparison with the original PVA (Table 1).

It was reported that the oxidation of PVA by in alkaline solutions occurs through formation of two intermediate complexes (1) and/or (2) (9):

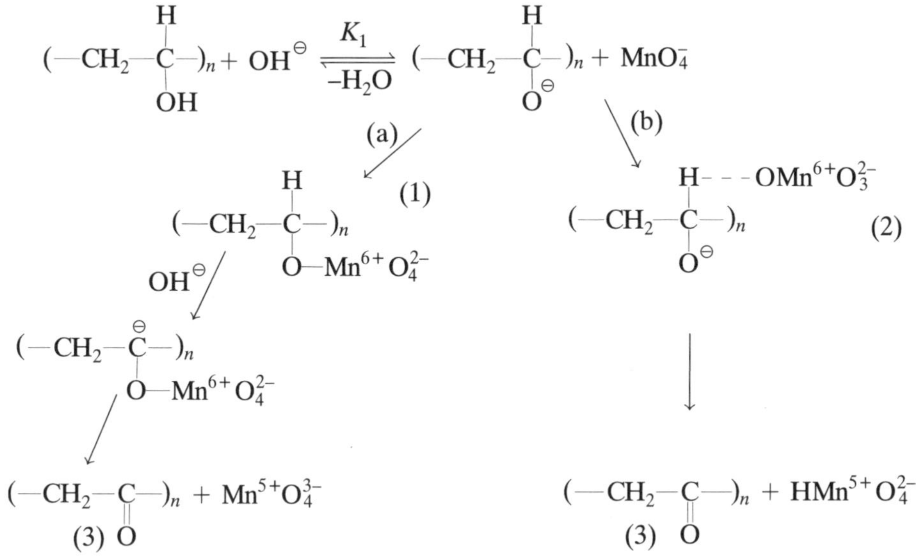

The reactions (a) and (b) lead to the formation of poly(vinyl ketone) (3) as a final product of oxidation of the substrate.

Preliminary Cone tests for PVA and PVA oxidized by $KMnO_4$ (Table 1) clearly indicated the substantial improvement of fire resistance characteristics for PVA oxidized by $KMnO_4$ in comparison with PVA. PVA oxidized by $KMnO_4$ gives about half the peak of heat release rate (Peak R.H.R kW/m^2), when compared with pure PVA. Even at 50 kw/m^2, the yield of char residue for PVA oxidized by $KMnO_4$ was 9.1%. One reason for this phenomenon may be explained by the ability for PVA oxidized by $KMnO_4$—(polyvinyl ketone structures) to act as a neutral (structure 1) and/or monobasic (structure 2) bidentate ligand.[7]

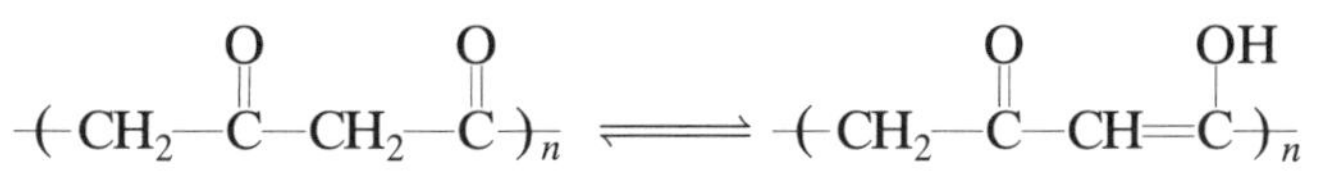

1 2

The experimental results of others (IR and electronic spectra)[8] provided strong evidence of coordination of the ligand (some metal ions Cu^{2+}, Ni^{2+}, Co^{2+}, Cd^{2+}, Hg^{2+}) through the monobasic bidentate mode (structure 2). Based on the above the following structure can be proposed for the polymeric complexes:

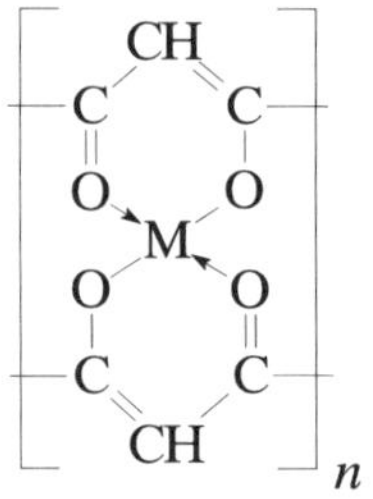

M—metal

The result of elemental analysis of PVA oxidized by $KMnO_4$ indicated the presence of 1.5% Mn remaining in this polymeric structure. Thus, we suggested that this catalytical amount of chelated Mn-structure incorporated in the polymer may provide the rapid high-temperature process of carbonization and formation of char.

The fire tests at 50 kW/m^2 for Nylon 6,6 and PVA (80:20%) compositions (typical rate of heat release curves for each sample is shown in Table 1 confirmed the assumption of the synergistic effect of carbonization.[7] Each of the individual polymers is less fire resistant than their composition. The sample with PVA oxidized by $KMnO_4$ displayed even better flame retardant properties due to the catalytical effect of Mn-chelate fragments on the formation of char.

Thus, the polymeric char former such as PVA, starch, glucose derivatives and polyfunctional alcohols may present a new trend in the global search for the type of ecologically-safe flame retardant systems.

LOW-MELTING GLASSES

The second example has been developed on the basis of an original concept of a low-melting phases (glasses) as a polymer additive.[9,10]

In principle, low-melting glasses can improve the thermal stability and flammability characteristics of polymers by:

1. Providing a thermal barrier for both undecomposed polymer and the char, if any, which forms as a combustion product.
2. Providing an oxidation barrier to retard oxidation of the thermally degrading polymer and its combustion char residue.
3. Providing a "glue" to hold the combustion char together and give it structural integrity.
4. Providing a coating to cover over, or fill in voids in the char, thus providing a more continuous external surface with a lower surface area.
5. Creating the potentially useful components of intumescent polymer additive systems.

W.J. Kroenke been developed a low-melting glass flame retardant system for PVC based on $ZnSO_4$–K_2SO_4–Na_2SO_4.[9] This system prove to be an excellent char former and a smoke depressant. Also tested were the FR-Low-melting—glasses systems with transition metals: Al, Ca, Ce, Ni, Mn, Co, V.

In the paper of J. Gilman it has been shown that silica gel in combination with potassium carbonate is an effective fire retardant for a wide variety of common polymers (at mass fraction of only 10% total additive) such as polypropylene, nylon, polymethylmethacrylate, poly (vinyl alcohol), cellulose, and to a lesser extent polystyrene and styrene-acrylonitrile.[13] The Cone Calorimeter data indicated that the peak heat release rate is reduced about two times without significantly increasing the smoke or carbon monoxide levels during the combustion. The efficacy of the additives in each of these inherently non-char-forming thermoplastic polymers (PP, PS, Nylon-6,6 and PMMA) depends on the polymer (PP > Nylon-6,6 PMMA > PS). The authors proposed a mechanism of action for these additives through the formation of a potassium silicate glass during the combustion. The pertinent phase diagrams do not show potassium silicate formation until 725°C. However, if sodium salts are present this temperature drops to 400°C–500°C. Other work on inorganic glass forming fire retardants examined an analogous borate/carbonate system; B_2O_3/MCO_3. These formulations were found to form an inorganic glassy foam as a surface barrier which insulated and slowed the escape of volatile decomposition gasses.[14]

POLYMER MORPHOLOGY MODIFICATION

The last representative of new trend in flame retardation is a modification of polymer physical structure (morphology) by means of polymer-polymer blends. We have found an extremal combustion behavior for a system polypropylene-polypropylene-co-polyethylene.[15] Which can be explained in terms of oxidative degradation of polymer materials. We studied the features of autooxidation and combustibility of blends of isotactic polypropylene (PP) and ethylene-propylene copolymers (PP-co-PE) as the thin films (50–80 μ). ASTM D2863 (ISO 4589 Part 2) was used to determine the oxygen index (LOI) for polymer films 140 by 52 mm.

The correlation between a polymer thermal oxidative degradation and its combustion under diffusion flames condition may represent an interesting specific application. In general, the solid phase polymer reaction can play the very important role in reduction of polymer combustibility. If we can decrease the reaction ability of a polymer relatively to oxygen, the critical conditions of the diffusion flame stability would change. Such a polymer will have a different fire behaviour. The LOI method should be a sensitive one to these transformations.

The kinetics of oxygen consumption for PP/PP-co-PE compositions is shown in Figure 1. It's clearly seen the composition of PP/PP-co-PE (62:38) has the highest induction period of auto-oxidation.

In this circumstances it has been proposed a theoretical model of a preliminary oxidation localization in interphaseous zone of a sample.[16] Apparently, the reaction ability of the compositions depends on the chemical structure of the interphaseous zone. It was shown the increase of PP concentration in the PP/PP-co-PE composition from 38 to 62% leads to the lowering of reaction ability of samples. The process of

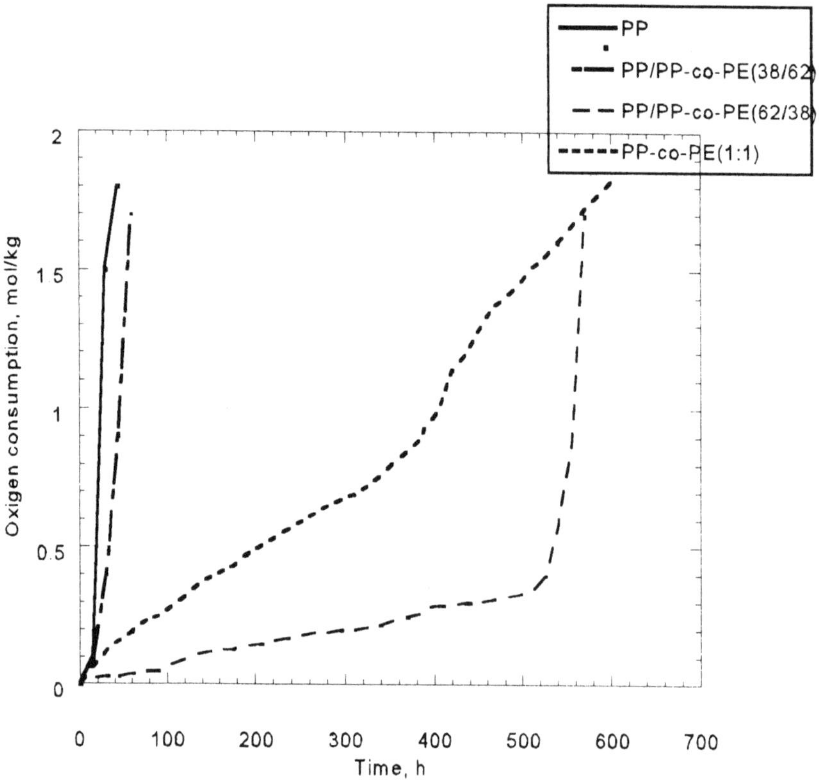

Figure 1 Kinetic curves of the oxygen consumption vs. time for PP/PP-co-PE compositions.

TABLE 2
LOI and char yield for PP/PP-co-PE compositions.

Composition	LOI	Char yield, % wt.
PP	17	0
PP/PP-co-PE—37,5/62,5	19.5	1.5
PP/PP-co-PE—61,5/38,5	21	3.4
PP-co-PE	18.5	0.5

auto-oxidation begins from the most active ingredient of a polymer composition, PP or PP-co-PE. Interphaseous zone decelerates the polymer oxidation. Otherwise, we simply have a different polymeric system with the different kinetic parameters of an oxidation and different mechanism of the solid phase reactions.

The combustibility tests confirm this hypothesis (Table 2). The sample with the minimal reaction activity, PP/PP-co-PE (62:38), has the highest values of LOI (21) and the char yield (3.4%).

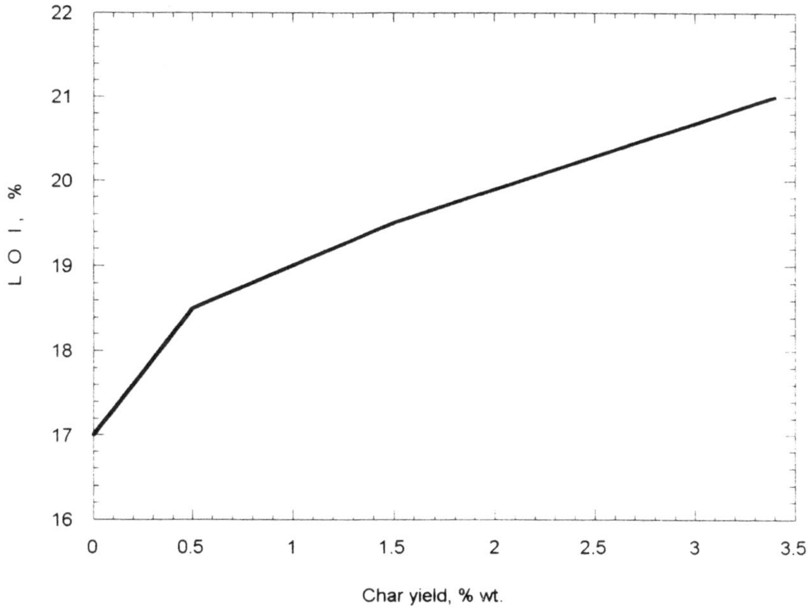

Figure 2 LOI vs. char yield for PP/PP-co-PE compositions.

A correlation between LOI and a char yield for studied polymer compositions is given in Figure 2. This data indicate the solid phase nature of the flame retardancy in PP/PP-co-PE compositions. The morphology modifications in the polymeric system lead to the desirable changes in combustibility.

REFERENCES

1. U.G. Ahlborg, G.C. Becking, L.S. Birnbaum, A. Brouwer, H. Derks, M. Freeley, G. Golor, A. Hanberg, J.C. Larsen, A. Liem, S.H. Safe, C. Schlatter, R. Waern and M. Younes, *Chemosphere*, 1994, **28**(6), p. 1049.
2. H. Beck, A. Dross and W. Mathar, *Environ. Health Perspect.*, **102** (Suppl 1), pp. 173–185.
3. R.E. Alcock and K.C. Jones, *Environmental Science & Technology*, 1996, **30**(11), p. 3133.
4. *US Environmental Protection Agency*, EPA/600, v. 1,2,3, 1994, Washington, DC.
5. G.E. Zaikov and S.M. Lomakin, ACS Symposium Series, *'Fire and Materials'*, Washington DC, 1995 **559**, p. 186.
6. G.E. Zaikov and S.M. Lomakin, *Polymer Degradation and Stability*, 1996, **54**(2–3), p. 223.
7. R.M. Hassan, *Polymer International*, 1993, **30**, p. 5.
8. R.M. Hassan, S.A. El-Gaiar and A.M. El-Summan, *Polymer International*, 1993, **32**, p. 39.
9. W.J. Kroenke, *Journal of Mat. Sci.*, 1986, **21**, p. 1123.
10. J.W. Gilman, S.J. Ritchie, Takashi Kashiwagi and S.M. Lomakin, *Fire and Materials*, 1997, **21**.
11. R.E. Myers and E. Licursi, *Journal of Fire Science*, 1985, **3**, p. 415.
12. S.M. Lomakin, L.S. Shibryaeva and G.E. Zaikov, *Chemical Physics*, (in Russian), 1997, in press.
13. L.S. Shibryaeva, A.A. Veretennikova, A.A. popov and T.A. Gugueva, *Visokomolec. Soed.*, 1997, (In Russian), in press.

Some Aspects of the Thermal Degradation of Poly(Vinyl Chloride)

B.B. TROITSKII and L.S. TROITSKAYA

Razuvaev Institute of Organometallic Chemistry, Russian Academy of Sciences, 49, Tropinina Street, 603600, Nizhny Novgorod, Russia

The kinetic factors and mechanism of the nonautocatalytic thermal degradation of PVC with effective removal of HCl are discussed. The papers which are concerned with the mathematical models of the initial stage of the nonautocatalytic thermal dehydrochlorination of idealized PVC, i.e., PVC having no abnormal fragments. The polymer, containing VC units and abnormal groups and the polymer having macromolecules with various stereoregularity, are considered. Mechanism of the autocatalytic thermal degradation of PVC in the presence of HCl is discussed.

INTRODUCTION

Poly(vinyl chloride) (PVC) is one of the most important commercial polymers. But PVC still poses many problems. Its rather low stability to the influence of heat and light requires stabilization of the polymer for practically all technical applications. The thermal degradation of PVC begins at temperatures above 100°C. PVC is one of the polymers, which decompose with isolation of side fragments from macromolecules. This leads to formation of HCl (> 90%) and polyenes:

$$\sim(CH_2{-}CHCl)_n\sim \longrightarrow m\mathrm{HCl} + \sim(CH_2{-}CHCl)_{n-m}{-}(CH{=}CH)_m\sim \qquad (1)$$

where $n > m$.

In spite of apparent simplicity of this summary reaction (1) the mechanism of the thermal degradation of PVC is very complicate. Besides units of vinyl chloride (VC) PVC macromolecules have abnormal fragments which appear due to peculiarities of radical polymerization of VC. At elevated temperatures polyenes, which form in the thermal degradation of PVC, may take part in the secondary reactions with each other, with HCl and so on. The thermal degradation of PVC is complicated by the catalytic effect of evolving HCl.

Effort to solve the degradation problems have led to the performance of many researches beginning with the papers cited in [1–3]. In recent years, the mechanism of the thermal degradation of PVC is intensively studied.[4–14]

It is well known[3–14] that the initial rate of the nonautocatalytic degradation of PVC with effective removal of HCl is much more than that of chlorohydrocarbons which are the low molecular weight models of the normal units of the polymer. It is generally assumed that structural abnormalities in the PVC chains are mainly responsible for the low thermal stability of the polymer.[3–14] There is considerable discussion about the nature and concentration of unstable fragments of PVC macromolecules and about their influence on the initial stage of polymer degradation.[3–14] The most important reason behind this is the difficulty in identifying and quantifying of the structural irregularities. The level of these abnormalities in the polymer is extremely low.

It has been shown that PVC contains 0.1–0.5 mol% of double bonds, 0.01–0.05 mol% of the internal chloroallylic fragments, 0.01–0.3 mol% of branching groups having the chlorine atom near the tertiary carbon atom, ~0.01 mol% of peroxide and hydroperoxide groups, up to 0.02 mol% of the internal "head-to-head" structures.[3–14] The authors of the paper [9] assume all the internal chloroallylic fragments to be conjugated ketoallylic groups.

Studies of the thermal degradation of the low molecular weight chlorohydrocarbons have shown that the internal chloroallylic structures, fragments with the chlorine atom near the tertiary carbon atom are unstable groups of PVC macromolecules.[3–15] Macromodels of PVC, containing known amounts of different unstable groups, have also been investigated. It has been demonstrated that an increase in concentration of the internal chloroallylic fragments, branching groups having the chlorine atom near the tertiary carbon atom, peroxide and hydroperoxide fragments leads to considerable increase of the initial rate of the thermal degradation of PVC.[4–14]

On the other hand, it is proposed that tacticity of macromolecules are mainly responsible for the low thermal stability of PVC.[5,12,13]

It is assumed[16–25] that one of the reason of the low thermal stability of PVC in comparison with the low molecular weight models of the normal units of the polymer is that PVC macromolecules contain much longer chains of VC units than investigated chlorohydrocarbons. The thermal degradation of low molecular weight model chlorohydrocarbons having only 1–2 units of VC has been studied in the liquid phase.[14,15]

The present review is concerned with several aspects of the thermal dehydrochlorination of PVC which have been studied recently by the authors and their collegues. Most of this work has been directed towards a detailed understanding of the kinetic peculiarities and mechanism of the nonautocatalytic degradation of PVC with effective removal of HCl and it has been greatly assisted by the use of the method of the mathematical models. In this review the mathematical models of the initial stage of the nonautocatalytic thermal degradation of idealized PVC, i.e., PVC having no abnormal fragments, the polymer which contains VC units and abnormal groups and the polymer having macromolecules with various stereoregularity, are considered. Mechanism of the autocatalytic thermal degradation of PVC in the presence of HCl is discussed.

1 KINETIC PECULIARITIES OF THE INITIAL STAGE OF THE NONAUTOCATALYTIC THERMAL DEGRADATION OF PVC WITH EFFECTIVE REMOVAL OF HCl

It is known[4–14] that in the presence of volatile products the thermal dehydrochlorination of PVC has an autocatalytic character, connected with the accelerating effect of HCl. The thermal degradation of PVC proceeds at different concentrations of HCl in the polymer depending on conditions in which experiment is carried out. In the paper [25] it has been discussed two extreme cases between which one can place many intermediate versions of the thermal degradation of PVC:

(i) A thin layer of twice precipitated PVC is decomposed in high vacuo with continuous and effective removal of HCl or a dilute solution of PVC in inert solvent is degraded with continuous and effective removal of HCl by stream of inert gas.
(ii) PVC is degraded in closed reaction vessel. HCl is not removed.

In the first case, the dehydrochlorination rate has a maximum value at the beginning and then decreases during the early stage and become principally steady up to some per cent of conversion (Figure 1, curve 1).[10,11,16,17,21,24–43]

In the second case, the kinetic curves of PVC dehydrochlorination have an autocatalytic character.[10,25,27,29,32,33,35–37]

In the papers [38, 39] critical phenomena which are observed in the thermal degradation of the polymer with continuous and effective removal of HCl, have been investigated. It has been obtained the value of critical thickness of PVC film, i.e., maximum thickness of the polymer film at which the thermal degradation of the polymer with effective removal of volatile products proceeds without autocatalysis. It is equal to 0.24, 0.18 and 0.15 mm at 190, 200 and 210°C respectively.[39]

The influence of reprecipitation of PVC samples on the thermal degradation of the polymer with effective removal of HCl has been discussed.[25]

Sections 1–4 of this review deals with the first case of the thermal degradation of PVC with continuous and effective removal of HCl. In section 5, the mechanism of

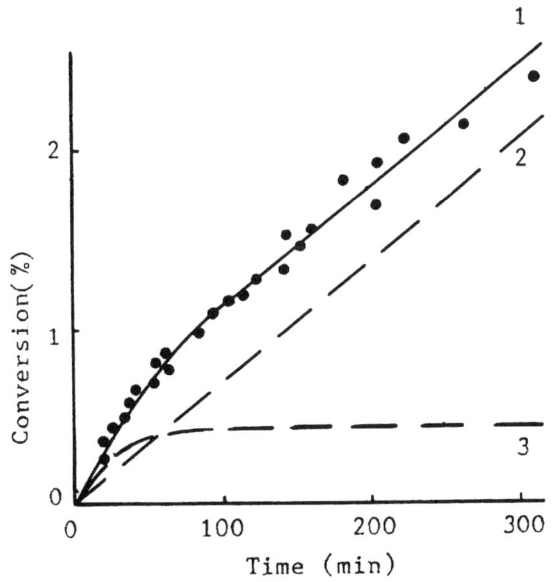

Figure 1 Kinetic curve of dehydrochlorination of PVC in vacuo ($\sim 10^{-4}$ mmHg) with continuous removal of HCl by freezing at 200°C (1), separated into curves 2 and 3.[29]

the autocatalytic thermal degradation of PVC in the presence of HCl is considered. It has been shown[29,36,37,40,41,43] that the kinetic curves of the initial stage (up to 10% conversion) of the nonautocatalytic thermal dehydrochlorination of PVC with effective removal of HCl at 180–210°C (Figure 1, curve 1) may be separated into two curves (curves 2 and 3) which are described by the equations for first-order reactions with different rate constants. The supposition has been made that the overall process of PVC dehydrochlorination consists of two processes which proceed simultaneously.[10,29,36,37,40,41,43] It has been proposed that curve 3 corresponds to the thermal dehydrochlorination of unstable fragments, present in the original polymer, and curve 2 corresponds to the thermal degradation of PVC initiated by dehydrochlorination of the normal units of macromolecules (Figure 1). As can be seen from Figure 1 (curve 3), unstable fragments, present in the original polymer, degrade completely during the early stage of PVC dehydrochlorination (less than 2% conversion). From the half-conversion period, $\tau_{1/2}$, (Figure 1, curve 3) the effective constants of rates of degradation of unstable fragments, k^{ef}_{unstab}, has been calculated for various samples of PVC[36,37,40,41,44] (Table 1). For the sample B (Table 1) the thermal degradation of unstable fragments, present in the original polymer, has been described by the equation for first-order reaction with the following effective rate constant:[29,36,37,40,43]

$$k^{ef}_{unst} = 10^{9.6 \pm 0.5} \times e^{-28000 \pm 1000/RT} \text{ sec}^{-1} \tag{2}$$

Above ~2–3% conversion the thermal degradation of PVC is initiated by the statistical degradation of the normal units of the polymer (Figure 1).[10,29,36,37,40,41,43]

In the papers [29, 40, 41] the thermal degradation of PVC has been carried out at higher temperatures, viz., 220–250°C and up to a higher per cent of conversion, viz., 25–70%. The kinetic curves for PVC degradation at 220–250°C are described by the equation for first-order reaction up to ~40% conversion. Above ~40% conversion the rate of PVC dehydrochlorination decreases more quickly than that calculated from the equation for first-order reaction.

The following Arrhenius expression for the effective constant of the rate of the thermal dehydrochlorination of PVC initiated by the statistical degradation of the

TABLE 1
The values of the effective rate constants of the thermal degradation of unstable fragments of various samples of PVC, k^{ef}_{unstab}, at 200°C calculated in [44] by method from [36, 37, 40, 41].

Number	Sample of PVC	$k^{ef}_{unst} \times 10^4$, sec^{-1}
1.	A	4.44
2.	B	6.24
3.	C	2.96
4.	D	3.6
5.	H	2.31
6.	K	2.31

Note: A, B, C and D are samples from Ref. 25; H and K are samples from Ref. 28.

normal units of the polymer, k_0^{ef}, has been obtained from the dependence of the logarithm of the initial rate of this reaction on $1/T$ at 180–250°C:[29,40,41]

$$k_0^{ef} = 10^{11.8 \pm 0.5} \times e^{-38000 \pm 1000/RT} \text{ sec}^{-1}. \tag{3}$$

It is shown[29,43] that

$$k_0^{ef} = k_0 l_{av} \text{ and } k_0 = k_0^{ef}/l_{av} \tag{4}$$

where k_0 is the constant of the rate of the thermal degradation of the normal units of PVC; l_{av} represents the average length of kinetic chain of PVC dehydrochlorination. The value of l_{av} has been determined to be equal to 8–15.[28–30,45]

From the equations (3) and (4) at $l_{av} = 8$[29,30] the following expression for k_0 has been obtained:[43]

$$k_0 = 10^{11.0 \pm 0.5} \times e^{-38000 \pm 1000/RT} \text{ sec}^{-1}. \tag{5}$$

2 MATHEMATICAL MODELS OF THE INITIAL STAGE OF THE THERMAL DEGRADATION OF PVC OBTAINED BY THE USE OF THE THEORY OF PROBABILITY AND THE THEORY OF THE CONSECUTIVE REACTIONS

In the papers [16–24], the mathematical models of the initial stage (up to 10% conversion) of the thermal dehydrochlorination of PVC has been proposed using the theory of probability and the theory of the consecutive reactions[46] by means of consideration of the degradation of the low molecular weight models for various fragments of PVC macromolecules by molecular mechanism in inert atmosphere in the absence of catalytic effect of HCl without consideration of peculiarities of the stereochemical structure of model chlorohydrocarbons in the assumption that $k_0 \ll k_1 \ll k_2 \cong k_3 \cong \ldots \cong k_{n-1}$, where $k_1, k_2, \ldots, k_{n-1}$ represent the effective constants of rates of dehydrochlorination of fragments with 1, 2, 3, ..., $n-1$ double bonds respectively; n is the number of VC units in chlorohydrocarbon. The values of k_0, k_1 and k_2 which have been obtained in the thermal degradation of chlorohydrocarbons in the liquid phase in the absence of HCl[15] have been used.

2.1 The Thermal Degradation of Low Molecular Weight Chlorohydrocarbons Containing only VC Units

It has been shown,[18,23,24] that the initial stage of the thermal degradation of model chlorohydrocarbons containing only VC units and having "head-to-tail" structure may be described by the following expressions:

$$[\text{HCl}]_{\text{norm}} = l_{av}C_0^0(1 - e^{-k_0 t}) - (l_{av} - 1)C_0^0\frac{k_0}{k_1}(1 - e^{-k_1 t}). \tag{6}$$

$$\text{V}_{\text{norm}} = [l_{av}k_0 e^{-k_0 t} - (l_{av} - 1)k_0 e^{-k_1 t}]C_0^0. \tag{7}$$

where C_0^0 represents the initial concentration of chlorohydrocarbon; t is the time of degradation.

For statistical initiation l_{av} may be defined as:[23]

$$l_{av} = \sum_{i=1}^{n} \frac{l_i}{n} = \frac{1}{2}(n+1) \tag{8}$$

Figure 2 shows the calculated values from equation (7), the curves of the dependence of the dehydrochlorination rate on time for degradation of chlorohydrocarbons have a different number of VC units at 200°C.[18] It is seen that the rates of degradation of compounds with $n \geq 2$ increase in the early stage and then become practically steady. In the stationary part of dehydrochlorination curves the rate of degradation, V_{stat}, may be described by the following equation which is typical for the unbranching chain reactions:[23,24]

$$V_{stat} = V_{init}\, l_{av} = k_0 C_0 l_{av}, \tag{9}$$

where V_{init} is the rate of initiation.

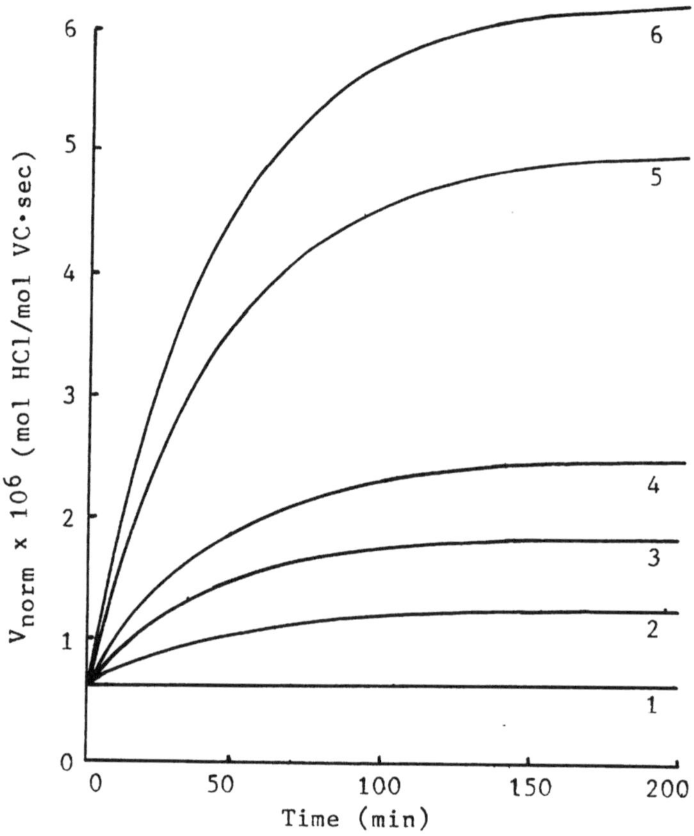

Figure 2 Calculated from equation (7) curves of the dependence of dehydrochlorination rate on time for the thermal degradation of chlorohydrocarbons, having different number of VC units (n), at 200°C: (1) $n = 1$; (2) $n = 3$; (3) $n = 5$; (4) $n = 7$; (5) $n = 15$; (6) $n = 19$.[18]

As can be seen from equations (6)–(9) and Figure 2, the value of l_{av} is of particular importance in the initial stage of the thermal degradation of chlorohydrocarbons. The less the number of VC units in the chlorohydrocarbon, the more stable it is.

It has been shown[18,23,24] that the equations (6) and (7) may be used for the initial stage of the thermal degradation of idealized PVC if the values of l_{av} for the thermal dehydrochlorination of PVC and the model compounds are equal to each other.

In the paper [23], the possible termination reactions of the chain of the thermal dehydrochlorination of chlorohydrocarbons, such as intermolecular Diels-Alder reaction between generated polyenes and the reaction of intramolecular cyclization of formed trienes and tetraenes, have been examined. The rates of reactions of chain termination have been compared with the rate of dehydrochlorination quantitatively.[23]

It has been shown that the termination of dehydrochlorination chain of chlorohydrocarbons occurs most probably due to the reaction of intramolecular cyclization of generated tetraenes and in the thermal degradation of chlorohydrocarbons having $n \geq 7$, $l_{av} \geq 4$.

As mentioned above, in the thermal degradation of PVC the value of l_{av} has been determined to be equal to 8–15.[28–30,45] Substitution of these values of l_{av} into equation (8) shows that low molecular weight chlorohydrocarbons, which may serve as models for PVC macromolecules, must contain 15 units of VC at a minimum.

Except the reaction of intramolecular cyclization of tetraenes, there are other reactions which may lead to the termination of dehydrochlorination of chlorohydrocarbons. The termination of dehydrochlorination chain may take place due to stereochemical reasons, when there is no conjugation of the double bond formed with conjugated double bonds which have been generated before.[27] The termination of chain may result from the reaction of formation of allene fragments by the following equation too:

$$\sim CH{=}CH{-}CH{=}CH{-}\underset{\displaystyle Cl}{\underset{|}{CH}}{-}CH_2\sim \longrightarrow \sim CH{=}CH{-}CH{=}C{=}CH{-}CH_2\sim + HCl \qquad (10)$$

2.2 The Thermal Degradation of Low Molecular Weight Hydrocarbons Containing VC Units and Unstable Fragments

The mathematical models of the thermal degradation of these model compounds have been considered under the following additional conditions:[17,21,24]

(i) The reaction of initiation, i.e., elimination of the first molecule of HCl, always occurs from the unstable fragment.
(ii) The termination of dehydrochlorination chain occurs due to the reaction of intramolecular cyclization of the generated tetraenes.

2.2.1 *The thermal degradation of low molecular weight chlorohydrocarbons having VC units and branching fragments with the chlorine atom near the tertiary carbon atom*

The thermal degradation of these chlorohydrocarbons may be described by the following equations:

Initiation:

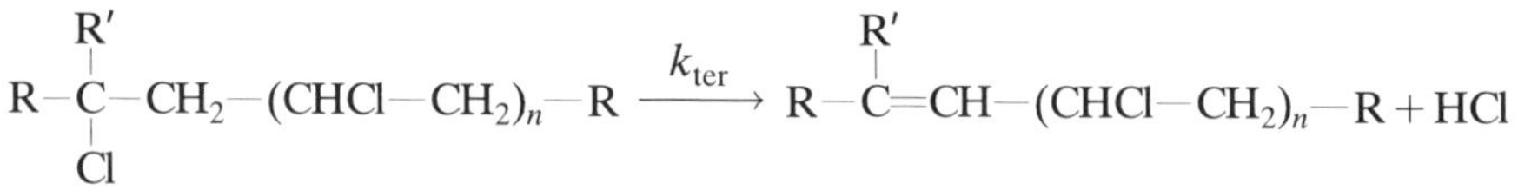

(11)

Propagation:

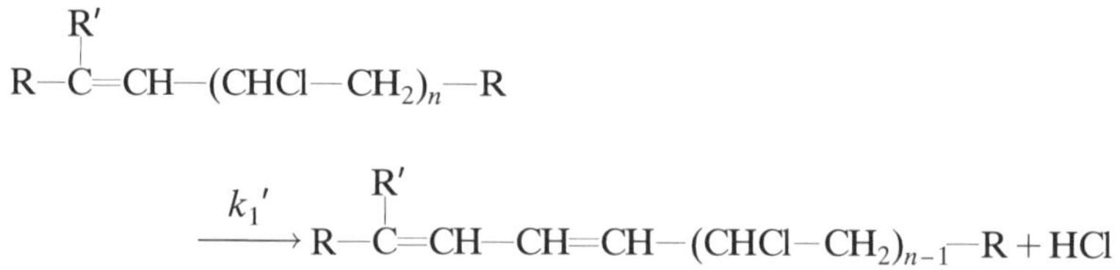

(12)

Termination:

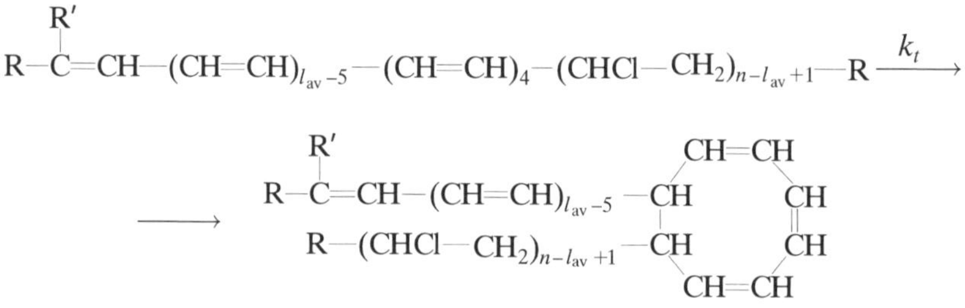

(13)

where R is alkyl; k_{ter} represents the effective constant of rate of dehydrochlorination of the branching fragments with the chlorine atom near the tertiary carbon atom; k_t is the constant of the rate of termination of dehydrochlorination chain.

The following expressions for the initial stage of degradation of model chlorohydrocarbons containing VC units and fragments with the chlorine atom near the tertiary carbon atom have been deduced:[21,24]

$$V_{ter} = k_{ter}C^0_{ter}\left[e^{-k_{ter}t} + (l_{av} - 1)\frac{k'_1}{k_{ter} - k'_1}(e^{-k'_1 t} - e^{-k_{ter}t})\right] \quad (14)$$

$$[HCl]_{ter} = C^0_{ter}(1 - e^{-k_{ter}t}) - (l_{av} - 1)C^0_{ter}\frac{k'_1}{k_{ter} - k'_1}(1 - e^{-k_{ter}t}) + (l_{av} - 1)C^0_{ter} \times \frac{k_{ter}}{k_{ter} - k_j}(1 - e^{-k'_1 t}) \quad (15)$$

where C^0_{ter} represents the initial concentration of chlorohydrocarbon having fragment with the chlorine atom near the tertiary carbon atom.

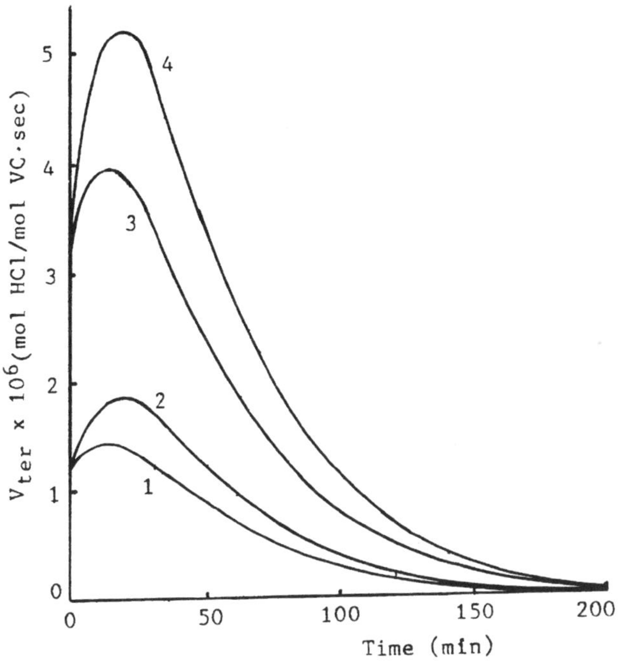

Figure 3 Calculated from equation (14) curves of the dependence of dehydrochlorination rate on time for the thermal degradation of chlorohydrocarbons, having VC units and fragment with the chlorine atom near the tertiary carbon atom, at different l_{av} and C^0_{ter} at 200°C in inert solvent: (1) and (3) $l_{av} = 6$; (2) and (4) $l_{av} = 8$; (1) and (2) $C^0_{ter} = 0.1$ mol%; (3) and (4) $C^0_{ter} = 0.28$ mol%.[21]

Figure 3 shows calculated values from equation (14) for the dependence of the rate on time for the thermal degradation of these chlorohydrocarbons at 200°C. The value of k_{ter} used was obtained for the thermal degradation of low molecular weight chlorohydrocarbon in the liquid phase [47]. As can be seen from Figure 3, the dependences of rate of dehydrochlorination of chlorohydrocarbons on time has a maximum at short times of degradation. The greater l_{av} and C^0_{ter}, the more considerable the maximum becomes. Then the dehydrochlorination rate decreases then to a small value. Figure 3 demonstrates that low molecular weight model chlorohydrocarbons having branching fragments with the chlorine atom near the tertiary carbon atom degrade completely after ~200 min at 200°C.

2.2.2 The thermal degradation of low molecular weight chlorohydrocarbons having VC links and the internal chloroallylic fragments

The thermal degradation of these chlorohydrocarbons may be represented by the following equations:

Initiation:

$$\mathrm{R{-}CH{=}CH{-}(CHCl{-}CH_2)_n{-}R} \xrightarrow{k_1} \mathrm{R{-}(CH{=}CH)_2{-}(CHCl{-}CH_2)_{n-1}{-}R + HCl} \qquad (16)$$

Propagation:

$$\mathrm{R{-}(CH{=}CH)_2{-}(CHCl{-}CH_2)_{\mathit{n}-1}{-}R} \xrightarrow{k_2} \mathrm{R{-}(CH{=}CH)_3{-}(CHCl{-}CH_2)_{\mathit{n}-2}{-}R + HCl} \tag{17}$$

Termination:

$$\mathrm{R{-}(CH{=}CH)_{\mathit{l}_{av}-3}{-}(CH{=}CH)_4{-}(CHCl{-}CH_2)_{\mathit{n}-\mathit{l}_{av}}{-}R}$$

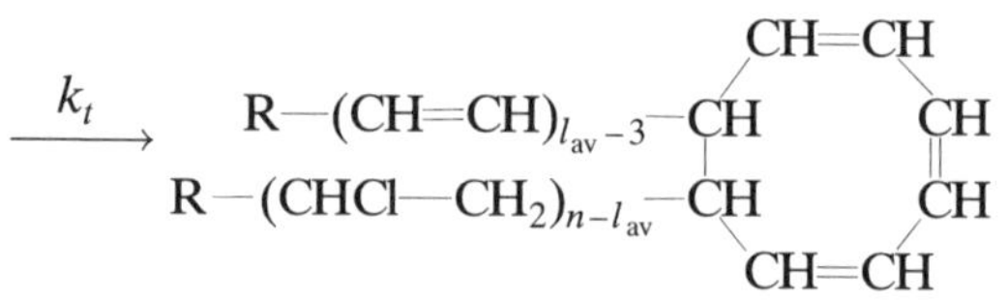

(18)

It has been shown that the initial stage of the thermal degradation of these model chlorohydrocarbons may be described by the following expressions:[21,24]

$$V_{\mathrm{all}} = k_1 C^0_{\mathrm{all}} \mathrm{e}^{-k_1 t} l_{\mathrm{av}} \tag{19}$$

$$[\mathrm{HCl}]_{\mathrm{all}} = C^0_{\mathrm{all}} (l - \mathrm{e}^{-k_1 t}) l_{\mathrm{av}} \tag{20}$$

where C^0_{all} represents the initial concentration of chlorohydrocarbon containing the internal chloroallylic fragment.

Figure 4 shows values calculated from equation (19) for the dependence of the rate on time for the thermal degradation of these chlorohydrocarbons at 200°C. As can be seen, the initial rate of degradation of chlorohydrocarbons is in direct proportion to concentration of chloroallylic fragments and l_{av}. The time for full degradation of the model compound containing the chloroallylic groups is equal to ~200 min at 200°C (Figure 4).[21,24]

2.3 Comparison of the Kinetic Curves for the Thermal Dehydrochlorination of PVC with Effective Removal of HCl with the Theoretical Curves of the Thermal Degradation of the Low Molecular Weight Models of PVC Macromolecules

2.3.1 Comparison of the kinetic curves for PVC degradation with the theoretical curves for decomposition of chlorohydrocarbons containing only VC units

In the paper [25], a comparison of the experimental curves of the dependence of the dehydrochlorination rate on time which have been obtained by different authors[25,28,32,38] for the initial stage (up to 10% conversion) of the thermal degradation of more than 20 various samples of PVC with effective removal of HCl at

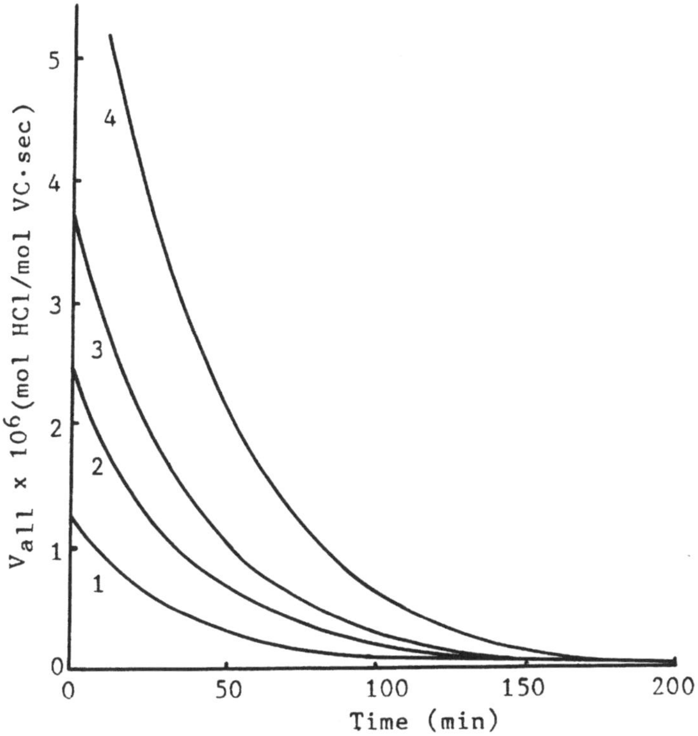

Figure 4 Calculated from equation (19) curves of the dependence of dehydrochlorination rate on time for the thermal degradation of chlorohydrocarbons, having VC units and the internal chloroallylic fragment, at different l_{av} and C^0_{all} at 200°C in inert solvent: (1) and (3) $l_{av} = 4$; (2) and (4) $l_{av} = 7$; (1) and (2) $C^0_{all} = 0.1$ mol%; (3) and (4) $C^0_{all} = 0.3$ mol%.[21]

180–210°C are presented. The theoretical curves for the thermal degradation of chlorohydrocarbons containing only VC units, which are the low molecular weight model compounds for idealized PVC are also presented. The theoretical curves have been calculated from the equation (7) using the values of k_0 and k_1 which have been determined for the thermal degradation of chlorohydrocarbons in the liquid phase with removal of HCl.[14,15] Data obtained in the paper [25], show clearly that the initial rates of degradation of the various samples of PVC (at $t \to 0$) are 3–30 (and more) times greater than the initial rates of the dehydrochlorination of model chlorohydrocarbons having only VC units. This indicates that the thermal degradation of unstable fragments, present in the original polymer, make the main contribution to the initial rate of degradation of PVC (at $t \to 0$). After a definite period of time ($\sim 100 - 150$ min at 200°C) unstable groups, present in the original PVC, decompose and the stationary rate of dehydrochlorination of PVC samples is determined only by the rate of degradation of the normal units of macromolecules.[25] It has been shown[25] that the stationary rates of dehydrochlorination of the various samples of PVC are not equal to each other and at most three times different from one another. But discrepancy between the stationary rates is considerably less than between the initial rates.

It has been considered that there are two reasons which may lead to deviation of the values of the stationary rates of degradation of the various samples of PVC.[25] First, the concentration of HCl in the polymer particles of the various samples of PVC having complicated morphological structure, various sizes and density may differ from one another due to the different rates of diffusion of HCl from them. Secondly, the results show that the higher the initial rate of PVC dehydrochlorination, the greater the stationary one.[25] It has been proposed[25] that the more HCl eliminated at the beginning of PVC dehydrochlorination, the greater is the effect of HCl on the stationary rate. One can also assume that in the initial stage of the thermal degradation of PVC samples having increased values of the stationary rates, the new structures, which initiate the dehydrochlorination of the normal units of PVC macromolecules, form [48]. This will be discussed in detail below in section 4.

Data, obtained in the paper [25], show that the stationary rates for the thermal dehydrochlorination of three different samples of PVC, namely of finely dispersed PVC powder (sample B), thin polymer film (sample I) and 1% 1,2,4-trichlorobenzene solution of PVC (sample H), which were decomposed with continuous and effective removal of HCl at 200°C at various conditions by different investigators,[25,28,38] are practically the same and have the least value, $V^{\min}_{\text{stat}} = 8 \times 10^{-7}$–$10 \times 10^{-7}$ mol HCl/

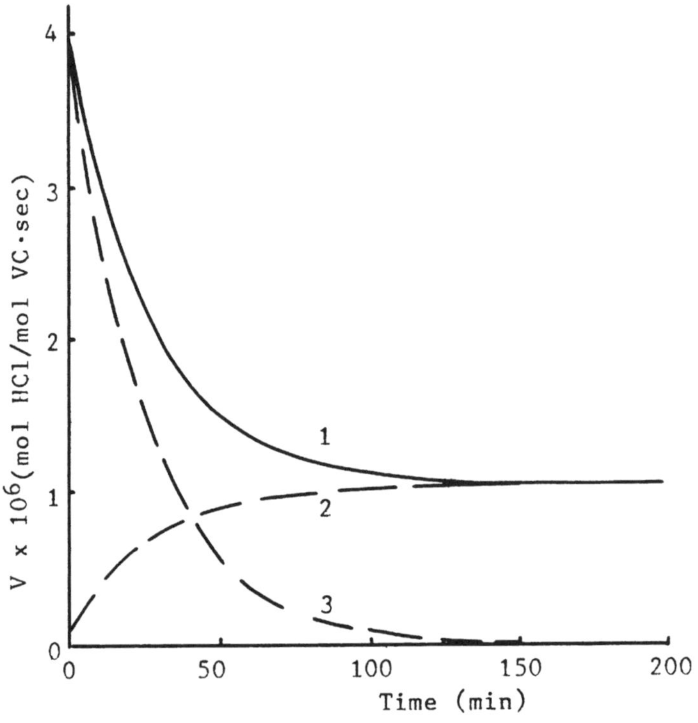

Figure 5 Dependence of dehydrochlorination rate on time at 200°C for thermal degradation of (1) PVC sample B in vacuo ($\sim 10^{-4}$ mmHg) with continuous removal of HCl by freezing; (2) idealized PVC containing only VC units; (3) unstable fragments present in original PVC sample B.[44] Curve 2 is calculated from equation (7) at the meanings of parameters obtained for PVC sample B. Curve 3 is obtained by geometrical substraction of curve 2 from curve 1. B is sample from Ref. 25.

mol VC sec. It has been concluded[25] that V_{stat}^{min} characterize the thermal degradation of PVC initiated by dehydrochlorination of normal units of macromolecules without influence of HCl.

The value of V_{stat}^{min} coincides with the calculated meaning of the stationary rate for degradation of model chlorohydrocarbons, containing only VC units, at $l_{av} \cong 0.9$–1.3.[25] But one must bear in mind that for calculations of the rate of degradation of model chlorohydrocarbons the value of $k_0 = 8.27 \times 10^{-7}\ sec^{-1}$, which has been obtained for the thermal dehydrochlorination of 8-chlorohexadecane at 200°C in liquid phase,[15] has been used (see section 2.1.). It has been shown that $l_{av} = 8$ for sample B[30] and $l_{av} = 10.4$ for sample H.[28] Using these experimental values of l_{av} and the value of V_{stat}^{min}, from the equation (9) one can obtain at 200°C, k_0 is equal to $1.3 \times 10^{-7}\ sec^{-1}$ and $7.4 \times 10^{-8}\ sec^{-1}$ for degradation of samples B and H respectively. Comparison of these values of k_0 with the value of k_0 for dehydrochlorination of 8-chlorohexadecane at 200°C shows that the latter is 6–11 times greater than the value of k_0 for degradation of VC units in PVC macromolecule.

Figures 5 and 6 represent the experimental curves of the dependence of the dehydrochlorination rate on time for degradation of samples B (Figure 5) and H (Figure 6) at 200°C and the calculated from the equation (7) curves of the dependence of the dehydrochlorination rate on time for degradation of model chlorohydrocarbons, containing only VC units, at the values of k_0, k_1 and l_{av}, which were

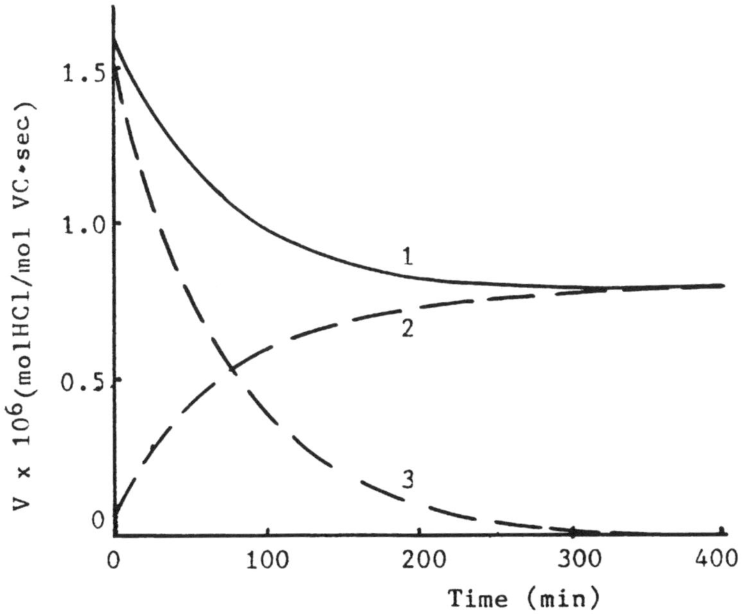

Figure 6 Dependence of dehydrochlorination rate on time at 200°C for thermal degradation of (1) 1% solution of PVC in 1,2,4-trichlorobenzene (sample H) with continuous removal of HCl by stream of inert gas; (2) idealized PVC containing only VC units; (3) unstable fragments present in original PVC sample H.[44] Curve 2 is calculated from equation (7) at the meaning of parameters obtained for PVC sample H. Curve 3 is obtained by geometrical substraction of curve 2 from curve 1. H is sample from Ref. 28.

obtained for samples B and H for the condition that $k_1 = k^{ef}_{unstab}$.[44] The values of k_1 were taken from Table 1.

It has been concluded[25] that comparison of the kinetic curves of the initial stage of the thermal degradation of PVC samples with the theoretical ones for decomposition of model compounds, containing only VC units, makes it possible to evaluate the summary contribution of degradation of unstable fragments present in the original PVC to the initial rate of dehydrochlorination of specific samples of PVC at $t \to 0$ quantitatively. This effect is seen from Figures 5 and 6.

2.3.2 *Comparison of the kinetic curves for PVC degradation with the theoretical curves for decomposition of mixture of chlorohydrocarbon having only VC units with compound containing VC units and unstable fragment*

Using the equations (6) and (20) and the expressions (7) and (19), one can obtain the following equations (21) and (22) which describe the initial stage of degradation of mixtures of chlorohydrocarbon, containing only VC units, with model compound having VC units and the internal chloroallylic fragment:

$$[\mathrm{HCl}]_1 = [\mathrm{HCl}]_{norm} + [\mathrm{HCl}]_{all} \tag{21}$$

$$V_1 = V_{norm} + V_{all} \tag{22}$$

The equations (23) and (24) which were obtained from equations (6) and (15) and equations (7) and (14), describe the initial stage of the thermal degradation of mixture of chlorohydrocarbon, containing only VC units, with model compound having VC units and the branching fragment with the chlorine atom near the tertiary carbon atom:

$$[\mathrm{HCl}]_2 = [\mathrm{HCl}]_{norm} + [\mathrm{HCl}]_{ter} \tag{23}$$

$$V_2 = V_{norm} + V_{ter} \tag{24}$$

The summation of equations (6), (15) and (20) and equations (7), (14) and (19) gives the expressions (25) and (26) which describe the initial stage of decomposition of the triple mixture of model chlorohydrocarbons, containing only VC inits, VC units and the internal chloroallylic group and VC units and the branching fragment with the chlorine atom near the tertiary carbon atom, in any ratio:

$$[\mathrm{HCl}]_3 = [\mathrm{HCl}]_{norm} + [\mathrm{HCl}]_{all} + [\mathrm{HCl}]_{ter} \tag{25}$$

$$V_3 = V_{norm} + V_{all} + V_{ter} \tag{26}$$

Using equations (15) and (20) and equations (14) and (19), one can obtain the expressions (27) and (28) which describe the initial stage of degradation of mixture of model chlorohydrocarbon, containing VC units and the internal chloroallylic group, with model compound having VC units and fragment with the chlorine atom near the tertiary carbon atom:

$$[\mathrm{HCl}]_4 = [\mathrm{HCl}]_{all} + [\mathrm{HCl}]_{ter} \tag{27}$$

$$V_4 = V_{all} + V_{ter} \tag{28}$$

In the papers [21,24], satisfactory coincidence of the theoretical curves of the thermal degradation of PVC calculated from expressions (21) and (23) with experimental ones, has been obtained. In the papers [44,49], good coincidence has been attained between the theoretical curves of the thermal dehydrochlorination of various samples of PVC which were calculated from equations (21)–(28), with the experimental curves. In the paper [49], integral and differential kinetic curves for the initial stage of the thermal degradation of nine samples of PVC in vacuo with continuous removal of HCl at 200°C have been obtained. It has been shown that these kinetic curves are well described by the expressions (21) and (22) respectively. The values of k^{ef}_{unstab} were calculated from the experimental curves of dehydrochlorination of PVC samples by the method proposed before.[36,37,40,41] At 200°C they are equal to 2.8×10^{-4}–$4.6 \times 10^{-4}\,sec^{-1}$. The investigated samples of PVC were calculated to contain 0.1–0.3 mol% of unstable fragments. There is the correlation between the total concentration of unstable groups in PVC samples and the initial rate of degradation of the polymers.[49] The obtained values of k^{ef}_{unstab} for PVC samples are close to the rate constants for the thermal degradation of the low molecular weight model chlorohydrocarbons having the branching groups with the chlorine atom near the tertiary carbon atom or the internal chloroallylic fragments in the liquid phase.[14,15,47] It has been concluded that these groups may be the main unstable fragments of PVC macromolecules.[49]

It is of interest to consider data which has been obtained for PVC samples having known quantity of unstable fragments.[44] In the paper [28], the series of PVC samples, containing various quantity of the internal chloroallylic groups, have been prepared by controlled chemical dehydrochlorination of the same sample of PVC (sample H) at low temperature. The thermal degradation of 1% 1,2,4-trichlorobenzene solution of these samples has been studied with effective removal of HCl. By geometrical substraction of the kinetic curve of dehydrochlorination of sample H having $C^0_{all} = 6 \times 10^{-5}$mol/mol VC from the kinetic curve of degradation of sample K having $C^0_{all} = 1.07 \times 10^{-3}$mol/mol VC, the kinetic curve of dehydrochlorination of PVC initiated by degradation of the internal chloroallylic fragments has been obtained at $C^0_{all} = 1.01 \times 10^{-3}$mol/mol VC (Figure 7, curve 1).[44] Figure 7 (curve 2) shows the theoretical curve of PVC dehydrochlorination initiated by degradation of the internal chloroallylic groups which was calculated from the equation (20) at the same value of C^0_{all} and at $k_1 = 2.55 \times 10^{-4}\,sec^{-1}$ and $l_{av} = 11.045$. In the paper [28], practically the same values of l_{av} have been determined for sample H ($l_{av} = 10.4$) and sample K ($l_{av} = 11.6$). From curve 1 (Figure 7) one can obtain the value of $\tau_{1/2}$. Using this value of $\tau_{1/2}$ it is possible to calculate $k^{ef}_{unstab} = 2.6 \times 10^{-4}\,sec^{-1}$ at 200°C. In this case k^{ef}_{unstab} is k_1, i.e., the constant of the rate of degradation of the internal chloroallylic fragments of PVC macromolecules. Thus, data, obtained in the papers [28,44], make it possible to evaluate k_1 in the thermal degradation of PVC.

Figure 8 represents the integral [Figure 8(a)] and differential [Figure 8(b)] kinetic curves of dehydrochlorination of sample H at 200°C (curves 1). The theoretical curves 1′, 2 and 3 were obtained under the assumption that sample H has only the internal chloroallylic groups as unstable fragments.[44] The curves 1′, 2 and 3 were calculated at the same values of parameters from the equations (21) [Figure 8(a)] and (22) [Figure 8(b)], the expressions (6) [Figure 8(a)] and (7) [Figure 8(b)] and the equations (20) [Figure 8(a)] and (19) [Figure 8(b)], respectively. Curve 1′

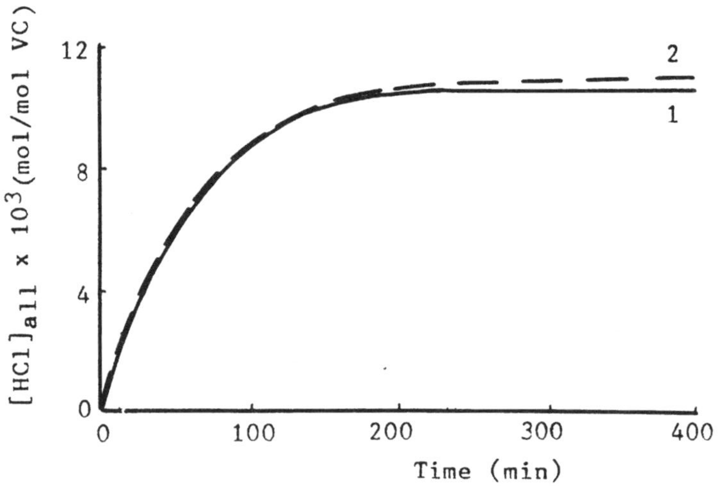

Figure 7 Kinetic curve of dehydrochlorination of internal chloroallylic fragments of PVC at 200°C (1). Curve 2 is calculated from equation (20).[44]

corresponds to the geometrical sum of curves 2 and 3. The theoretical curve 1′ coincides with the experimental curve 1 at the following values of parameters: $k_0 = 7 \times 10^{-8}\,\text{sec}^{-1}$, $C^0_{\text{all}} = 6 \times 10^{-4}$mol/mol VC, $l_{\text{av}} = 11.045$ and $k_1 = 2.3 \times 10^{-4}\,\text{sec}^{-1}$. It is necessary to note that the value of k_1 corresponds to the value of $k^{\text{ef}}_{\text{unstab}}$ which was determined for sample H from the value of $\tau_{1/2}$ (Table 1). The meanings of k_0 and l_{av} coincide practically with the meanings of these parameters obtained in the paper [28]. But the value of C^0_{all} which was chosen for coincidence of the theoretical curve 1′ with the experimental curve 1, is 10 times greater than that determined for sample H in the paper [28]. One may assume that sample H has not only the internal chloroallylic fragments but other unstable groups as well.

Figure 9 shows the theoretical curves of PVC dehydrochlorination (curves 1′, 2 and 3) which were obtained under the assumption that in sample H there are the internal chloroallylic fragments and the branching groups with the chlorine atom near the tertiary carbon atom, the concentration of the internal chloroallylic fragments being equal to that determined in the paper [28]. The theoretical curves 1′, 2 and 3 were calculated at the same meanings of parameters from the equations (25) [Figure 9(a)] and (26) [Figure 9(b)], the equations (6) [Figure 9(a)] and (7) [Figure 9(b)] and the equations (27) [Figure 9(a)] and (28) [Figure 9(b)], respectively. The coincidence of the experimental curve 1, with the theoretical curve 1′ is observed at the following meanings of parameters: $k_0 = 7 \times 10^{-8}\,\text{sec}^{-1}$, $C^0_{\text{all}} = 6 \times 10^{-5}$ mol/mol VC, $k_1 = 2.3 \times 10^{-4}\,\text{sec}^{-1}$, $C^0_{\text{ter}} = 5.45 \times 10^{-4}$ mol/mol VC, $k_{\text{ter}} = 2.31 \times 10^{-4}\,\text{sec}^{-1}$ and $l_{\text{av}} = 11.045$. From Figure 9(b) one can see that in this case the differential theoretical curves 1′ and 3 have maximum at small times of degradation. Thus, it has been shown that the initial stage (up to ~10% conversion) of the thermal dehydrochlorination of PVC may be described by the equations (21)–(26) which have been deduced under the supposition that the thermal degradation of PVC initiates by decomposition of normal units and unstable fragments such as the internal

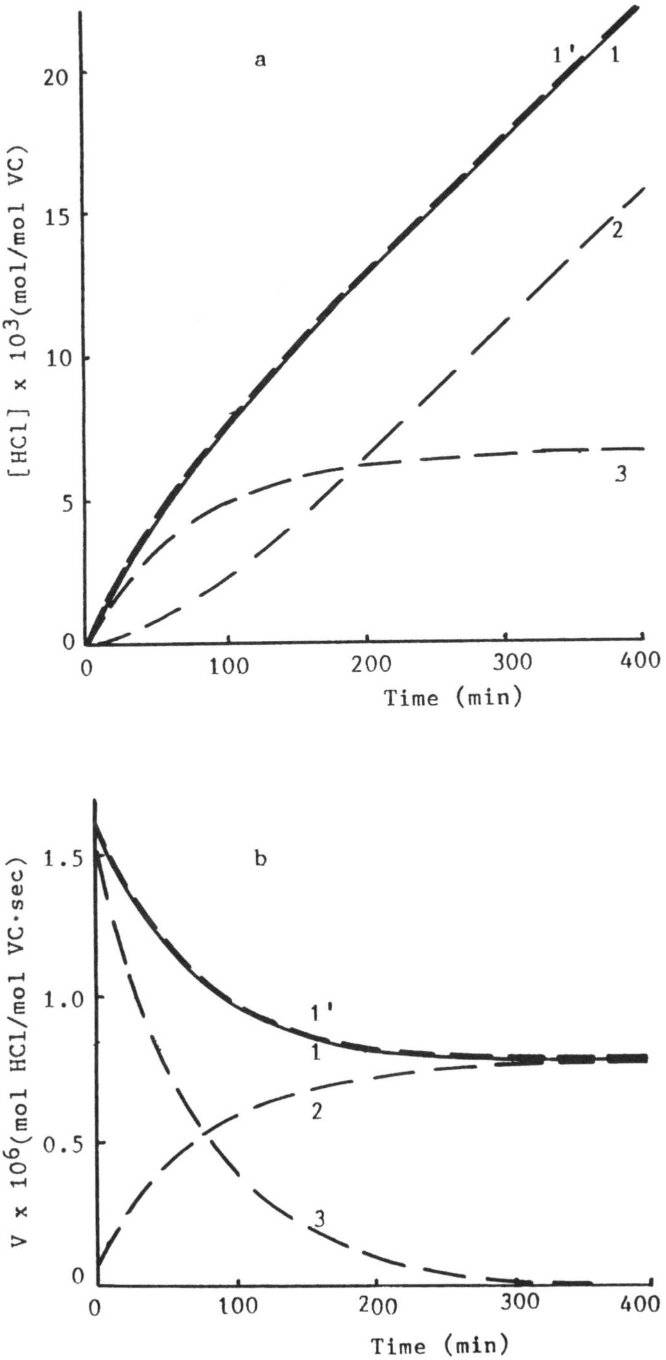

Figure 8 Integral (a) and differential (b) kinetic curve of dehydrochlorination of 1% solution of PVC in 1,2,4-trichlorobenzene (sample H) with continuous removal of HCl by stream of inert gas at 200°C (1). Curves 1′, 2 and 3 are calculated from equations (21a) and (22b); equations (6a) and (7b); equations (20a) and (19b) respectively.[44] H is sample from Ref. 28.

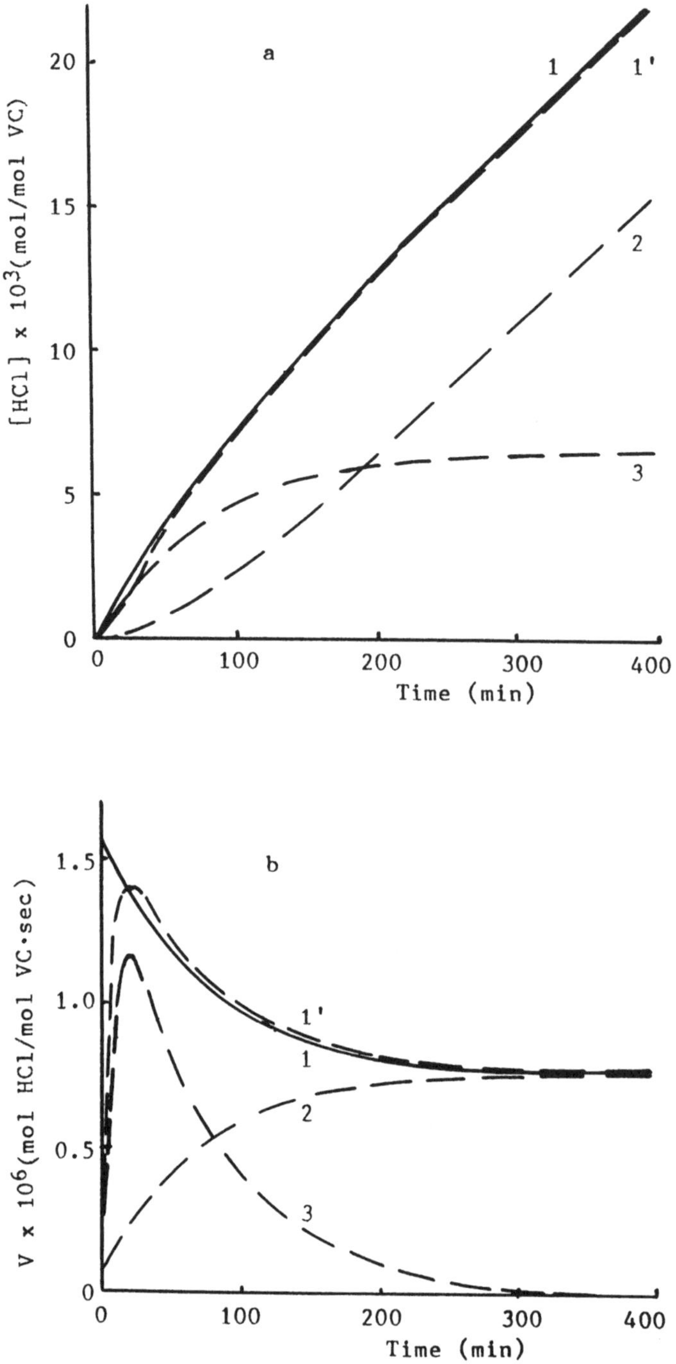

Figure 9 Integral (a) and differential (b) kinetic curve of dehydrochlorination of 1% solution of PVC in 1,2,4-trichlorobenzene (sample H) with continuous removal of HCl by stream of inert gas at 200°C (1). Curves 1′, 2 and 3 are calculated from equations (25a) and (26b); equations (6a) and (7b); equations (27a) and (28b) respectively.[44] H is sample from Ref. 28.

chloroallylic groups and the branching fragments with the chlorine atom near the tertiary carbon atom.

3 MATHEMATICAL MODELS OF THE INITIAL STAGE OF THE THERMAL DEGRADATION OF PVC OBTAINED BY MEANS OF NUMERICAL SOLUTION OF THE SYSTEMS OF THE DIFFERENTIAL EQUATIONS

3.1 The Thermal Degradation of PVC Initiated by Decomposition of Normal Units and the Internal Chloroallylic Fragments

In the paper [26], the mathematical models for the initial stage of the thermal degradation of PVC have been examined using the program given in the book [50] for solution of the systems of the differential equations according to Euler's method with a computer under the same assumptions as in section 2.

The mathematical models for the thermal degradation of PVC initiated by decomposition of normal units and the internal chloroallylic fragments, have been considered.[26] The theoretical curves for PVC dehydrochlorination at 200, 240 and 250°C have been calculated. It has been shown that these curves coincide with the experimental ones up to $\sim$30–40% conversion. It has been demonstrated that there is coincidence of these theoretical curves with curves calculated from the equation (21) at the same values of k_0, k_1 and C^0_{all}. Results obtained in the paper [26] give the evidence of the validity of the equations which have been previously[16–24] deduced for the initial stage (up to $\sim$10% conversion) of PVC degradation initiated by decomposition of normal units and unstable fragments such as the internal chloroallylic groups, the branching fragments with the chlorine atom near the tertiary carbon atom or sum of these fragments in all proportions [the equations (21)–(26)]. The mathematical models proposed in the paper[26] make it possible to describe the initial stage of the thermal degradation of PVC up to $\sim 30-40\%$ conversion.

3.2 Influence of Tacticity of Macromolecules on the Thermal Degradation of PVC

Only a few papers have dealt with the influence of tacticity of macromolecules on the thermal degradation of PVC.[5,26,49,51–53] It has been shown[52] that in the thermal degradation of PVC above the glass transition temperature, the polyene length distribution is characterized by a high amount of very short polyenes. Below the glass transition temperature the formation of much long polyenes is observed due to degradation of highly syndiotactic sequences in macromolecules.[52] It has been established[53] that the bulk and suspension polymers prepared at very low conversions (0.1–2%) differ from those obtained at high conversions (70%). The former polymers have more syndiotactic sequences and are less thermostable at 190°C, more long polyenes form in the thermal degradation of these polymers. On the other hand, it has been proposed[51] that the thermal degradation of PVC is the stereoselective reaction, and isotactic triads (mm) decompose with a greater rate than syndio (rr) or heterotactic (rm) triads. The reactivity of isotactic triads is higher as the length of the isotactic sequence ending with -mmr-, increases. The conclusion has been drawn[51] that the very labile structures in PVC are chlorine atoms located mainly at the normal GTTG* isotactic triad conformation in the -mmr- structures which are at the end of some definite isotactic sequences. The content of this conformation has been estimated to lie between 0.2 and 0.8% depending on the overall isotactic content of the sample of PVC.[51]

In the paper [49], the tacticity of nine various samples of suspension PVC has been measured by ^{13}C NMR spectroscopy. Configuration of PVC macromolecules is described by Bernoullian statistics of chain growth and is determined by probability of meso-addition, P_m.[54] In the paper [49] using ^{13}C NMR data, the values of P_m were calculated and the contents of tactic sequences were evaluated in PVC samples. The dehydrochlorination of PVC samples under vacuum with continuous removal of HCl has been studied at 200°C. The total concentration of unstable groups in PVC samples has been determined. It has been established that only the contents of isotactic nonads may be compared with the values of the concentrations of the unstable fragments in the samples. There is no correlation between the initial rate of PVC degradation and the content of isotactic triads or nonads in the samples.[49] It is interesting to note that the correlation between V_{stat} and the content of isotactic triads is absent too.[49] It has been shown[49] that the values of rate constants for the thermal degradation of two stereoisomers, *d,l*-2,4-dichloropentane and *meso*-2,4-dichloropentane, in the liquid phase at 200°C are practically the same and do not depend on stereoisomery of compounds. The results obtained in the paper [49], give evidence that the tacticity of macromolecules has no significant influence on the initial stage of the thermal degradation of PVC.

The mathematical model for the initial stage of the thermal degradation of PVC has been proposed at the assumption that tacticity of macromolecules has the greatest influence on the thermal stability of the polymer.[26] It has been supposed that the PVC degradation is initiated by decomposition of normal units and the unstable conformer of the definite isotactic isomer (isotactic heptad, octad or nonad). It has been shown that there is no coincidence between the experimental kinetic curve for PVC dehydrochlorination and the theoretical ones. The theoretical curves of PVC degradation are S-shaped ones. The greater the concentration of the isotactic isomer, the greater the discrepancy between the theoretical curves of PVC dehydrochlorination and the experimental one. The conclusion has been made that at elevated temperatures the thermal degradation of PVC is not a stereoselective reaction.[26]

4 MECHANISM OF THE NONAUTOCATALYTIC THERMAL DEGRADATION OF PVC

Two theories have been offered for the nonautocatalytic thermal degradation of PVC with effective removal of HCl: the molecular and the radical theories.[3–10,12–14,27,55,56]

In accordance with the radical theory, the chlorine atoms and macroradicals are the main active particles in the thermal degradation of PVC. It is well known that metals are the effective acceptors of the chlorine atoms. It has been established[36,37] that some metals (mercury, silver) which do not react with HCl, do not have an influence on the rate of the nonautocatalytic thermal degradation of PVC with effective removal of HCl. Recently[57] it has been shown that fullerene C_{60} retards the thermal depolymerization of poly(methyl methacrylate) (PMMA) and does not influence the nonautocatalytic thermal dehydrochlorination of PVC with effective removal of HCl. It is well known[58] that C_{60} reacts easily with low molecular weight free radicals with formation of relatively stable particles. The thermal depolymerization of PMMA is the chain radical reaction.[59] It is assumed[57] that the inhibiting influence of C_{60} on PMMA in its thermal degradation is connected with interaction of fullerene with macroradicals. These data indicate that the nonautocatalytic PVC degradation with effective removal of HCl proceeds mostly by the molecular mechanism. On the basis of the numerous experimental data concerning the thermal degradation of the low molecular weight model chlorohydrocarbons, the molecular mechanism has been proposed for this process.[14,60,61] This supports the molecular mechanism of the nonautocatalytic thermal degradation of PVC too.

The following data confirm that in the nonautocatalytic PVC degradation radical processes take place. It is well known that in the thermal degradation of PVC at 180–210°C benzene evolves in small quantities (100–1000 times less than the quantity of HCl).[4–10,29,34,37,56] Inhibitors of free radical reactions, such as nitrogen oxide and α-naphthol decrease the rate of its formation in the nonautocatalytic degradation of PVC with effective removal of HCl.[34,56] Peroxides and hydroperoxides which are present in PVC in small quantities, increase the initial rate of PVC dehydrochlorination.[3,5,55,62–64] In the papers [10,11,27,29,35], it has been suggested that the nonautocatalytic thermal degradation of PVC mostly proceeds by a molecular mechanism complicated by radical reactions. In the papers [35,48,65], the more probable reactions of initiation of the nonautocatalytic thermal degradation of PVC by the radical mechanism have been proposed. The role of thermally excited states of polyenes and polyenyl carbocations in the thermal degradation of PVC has been discussed. Data concerning dependences of energies of electron transitions from the basic level (S_0) to the first excited singlet level (S_1) and from S_0 to the first triplet level (T_1) and of energy barriers for rotation about central double bond in polyenes and polyenyl carbocations on n have been considered.[48] It is known that cis-trans rearrangement of polyenes is one of the reactions which characterize their reactivity. The thermal monomolecular reaction of cis-trans rearrangement of the polyenes proceeds via excited triplet state:[66–68]

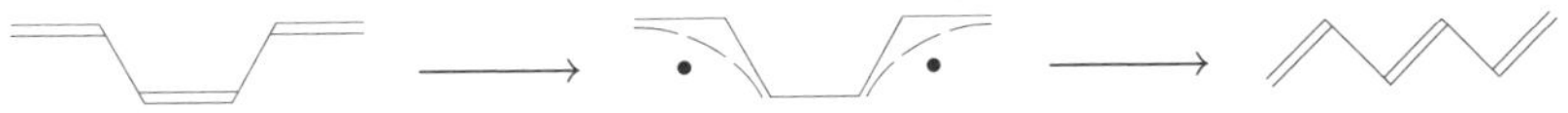 (29)

Using experimental data[66–68] concerning the thermal cis-trans rearrangement of all-trans-β-carotene, the low molecular weight model of polyene fragments of PVC, it has been shown[48] that at 180–200°C reactivity of polyenes having ≥ 8 conjugated double bonds is great. The assumption has been made that in PVC degradation polyenes in the excited triplet state (biradical state) may take part in different radical reactions, in particular, in the reaction of initiation of polymer dehydrochlorination:[35,48,65]

$$\sim(\mathrm{CH{=}CH})_n\sim \longrightarrow \sim[\dot{\mathrm{C}}\mathrm{H}-(\mathrm{CH{=}CH})_{n-1}-\dot{\mathrm{C}}\mathrm{H}]\sim^* \quad (30)$$

$$\sim[\dot{\mathrm{C}}\mathrm{H}-(\mathrm{CH{=}CH})_{n-1}-\dot{\mathrm{C}}\mathrm{H}]\sim^* + \sim\mathrm{CH_2}-\mathrm{CHCl}\sim \longrightarrow \sim\dot{\mathrm{C}}\mathrm{H}-(\mathrm{CH{=}CH})_{n-1}-\mathrm{CH_2}\sim + \sim\dot{\mathrm{C}}\mathrm{H}-\mathrm{CHCl}\sim \quad (31)$$

$$\sim\dot{\mathrm{C}}\mathrm{H}-\mathrm{CHCl}\sim \begin{cases} \longrightarrow \mathrm{Cl}\bullet + \sim\mathrm{CH{=}CH}\sim \\ \longrightarrow \sim\dot{\mathrm{C}}\mathrm{H}-(\mathrm{CH{=}CH})-\mathrm{CHCl}\sim + \mathrm{HCl} \end{cases} \quad (32)$$

Reactivity of polyenyl carbocations is greater than that of polyenes because the energy of excitation of them into triplet state is less. It has been shown[48] that the activation energies of the thermal decomposition of the low molecular weight model chlorohydrocarbons having one or two conjugated double bonds, in the liquid phase with removal of HCl agree closely with the energies of $S_0 \rightarrow T_1$ electron transitions in polyenyl carbocations. In the excited triplet state, polyenyl carbocation is the carbocation-biradical. The following reaction of the thermal dehydrochlorination of polyenyl fragment has been proposed under the assumption that the main elementary act of the reaction is intramolecular transference of electron.[48,65]

$$\sim(\mathrm{CH{=}CH})_n-\underset{\mathrm{Cl}^{\sigma-}}{\overset{\delta+}{\mathrm{CH}}}-\mathrm{CH_2}\sim \rightleftharpoons \left| \sim(\dot{\mathrm{C}}\mathrm{H}\overset{+}{=}\mathrm{CH})_n-\underset{\mathrm{Cl}^-}{\dot{\mathrm{C}}\mathrm{H}}-\mathrm{CH_2}\sim \right| \quad (33)$$

Then subsequent transformation of ion-biradical pair into biradical may occur:[48,65]

$$\left| \sim(\dot{\mathrm{C}}\mathrm{H}\overset{+}{=}\mathrm{CH})_n-\underset{\mathrm{Cl}^-}{\dot{\mathrm{C}}\mathrm{H}}-\mathrm{CH_2}\sim \right| \longrightarrow \sim\dot{\mathrm{C}}\mathrm{H}-(\mathrm{CH{=}CH})_n-\dot{\mathrm{C}}\mathrm{H}\sim + \mathrm{HCl} \quad (34)$$

Forming biradical may initiate the thermal degradation of PVC by the radical mechanism equations (31) and (32).[48,65]

The expressions (31)–(34) represent the most probable reactions of the initiation of the degenerated branching of chain in the thermal degradation of PVC with removal of HCl. It follows that this process must be an autocatalytic one. In fact in the thermal dehydrochlorination of PVC with effective removal of HCl autocatalysis is not observed (see section 1). As discussed in the paper [48], the reactions of cyclization decrease the concentration of long polyenes and increase the concentration of short ones. As mentioned above, in the thermal degradation of PVC with effective removal of HCl $l_{av} = 8$–15,[28–30,45] the average number of conjugated double bonds in the polyenes formed, has been determined by the use of absorption spectra of degraded PVC, is equal to 3–10.[5,28,69] The energy of excitation of short polyenes to the triplet state is more than long ones.[48] It has been concluded[48,65] that in the thermal degradation of PVC with effective removal of HCl probability of the reactions (31)–(34) is little therefore the degenerated branching of chain proceeds with a small rate. One cannot also exclude the possibility of removal of active particles—atomic chlorine from the zone of the reaction in the thermal degradation of PVC with effective removal of HCl.[35]

5 MECHANISM OF AUTOCATALYTIC THERMAL DEGRADATION OF PVC

As mentioned above (see section 1), the thermal degradation of PVC is complicated by the catalytic effect of evolving HCl. In the presence of HCl the thermal dehydrochlorination of the polymer has an autocatalytic character.[10,25,27,29,32,33,35–37] The initial rate of degradation has a minimum value and then the rate of PVC dehydrochlorination increases up to a maximum value. The maximum rate is some 10 times greater than the initial one.

The thermal degradation of PVC in the presence of HCl is generally believed to proceed by an ionic or molecular mechanism.[5,9–14,27,33,35,70–73] Some reaction schemes have been offered, equations (35)–(41):

$$\sim CH_2{-}\underset{\underset{H-Cl}{Cl}}{CH}{-}\underset{H}{CH}{-}CHCl\sim \longrightarrow \sim CH_2{-}CH{=}CH{-}CHCl\sim + HCl \quad [70] \tag{35}$$

$$\sim(CH{-}CH)_n{-}\underset{\underset{H}{Cl}}{CH}{-}\underset{\underset{Cl}{H}}{CH}\sim \longrightarrow \sim(CH{=}CH)_{n+1}\sim + 2HCl \quad [33,35] \tag{36}$$

$$2HCl \rightleftharpoons H^+HCl_2^- \rightleftharpoons H^+ + HCl_2^- \quad [73] \tag{37}$$

$$RCl + HCl \rightleftharpoons R^+HCl_2^- \rightleftharpoons R^+ + HCl_2^- \quad [14] \tag{38}$$

$$\sim(CH{=}CH)_n\sim + HCl \longrightarrow \sim \underset{Cl^-}{\overset{+}{CH}}{-}(CH{=}CH)_{n-1}\sim \quad [72] \tag{39}$$

$$\sim CH_2{-}(CH{-}CH)_n{-}\underset{Cl}{CH}\sim + HCl \rightleftharpoons \sim CH_2{-}(CH{=}CH)_n{-}\overset{+}{CH}\sim \; [HCl_2]^- \quad [27,35] \tag{40}$$

$$\sim(CH{=}CH)_n{-}\underset{[HCl_2]^-}{\overset{+}{CH}}\sim \rightleftharpoons \sim(CH{=}CH)_n{-}\overset{+}{CH}\sim + [HCl_2]^- \quad [27,35] \tag{41}$$

It is necessary to note that PVC is a chlorohydrocarbon having small dielectric penetration.[4] In these media, the probability of dissociation of ionic pairs into free ions is small. Therefore in the initial stage of the autocatalytic thermal degradation of PVC (upto $\sim 10\%$ conversion) there is a small possibility of the presence of free ions in accordance with reactions (37)–(39) and (41). It is more probable to suppose that in the autocatalytic thermal degradation of PVC contact ionic pairs are active particles, equation (40). But there are numerous experimental data which testify that in the thermal degradation of PVC in the presence of HCl, radical reactions take place. These data are considered below.

5.1 Mathematical Models of the Initial Stage of the Autocatalytic Thermal Degradation of PVC

Several mathematical models for the initial stage of the thermal degradation of PVC in the presence of HCl have been proposed taking into consideration the different mechanisms for the autocatalytic degradation of the polymer.[74,75] The theoretical curves are compared with the kinetic curves for the thermal degradation of PVC. It has been shown[74,75] that the kinetic curves of PVC autocatalytic dehydrochlorination at a constant pressure of HCl during an experiment are described by the expression (42) at the value of the branching factor $\varphi = 1 - 1.5 \times 10^{-4}$:

$$[\mathrm{HCl}]_5 = [\mathrm{HCl}]_{\mathrm{norm}} + A(e^{\varphi t} - 1) \tag{42}$$

where $[\mathrm{HCl}]_5$ is the summary quantity of HCl evolving during nonautocatalytic and autocatalytic dehydrochlorination of PVC; $[\mathrm{HCl}]_{\mathrm{norm}}$ is calculated from equation (6). The expression $A(e^{\varphi t} - 1)$ is typical for the kinetics of branched chain reactions[76] where A and φ are constant values.

5.2 Retarding Effect of Compounds which do not React with HCl on the Autocatalytic Thermal Degradation of PVC

It has been established that maleic anhydride, active dienophil, which does not react with HCl and interacts easily with polyenes by the Diels-Alder reaction, suppresses the autocatalytic dehydrochlorination of PVC.[33,35,77–80] It has been concluded that the accelerating effect of HCl is marked when there are sections of conjugated double bonds in PVC macromolecules.[33,35,77–80] This conclusion is supported by the following experiments. It has been shown that the longer degradation in vacuo proceeded, the more polyene areas formed, and the higher the initial dehydrochlorination rate with the HCl addition became.[35,78] The thermal degradation of 8-chlorohexadecane and 8-chloro-6-tridecylene which are the low molecular weight model compounds for normal units of PVC and chloroallylic fragments respectively, in the liquid phase has been studied.[14,15] It has been shown that HCl has no influence on the thermal degradation of 8-chlorohexane and accelerates the thermal dehydrochlorination of 8-chloro-6-tridecylene. Consequently, one can propose that HCl does not affect the thermal degradation of normal units of PVC and increases the rate of dehydrochlorination of fragments having double (conjugated double) bonds, $\sim(CH{=}CH)_n{-}CHCl\sim$.

The autocatalytic dehydrochlorination of PVC is suppressed by triethyl silane which does not react with HCl under the conditions at which the thermal degradation of PVC is carried out.[81] In this process, the formation of H_2 ($\sim$0.1 part of the quantity of evolved HCl) takes place. The elimination of H_2 is proof of the presence of free radicals, equations (43) and (44):[81]

$$Cl^\bullet + Et_3SiH \longrightarrow Et_3SiCl + H^\bullet \tag{43}$$

$$H^\bullet + \sim CH_2{-}CHCl\sim \longrightarrow H_2 + \sim\dot{C}H{-}CHCl\sim \tag{44}$$

When the thermal degradation of PVC in the presence of Et_3SiH is carried out with addition of HCl, the rate of PVC dehydrochlorination does not increase, but in degraded polymer, the quantity of long polyenes decreases. The latter is supported by absorption spectra of degraded PVC.[81] It has been proposed that HCl is the catalyst of the reaction of Et_3SiH with polyene fragments, equations (40) and (45).[29]

$$\underset{[HCl_2]^-}{\sim(CH{=}CH)_n{-}CH\sim} + Et_3SiH \longrightarrow \sim(CH{=}CH)_n{-}CH_2\sim + HCl + Et_3SiCl \tag{45}$$

During PVC degradation in evacuated ampoules in the presence of mercury or silver, autocatalysis does not take place.[36,37,82] This metals do not interact with HCl, but react easily with atomic chlorine. Mercury may form two chlorides: $HgCl_2$ and Hg_2Cl_2. In the thermal degradation of PVC in the presence of mercury Hg_2Cl_2 was determined only.[36,37,82] It has been assumed that in this process the following reactions proceed:[36,37,82]

$$Cl^\bullet + Hg \longrightarrow {}^\bullet HgCl \tag{46}$$

$$2\dot{H}gCl \longrightarrow Hg_2Cl_2 \tag{47}$$

It has been shown[35,78] that triphenylmethane and toluene which are the inhibitors of the free radical reactions, decrease the rate of the autocatalytic dehydrochlorination of PVC. One can suggest that the following reactions may occur:

$$R^\bullet \text{ (or } Cl^\bullet) + C_6H_5CH_3 \longrightarrow RH \text{ (or HCl)} + C_6H_5\dot{C}H_2 \tag{48}$$

$$R^\bullet \text{ (or } Cl^\bullet) + (C_6H_5)_3CH \longrightarrow (C_6H_5)_3\dot{C} + RH \text{ (or HCl)} \tag{49}$$

The reaction (48) is supported by the following data. It has been established[83] that in the thermal degradation of PVC in the presence of toluene labeled with tritium ($C_6H_5CH_2T$), tritium is introduced into the polymer.

As mentioned above (see section 4), fullerene C_{60} retards the process of the radical thermal depolymerization of PMMA.[57] It has been shown[57] that fullerene C_{60} decreases the rate of the autocatalytic dehydrochlorination of PVC too. Experiments show that C_{60} does not react with HCl under the conditions of carrying out the autocatalytic degradation of PVC. It has been assumed that the retarding effect of C_{60} in the autocatalytic dehydrochlorination of PVC is connected with its interaction with free radicals:[57]

$$mR\bullet \text{ (or } mCl\bullet) + C_{60} \longrightarrow (mR)C_{60} \text{ [or } (mCl)C_{60}] \qquad (50)$$

It has been demonstrated that PVC mixed with other polymers initiates the radical reactions of the thermal degradation of these polymers.[84–88]

Intriguing data were obtained recently in the paper.[89] By ESR spectroscopy it has been shown that in thermally degraded PVC the concentration of stable paramagnetic centers increases considerably if the polymer is decomposed in the presence of HCl.

5.3 Autocatalytic Thermal Degradation of PVC as the Branched Chain Reaction with the Degenerated Branching of Chain

In the papers [48, 65, 74, 75, 89], a new theory is developed for the autocatalytic thermal degradation of PVC. It has been supposed that this process is the branched chain reaction with degenerated branching of the chain.

As mentioned above (see section 4), it has been shown[35,48,65] that the reactions with participation of polyenes and polyenyl carbocations excited into triplet state, equations (31)–(34), lead to the degenerate branching of the chain in the thermal degradation of PVC, but probability of them is low.

In the thermal degradation of PVC in the presence of HCl the reaction (51) which initiates the degenerated branching of chain, may take place [35]:

$$\begin{aligned} &\sim[\dot{C}H-(CH{=}CH)_{n-1}-\dot{C}H]^{*}\sim + HCl \\ &\longrightarrow \sim CH_2-(CH{=}CH)_{n-1}-\dot{C}H + Cl\bullet \end{aligned} \qquad (51)$$

It has been demonstrated[27,35,74,75] that two types of complexes of HCl (electrophilic agent) with polyenes are possible, equations (40) and (52).

$$\sim(CH{=}CH)_n\sim + HCl \rightleftharpoons \left\{ \begin{array}{c} \sim(CH\overset{\delta+}{=}CH)_n\sim \\ HCl^{\sigma-} \end{array} \right\} \qquad (52)$$

These complexes are the contact ionic pairs. The equation (52) demonstrates the formation of the charge transfer complex. The complex in equation (40) is a molecular one.

The reaction scheme of the autocatalytic thermal degradation of PVC initiated by equation (52) has been considered in the paper [89]. From this scheme, it follows that H_2 must form. But experiments have shown that during the thermal degradation of PVC in the presence of HCl, H_2 is not practically evolve.[89] The conclusion has been made that it is unlikely that initiation of the autocatalytic degradation of PVC proceeds by reaction (52).[89]

Consider now equation (40). In the paper [90] it has been shown that as a result of interaction of chlorine anion, Cl^-, with HCl with formation of $[HCl_2]^-$ the energy equal to ~14 kcal/mol is releases. It has been demonstrated[48] that the activation energies for the thermal degradation of low molecular weight models of polyenyl fragments of PVC macromolecules, which have one or two conjugated double bonds, in the liquid phase in the presence of HCl are in the field of triplet state of polyenyl carbocations. It has been concluded[48,65] that probability of reactions (53) and (54) is greater than the reactions (33) and (34).

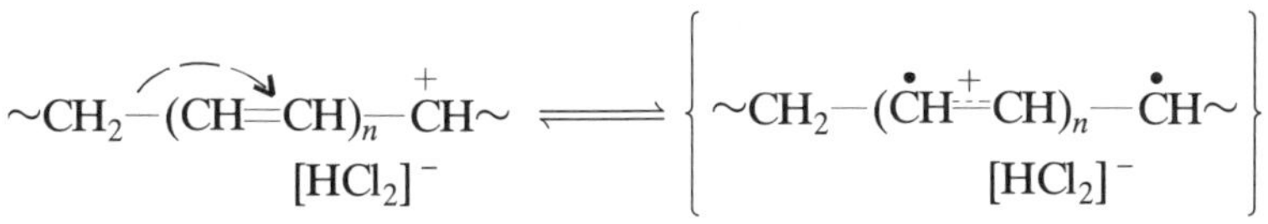
(53)

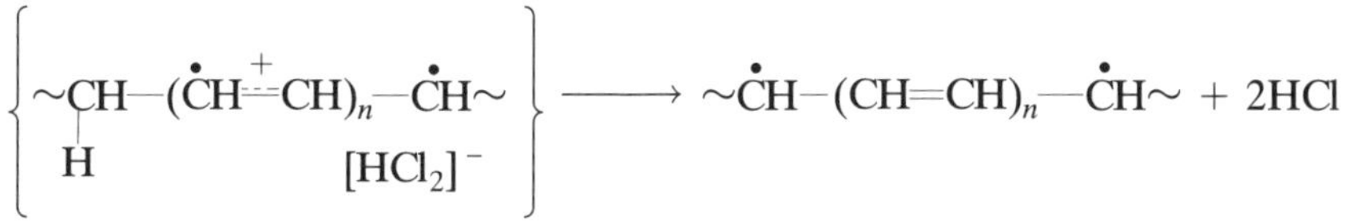
(54)

It has been supposed[48,65] that in the autocatalytic thermal degradation of PVC, the reactions (51), (53) and (54) make the principal contribution to the degenerate branching of the chain reaction. HCl acts as the catalyst for the degenerate branching reactions of the chain equations (51), (53) and (54) which proceed with a small rate in the nonautocatalytic thermal degradation of PVC equations (31)–(34).

CONCLUSION

The review demonstrates that in recent years there has been progress in some aspects of the thermal degradation of PVC. In the papers of recent years it has been shown that the mathematical models of the initial stage of the thermal decomposition of the low molecular weight model chlorohydrocarbons having only VC units and model compounds, containing VC units and unstable fragments, have made it possible:

—to investigate kinetic perculiarities of the initial stage (up to ~10% conversion) of the nonautocatalytic thermal dehydrochlorination of PVC quantitatively;
—to show that low molecular weight chlorohydrocarbons which may serve as models for PVC macromolecules, must contain 15 units of VC at the minimum;
—to evaluate the summary contribution of unstable fragments present in the original polymer to the initial rate of PVC degradation at $t \to 0$ quantitatively. It has been demonstrated that the internal chloroallylic fragments and branching groups with the chlorine atom near the tertiary carbon atom may be the main unstable fragments of PVC macromolecules. But one cannot exclude the influence of other unstable groups on the initial rate of the thermal degradation of PVC, such as

oxygen-containing fragments. The additional investigations are necessary in this direction.
—to show that above ~2–3% conversion the thermal dehydrochlorination of PVC is initiated by the statictical degradation of the normal units of the polymer;
—to show that at elevated temperatures (180–200°C) the thermal degradation of PVC is not a stereoselective reaction.

The mathematical models for the initial stage of the thermal degradation of PVC which give the possibility to describe this process up to ~30–40% conversion, have been proposed. The mathematical models for the PVC degradation may be used for investigation of the initial stage of decomposition of a wide range of polymers which degrade with the splitting out of side fragments from the macromolecules, equation (1), such as poly(vinyl bromide), poly(vinyl fluoride), poly(vinyl acetate), poly(vinyl alcohol), etc.

Early[10,11,27,29,35] on the basis of the numerous experimental data it has been suggested that the nonautocatalytic thermal degradation of PVC mostly proceeds by a molecular mechanism complicated by radical reactions. Recently[48,65] the most probable reactions of initiation of PVC dehydrochlorination by the radical mechanism have been proposed.

The new theory that the autocatalytic thermal degradation of PVC is the branched chain reaction with degenerate branching of the chain was developed. The reactions with the participation of polyenes and polyenyl carbocations excited into the triplet state, make the principal contribution to the degenerate branching of the chain. HCl acts as the catalyst of these reactions equations (51), (53) and (54) which proceed with the small rate in the nonautocatalytic thermal degradation of PVC equations (31)–(34).

ACKNOWLEDGEMENTS

The research described in this publication was made possible in part by grant No. NOX000 from the International Science Foundation and by grant No. NOX300 from the International Science Foundation and the Russian Government.

REFERENCES

1. N. Grassie, *Chemistry of High Polymer Degradation Processes*, Butterworths Scientific Publications, London, 1956.
2. S.L. Madorsky, *Thermal Degradation of Organic Polymers*, Interscience Publishers, New York, London, Sydney, 1964.
3. W.C. Geddes, *Rubber Chem. Technol.*, 1967, **40**, p. 177.
4. W.H. Starnes, Ir., *Developments in Polymer Degradation-3* (N. Grassie, ed.) Applied Science Publishers Ltd., London, 1981, p. 135.
5. D. Braun, *Developments in Polymer Degradation-3* (N. Grassie, ed.) Applied Science Publishers Ltd., London, 1981, p. 101.
6. A.A. Caraculacu, *Pure Appl. Chem.*, 1981, **53**, p. 385.
7. A. Guyot, M. Bert, P. Burille, M.-F. Llauro and A. Michel, *Pure Appl.Chem.*, 1981, **53**, p. 401.

8. G. Scott, *Developments in Polymer Degradation-1* (N. Grassie, ed.) Applied Science Publishers Ltd., London, 1977, p. 205.
9. K.S. Minsker, M.I. Abdullin, S.V. Kolesov and G.E. Zaikov, *Developments in Polymer Stabilization-6* (G. Scott, ed.) Applied Science Publishers Ltd., London, New York, 1983, p. 173.
10. B.B. Troitskii and L.S. Troitskaya, *Usp. Khim.*, 1985, **54**, p. 1287.
11. B.B. Troitskii and L.S. Troitskaya, *Organometallic Compounds and Radicals* (M.I. Kabachnik, ed.) Nauka, Moscow, 1985, p. 231, in Russian.
12. M.K. Nagvi, *J. Macromol. Sci., Rev. Macromol. Chem. Phys.*, 1985, **C25**, p. 119.
13. A.A. Yassin and M.W. Sabaa, *J. Macromol Sci., Rev. Macromol. Chem. Phys.*, 1990, **C30**, p. 491.
14. Z. Mayer, *J. Macromol Sci., Rev. Macromol Chem.*, 1974, **C10**, p. 263.
15. Z. Mayer, B. Obereigner and D. Lim, *J. Polym. Sci.*, 1971, **C33**, p. 289.
16. B.B. Troitskii and L.S. Troitskaya, *Prept. Int. 31 Microsymp. Macromol. "Polyvinyl Chloride"*, Prague, Czechoslovakia, 1988, p. 69.
17. B.B. Troitskii and L.S. Troitskaya, *Prept. Symp. Academies of Sciences of Socialist Countries on Degradation and Stabilization of Polymers*, Moscow, USSR, October 1988, p. 17.
18. B.B. Troitskii and L.S. Troitskaya, *Dokl. Akad.* Nauk USSR, 1988, **303**, p. 146.
19. B.B. Troitskii and L.S. Troitskaya, *Prept. Conference on Degradation and Stabilization of Polymers*, Dushanbe, USSR, October 1989, p. 69, in Russian.
20. B.B. Troitskii and L.S. Troitskaya, *Prept. X-th Anniversary Symposium Polymers '89*, Varna, Bolgaria, October 1989, P-4. 18, p. 279.
21. B.B. Troitskii and L.S. Troitskaya, *Dokl. Akad.* Nauk USSR, 1989, **305**, p. 664.
22. B.B. Troitskii and L.S. Troitskaya, *Prept. Conference "Polyvinyl Chlorde-91"*, Dzerzinsk, USSR, October 1991, p. 12, in Russian.
23. B.B. Troitskii and L.S. Troitskaya, *J. Polym. Sci. Part A: Polym. Chem.*, 1990, **28**, p. 2695.
24. B.B. Troitskii and L.S. Troitskaya, *Intern. J. Polymeric Mater.*, 1990, **13**, p. 173.
25. B.B. Troitskii and L.S. Troitskaya, *J. Polym. Sci. Part A: Polym. Chem.*, 1993, **31**, p. 75.
26. B.B. Troitskii and L.S. Troitskaya, *Eur. Polym. J.*, 1997, **33**, p. 1289.
27. B.B. Troitskii and L.S. Troitskaya, *Vysokomol. Soedin.*, 1978, **20A**, p. 1443.
28. B. Ivan, J.P. Kennedy, T. Kelen, F. Tudos, T.T. Nagy and B. Turcsanyi, *J. Polym. Sci., Polym. Chem. Ed.*, 1983, **21**, p. 2177.
29. B.B. Troitskii, *Dissertation Doct. Chem. Sci.*, 1978, Moscow University, Moscow.
30. B.B. Troitskii, L.S. Troitskaya, V.N. Denisova, M.A. Novikova and Z.B. Luzinova, *Eur. Polym. J.*, 1977, **13**, p. 1033.
31. G.A. Razuvaev, B.B. Troitskii and L.S. Troitskaya, *Prept. Int. Symp. Poly(vinyl Chloride)*, Lyon-Villeurbanne, France, 1976, Topic. VII, p. 261.
32. G. Talamini, G. Cinque and G. Palma, *Mat. Plast.*, 1964, **30**, p. 317.
33. L.S. Troitskaya, V.N. Myakov, B.B. Troitskii and G.A. Razuvaev, *Vysokomol. Soedin.*, 1967, **9A**, p. 2119.
34. M.B. Neiman, R.A. Papko and V.S. Pudov, *Vysokomol. Soedin.*, 1968, **10A**, p. 841.
35. G.A. Razuvaev, L.S. Troitskaya and B.B. Troitskii, *J. Polym. Sci. A-1*, 1971, **9**, p. 2673.
36. B.B. Troitskii, L.S. Troitskaya, V.N. Myakov and A.F. Lepaev, *Prept. Int. Symp. Macromol.*, Helsinki, 1972, **5**, p. 189.
37. B.B. Troitskii, L.S. Troitskaya, V.N. Myakov and A.F. Lepaev, *J. Polym. Sci. Polym. Symp.*, 1973, **42** Part 3, p. 1347.
38. V.S. Pudov and R.A. Papko, *Vysokomol. Soedin.*, 1970, **12B**, p. 218.
39. R.A. Papko and V.S. Pudov, *Vysokomol. Soedin.*, 1973, **15B**, p. 761.
40. B.B. Troitskii, L.S. Troitskaya and A.F. Lepaev, *Dokl. Akad.* Nauk USSR, 1973, **210**, p. 877.
41. B.B. Troitskii, V.A. Dozorov, F.F. Minchuk and L.S. Troitskaya, *Eur. Polym. J.*, 1975, **11**, p. 277.
42. B.B. Troitskii, *Chemistry and Technology of Macromolecules*, VINITI, Moscow, 1974, **5**, p. 172, in Russian.
43. B.B. Troitskii, L.S. Troitskaya, V.N. Denisova and Z.B. Luzinova, *Polym. J.*, 1978, **10**, p. 377.
44. B.B. Troitskii, L.S. Troitskaya, unpublished data.
45. W.C. Geddes, *Eur. Polym. J.*, 1967, **3**, p. 747.
46. N.M. Rodigin and E.N. Rodigina, *Consecutive Chemical Reactions. Mathematical Analysis and Calculation*, Akad. Nauk USSR, Moscow, 1960, in Russian.
47. S.L. Haynie, G.M. Villacorta, I.M. Plitz and W.H. Starnes, Ir., *Polym. Prepr.*, 1983, **24**, p. 3.
48. B.B. Troitskii and L.S. Troitskaya, *Eur. Polym. J.* submitted.

49. B.B. Troitskii, L.S. Troitskaya, Yu. A. Kurskii, A.G. Kronman, A.S. Yakhnov, M.A. Novikova, T.G. Ganyukhina and V.N. Denisova, *Eur. Polym. J.* (in press).
50. K. Ebert and H. Ederer, *Computeranwendungen in der Chemie*, VCH Verlagsgesellschaft mbH, Weinheim, 1985.
51. J. Millan, G. Martinez, M.L. Jimeno, P. Tiemblo, C. Mijangos and J.M. Gomez-Elvira, *Makromol. Chem. Macromol. Symp.*, 1991, 48/49, p. 403 and references cited herein.
52. J. Behnisch and H. Zimmermann, *Makromol. Chem.*, 1989, **190**, p. 2347.
53. M.J. Cuthbertson, H.J. Bowley, D.L. Gerrard, W.F. Maddams and J.S. Shapiro, *Makromol. Chem.*, 1987, **188**, p. 2801.
54. F.A. Bovey, *Pure Appl. Chem.*, 1971, **26**, p. 193.
55. W.C. Geddes, *Eur. Polym. J.*, 1967, **3**, p. 733.
56. R.A. Papko and V.S. Pudov, *Vysokomol. Soedin.*, 1974, **16A**, p. 1409.
57. B.B. Troitskii, L.S. Troitskaya, A.S. Yakhnov, M.A. Lopatin and M.A. Novikova, *Eur. Polym. J.* (in press).
58. J.R. Morton, K.F. Preston, P.J. Krusic, S.A. Hill and E. Wasserman, *J. Amer. Chem. Soc.*, 1992, **114**, p. 5454.
59. N. Grassie and G. Scott, *Polymer Degradation and Stabilization*, 1985, Cambridge University Press, Cambridge.
60. A. Maccol, *The Chemistry of Alkenes* S. Patai, ed. Interscience Publishers, London, New York, Sydney, 1964, Chap. 3.
61. K. Ingold, *Structure and Mechanism in Organic Chemistry*, Cornell University Press, Ithaca, London, 1969, 2nd ed.
62. V.I. Zegel'man, V.V. Lisitskii, V.A. Titiva, S.I. Miroshnichenko, A.P. Aleksandrov, V.N. Genkin and V.A. Popov, *Dokl. Akad.* Nauk USSR, 1984, **277**, p. 896.
63. D. Braun and D. Sonderhof, *Eur. Polym. J.*, 1982, **18**, p. 141.
64. B.B. Troitskii and L.S. Troitskaya, *Physicochemical Principles of Synthesis and Processing of Polymers*, Gorky University, Gorky, 1985, p. 3, in Russian.
65. B.B. Troitskii and L.S. Troitskaya, *Abstracts of II Conference on Modern Trends in Chemical Kinetics and Catalysis*, Novosibirsk, Russia, November 1995, **3**, p. 582.
66. K.W. Egger and T.L. James, *Trans. Faraday Soc.*, 1970, **66**, p. 410.
67. W.E. Doering and T. Kitagawa, *J. Amer. Chem. Soc.*, 1991, **113**, p. 4288.
68. W.E. Doering, Ch. Sotirion-Leventis and W.R. Roth, *J. Amer. Chem. Soc.*, 1995, **117**, p. 2747.
69. B. Vancso, T.T. Nagy, B. Turcsanyi, T. Kelen and F. Tudos, *Macromol. Chem. Rapid Communs.*, 1982, **3**, p. 527.
70. D. Braun and R.F. Bender, *Eur. Polym. J.*, 1969, **5**, p. 269.
71. L. Tvaroska, T. Bleha and L. Valko, *Polym. J.*, 1975, **7**, p. 34.
72. R. Schlimper, *Plast. Kautsch.*, 1966, **13**, p. 196.
73. S. van der Ven and W.F. Wit, *Angew. Makromol. Chem.*, 1969, **8**, p. 143.
74. B.B. Troitskii and L.S. Troitskaya, *Dokl. Russian Akad.* Nauk, 1994, **334**, p. 462.
75. B.B. Troitskii and L.S. Troitskaya, *Eur. Polym. J.*, 1995, **31**, p. 533.
76. N.N. Semenov, *Chain Reactions*, Nauka, Moscow 1986, in Russian.
77. G.A. Razuvaev, L.S. Troitskaya, V.N. Myakov and B.B. Troitskii, *Dokl. Akad.* Nauk USSR, 1966, **170**, p. 1342.
78. B.B. Troitskii, L.S. Troitskaya and G.A. Razuvaev, *Vysokomol. Soedin.*, 1971, **13A**, p. 1183.
79. B.B. Troitskii, V.N. Myakov and G.A. Razuvaev, *Vysokomol. Soedin.*, 1966, **8**, p. 2032.
80. B.B. Troitskii and V.N. Myakov, *Plast. Massy*, 1967, **3**, p. 13.
81. V.N. Myakov, B.B. Troitskii and G.A. Razuvaev, *Vysokomol. Soedin.*, 1969, **11B**, p. 661.
82. V.N. Myakov and B.B. Troitskii, *Vysokomol. Soedin.*, 1970, **12B**, p. 100.
83. C.H. Bamford and D.F. Fenton, *Polymer*, 1969, **10**, p. 63.
84. J.C. McNeill and D. Neil, *Makromol. Chem.*, 1968, **117**, p. 265.
85. J.C. McNeill and D. Neil, *Eur. Polym. J.*, 1970, **6**, p. 569.
86. D.L. Gardner and J.C. McNeill, *Eur. Polym. J.*, 1971, **7**, p. 603.
87. A. Guyot, M. Bert, A. Michel and J.C. McNeill, *Eur. Polym. J.*, 1971, **7**, p. 471.
88. J.C. McNeill, D. Neil, A. Guyot, M. Bert and A. Michel, *Eur. Polym. J.*, 1971, **7**, p. 453.
89. B.B. Troitskii, L.S. Troitskaya, A.S. Yakhnov, M.A. Novikova, V.N. Denisova, V.K. Cherkasov and M.P. Bubnov, *Poly. Deg. and Stab.* in press.
90. I.C. Evans and G.J.-S. Lo, *J. Phys. Chem.*, 1966, **70**, p. 11.

Reviews of Conferences

The Fifth Conference on "Physics and Chemistry of Elementary Chemical Processes" (Dedicated to the Memory of Prof. Vladislav V. Voevodskii)

G.E. ZAIKOV

Institute of Biochemical Physics, 4 Kosygin str., 117334 Moscow, Russia

The Fifth All-Russia Conference on Physics and Chemistry of Elementary Chemical Processes was held between Sept.29–Oct.3 (year 1997) at the Institute of Chemical Physics in Chernogolovka. The conferences dedicated to the memory of Prof. V.V. Voevodskii are organized every five years in turn by Moscow and Novosibirsk and are devoted to the current basic problems of the physics and chemistry of elementary chemical processes.

The main scientific topics at the fifth conference were:

—Kinetics and dynamics of elementary chemical processes, electron transport, weak interactions, effects of surrounding.
—Free radicals in liquid, gas and on surface; chain and catalytic reactions.
—Free radicals in solids, synthetic and natural polymers.
—Free radicals in high-energy chemical reactions (photo-, radiation, plasmo- and mechanochemistry).
—Free radicals in ecology, biology and medicine; molecular dynamics; spin labels and trups.
—New approaches and methods in ESR spectroscopy.

Professor V.I. Goldanskii was chairman of Organizing committee, Prof. Yu.D. Tsvetkov was vice-chairman. The scientific advisory board included the most famous Russian scientists in the field of ESR-methods and application:

About 300 scientists from 60 research centers of Russia, former Soviet Union and some countries of Europe, America and Asia took part in this conference. All the speakers and scientists who participated in the discussion emphasized that the research and ideas of Prof. V. Voevodskii defined the development of science in the area of chemistry and physics.

The Sixth European Meeting on "Fire Retardancy of Polymeric Materials"

G.E. ZAIKOV

Institute of Biochemical Physics, Russian Academy of Sciences, 4 Kosygin str., Moscow 117334, Russia

The Sixth European meeting on Fire Retardancy of Polymeric Materials was held in Lille (Cite Scientific) on the base of Ecoile Nationale Superieure de Chimie de Lille (ENSCL) France on September 22–24, 1997. The previous Fifth Conference was in Salford University (Manchester, England) in September 1995. Prof. Rene Delobel (ENSCL) was chairman of Organizing Committee and Drs. S. Bourbigot and M. Le Bras from ENSCL were members of General Secretariat. The international scientific committee included Prof. G. Camino (University of Torino, Italy), Dr. J.-M. Catala (Institut C. Sadron, Strasbourg, France), Dr. Dewitt (Solvay, Brussels, Belgium), Mr. F. Gensous (Elf Atochem, Lacq, France), Dr.M.-L. Hardy (Albermarle, Baton Rouge, USA), Prof. A.-R. Horrocks (Bolton Institute of Higher Education, UK), Prof. M. Lewin (Polytechnic University, NYC, USA), Prof. E. Marechal (Groupment Francais des Polymeres, France), Prof. R. Mulhaupt (University of Freiburg, Germany), Dr.D. Price (University of Salford, UK), Prof. J. Wang (Beijing Institute of Technology, China), Prof. G.E. Zaikov (Russian Academy of Sciences, Moscow, Russia).

Scientists from 25 countries (France, USA, Germany, Israel, China, Russia, Belorussia, Italy, UK, Japan, Belgium, The Netherlands, Austria, Croatia, Hungary, Sweden, Norway, India, Switzerland and Romania) contributed to the conference. Thirty five plenary lectures were presented at the conference which also included two sessions (I. Polymers, Composites—16 lectures, and II. Textiles, Wood, Fibres—15 lectures) as well as poster sessions (40 posters).

The meeting was opened with remarks of Prof. Rene Delobel, who emphasized the present interest of science and practice of the aforesaid problems. Mr. F. Henry from Assemblee Pleniere des Sosietes d'Assurances Dommages, Paris, France) gave the opening lecture with information about insurance system in France in case of fire.

The first main lecture of the conference was presented by Prof. Menachem Lewin (Herman F. Mark Polymer Research Institute, Polytechnic Universithy, Brooklyn, New York, USA) about physical and chemical mechanisms of flame retardancy of polymers. On behalf of scientific group L. Costa (Universita di Torino), J.M. Catala (Institute Charles Sadron, Strasbourg, France), K.M. Gibov (Research Institute for Chemical Science, Alma Aty, Kazakhstan), A.V. Gribanov (Research Institute for High Molecular Compounds, St. Petersburg, Russia), S.V. Levchik (Belorussian

University, Minsk, Belorussia), N.A. Khalturinskij (Research Institute for Synthetic Polymeric Materials, Moscow, Russia), Dr. Levchik spoke about the mechanism of action of halogen-free fire retardants and development approachs to design of new fire retardants with reduced environmental and health impact. Dr. D. Price gave information about Laser Pyrolysis/time-of-flight mass spectrometry studies pertinent to the behavior of flame retarded polymers in real fire situations. This report was prepared by scientifical group: F. Gao, J. Milness (both from Science Research Institute, University of Salford, Manchester, UK), B. Eling (International Research and Development, ICI Chemicals and Polymers Ltd., Cleveland, UK), C.I. Lindsay, P.T. McGrail (both from Composite Science Workshop, ICI Chemicals and Polymers Ltd., Cleveland, UK). The lecture of Dr. J.E.J. Staggs (University of Leeds, Novell, Leeds, UK) was devoted to Modelling the effect of solid-phase additives on thermal degradation of solids. On behalf of group of Russiuan scientist from Research Institute for Synthetic Polymeric Materials, Moscow, Russia (M.Yu. Yablokova, T.A. Rudakova, A.V. Antonov, N.A. Khalturinskiio), Dr. I.S. Reshetnikov presented the lecture "Special features of bubble formation during intumescent systems burning". Transition between regimes in the degradation of thermoplastic polymers was presented by Dr. C. Di Blasi (Universita di Napoli, Italy). Prof. J. Wang (Beijing Institute of Technology, Beiging, China) spoke about Studies of thermal degradation and charring of polymers by XPS/TGA Two the most important reports were presented by Drs. Takashi Kashiwagi and John W. Gilman (both from National Institute of Standards and Technology, Gaithersburg, USA). Dr. T. Kashiwagi was speaking about New flame retardant additives (coauthors J.W. Gilman, N.R. Nyden, S.M. Lomakin from the Institute of Biochemical Physic Russian Academy of Sciences), the topic of J.M. Gilman's lecture (coauthors T. Kashiwagi, J. Lichtenham from Philips Laboratory, Edwards Air Force Base, CA USA) was Nanocomposites: a revolutionary new flame retardant approach The lecture of Prof. G. Camino (coauthor P. Luda) reviwed work in the area of intumescence mechanisms. He showed that the "intumescent" behavior resulting from combination of charring and foaming of the surface of the burning polymers is being widely developed in fire retardancy because it is characterized by a low environmental impact. Application of polymer composites for Navale was discussed in the lecture of F. Le Lay and J. Gutierrez (DGA-DCNB, Constraction Navale, La Montagne, France). Group of scientists: S.V. Levchik A.I. Balabanovich, G.F. Levchik (Research Institute for Physical Chemical Problem, Byelorussian University, Minsk, Belorussia), Ch. Wilkie (Department of Chemistry, Marquette University, Baton-Rouge, USA), G. Camino (Universita di Torino, Italy) reported about the relationship cross-linking-charring-fire retardancy in high energy irradiated nylon 6. Photooxidation of fire retarded polypropylene was the topic of lecture of J.L. Gardette, C. Sinturel and J. Lemaire (Universite Blaise-Pascal, Laboratoire de Photochimie Moleculaire et Macromoleculaire, Aubiere, France). G. Anthony (FMC Corporation, Manchester, UK) spoke about kinetic and chemical studies of polymer cross-linking using thermal gravimetry and hyphenated methods. The report of I.G. Assovskii (Institute of Chemical Physics, Moscow, Russia) had dealt with thermal regimes of heterogeneous reaction in porous material, smoldering to combustion transition. Some aspects of mechanical stability of intumescent chars were presented in the lecture of Prof. A.A. Berlin (Institute of Chemical Physics, Moscow, Russia (coauthors I.S. Reshetnikov,

M.Yu. Yablokova, N.A. Khalturinskij—all from Research Institute for Synthetic Polymeric Materials, Moscow, Russia). The lectures of Prof. A.R. Horrocks (Bolton Institute of Higher Education, UK) and B.K. Kandola (Dept. of Textiles, Faculty of Technology, Bolton Institute, Bolton, UK) were dedicated to flame retardant cellulose textiles. Ecological Aspects of polymer flame retardancy were discussed in the lectures of Prof. G.E. Zaikov (Institute of Biochemical Physics), his coauthor S.M. Lomakin from the same institute. Participants of conference have discussed with great interest information presented in reports of Dr. R. Dewitt (Solvay, Brussels, Belgium) about the European regulations in the field of flammability of polymeric materials, Prof. M.L. Hardy (Albermarle Corporation, Baton Rouge, USA) about regulatory status and environmental properties of brominated flame retardant undergoing risk assessment in the EU and Drs. M. Checchini, C. Cecchini, B. Cellarosi, F.O. Sam (EniChem Research Centre, Porto Marghera, Venezia, Italy) about the use of cone calorimeter for evaluating of fire performances of polyurethane foams.

The next 4 reports were devoted to standards, tests and equipments of flammability study (J. Troitzsch, Fire and Environment, Protection Service, Wiesbaden, Germany), a cone calorimeter test for the measurment of flammability properties of insulated wire (P.J. Elliot, R.H. Whiteley Raychem Ltd., Corporate Technology Europe, Swindon, UK), combustibility and toxicity of board materials used for interior fittings and decorations (R. Kozlowski, D. Wesolek, M. Wladyka, Przybylak Institute of Natural Fibers Science Information Centre, Poznan, Poland), regulations on flammability in aeronautique (J.E. Petit, A. Mansuet, Toulouse, France).

Three last plenary lectures were devoted to problems of decreasing of flammability of polymeric materials (Prof. Rene Delobel), property evaluation of flame retardant polymeric materials using a range of instrumental techniques (J.P. Redfern, Rheomethric Scientific Ltd., Epsom, Surrey UK) and decreasing of flammability of polymeric materials for the space programme (D. Rebuffat, J.F. Petit, A. Mansuet, M. Ferie (DGA-CEAT, Toulouse, France); V. Cervantes, M. Vachon (BERTIN *et Cie*, Tarnos, France).

Between different topics which were discussed in the session I (Polymers and composites) we have first of all to show information about new flame retardant systems for styrenic plastics and method to prepare them, developments in the use of magnesium hydroxide as a fire retardant filler for thermoplastics, influence of the incorporation of several talcs in a PP-PE copolymer flame retarded by a brominated trimethylphenyl indane/antimony trioxide blend, halogen-free flame retarded thermosets, properties of flame retarded polystyrene, latest developments in the flame retardancy of engineering thermoplastics, thermal properties and flammability of polyarylenes and their modifying products, new ecological polyester resins with reduced flammability and smoke evolution capacity, brominated copolymers of reduced flammability, resorcinol bis (diphenyl phosphate), as a non-halogen flame retardant additive, the use of organophosphorus functionality to modify the thermal and fire retardant behavior of polyamides, use of zinc borate in the flame retardancy of some polymers.

The most important reports of the session II (Textiles, Wood, Fibers) were devoted to the flammability of Lyocell, novel fire resistant textiles—multisponsor approach, burning behaviour of tropical wood-the effect of flame retardants, flame retardant composites—a review—the use of intumescent/fibre composites, flame retardant treated plywood, mechanistic study on fire retardant action of fluorine-containing additives inb ABS, flame retardant alkyd paint, fire resistant ligno-cellulosic-mineral composite particleboards, heterocyclic additives and stabilizers to polymer materials.

The posters covered a very broad field of decreasing of flammability of polymers and copolymers.

Two hundred and fifty scientists from 100 research centres took part in this conference. Practically it was not European, but world conference, because the scientists from Europe, America, Asia and Africa took part in this meeting.

The conference was a very high level and showed that either fundamental research of polymer flammability or practical application of novel flame retardants successfully develop.

The next VII European meeting on Fire Retardancy of polymeric materials is scheduled on September 10–12, 1999 in University of Greenwich, London, England. The organizers of conference are Prof. Metcalfe from school of chemistry and life sciences, University of Greenwich, Wellington street, Woolwich, London SE186PE and Dr. Dennis Price from University of Salford, Salford, Manchester, UK. The main organizer of the next conference is Fire chemistry discussion group (UK).

Progress in Polymer Science in Japan

The reviews in this section cover papers presented at the 46th Annual Meeting (Spring) and Symposium on Macromolecules (Fall) of the Society of Polymer Science, Japan (SPSJ) which were held in the Tokyo Institute of Technology at Okayama on May 24–26, 1997 and the Nagoya Institute of Technology on October 1–3, 1997 respectively. There were 3,052 attendees and 1,798 presentations at the Spring Meeting, and 2,550 attendees and 1,569 presentations at the Fall Symposium.

The Spring Meeting covered general topics, functional polymers, high performance polymers, polymer structure, interfacial and surface properties, polymer engineering and technology, polymer synthesis, polymer reaction, bio-related polymers, physical properties of polymer solution, polymer dynamic and rheology, and physical properties of polymer solid.

The Fall Symposium covered 866 general topics and 9 invited lectures. The papers presented in the special topics covered 49 frontiers in radical polymerization, 21 metalocene catalysts, 63 organic photonics from materials to devices, 45 functional polymers for electronics, 47 polymer gels, 45 glycopolymers, 53 basic science of polymer alloys, 42 enhancements of performance of polymer alloys by structure control, 93 designs of supramolecules, 77 supramolecular systems and molecular recognition, 20 dispersion structures in polymer systems, 35 dynamics of glassy polymers and diffusion of small molecules in glassy polymeric membranes, 54 polymer characterizations, 43 computationals and 16 polyvinylchlorides.

Each review article concentrates on presentations made at both meetings. The support of the Board of Directors of the SPSJ, and in particular Mr Kenichi Shida, Secretary General of the SPSJ, is acknowledged by the Regional Editor.

REFERENCES

References which appear in brackets in the text are page numbers in Polymer Preprints Japan (Japanese edition), volume 46 (1997). Following the page numbers, E signifies the page number for the English abstract in Polymer Preprints, Japan (English edition) volume 46 (1997).

Any enquiry about the Meeting or References, please contact the SPSJ office on the following fax number: +81-3-3545-8560.

Computer Science of Polymers

KAZUYOSHI UEDA[1] and AKIRA IMAMURA[2]

[1]*Physical Chemistry Laboratory, Department of Material Science, Faculty of Engineering, Yokohama National University, Tokiwadai Hodogaya-ku, Yokohama, 240-8501, Japan*
[2]*Department of Chemistry, Faculty of Science, Hiroshima University, Kagamiyama, Higashi-hiroshima 739-8526, Japan*

1 POLYMER PROPERTY

1.1 Molecular Orbital Approach

Y. Kurihara, Y. Aoki *et al.* (3652, E882) studied the reversible interconversion between the two structures with different bond lengths in polydiacetylene single crystal induced by photoexcitation. The excitation energies of polydiacetylenes were calculated by the single excitation configuration interaction based on the localized molecular orbitals, which were obtained using the "Elongation method" at the CNDO/S approximation level. "Elongation method" is a MO program which was developed in their laboratory. As a first step, they assumed that the central unit of the oligomer composed of 7 units is changed by photo excitation. The differences between the energies around the phase transition in polydiacetylene were 0.6 eV for the ground state and 0.04 eV for the excited state. This implies a possibility that the photoinduced phase transition could arise between the acetylenic type structure and butatrienic type one.

T. Yamazaki, Y. Aoki *et al.* (3654, E882) proposed a convenient method to calculate the circular dichroism of organic molecules and polymers by using molecular orbital calculation. In the Davidson's CI method which has been widely used for obtaining excited states of molecules, the configuration state function (CSFs) that are not included in the CI calculations could make a great contribution to the transition moment. In order to improve this deficiency, they performed the CI calculations by including all the CSFs which could contribute to the transition moments. As a first step, they apply this treatment to peptide oligomers and discussed the reliability and applicability of their approach towards large polymers.

T. Kawaguchi, Y. Aoki *et al.* (3660, E883) provided a new method to design ferromagnetic organic polymers by using ab initio MO method. They proved that the linkage between starred and unstarred carbon atoms in a Non-bonding Molecular Orbital (NBMO) does not have an affect on the NBMO in the framework of the simple Huckel method. This suggests that this type of linkage between molecules could provide an NBMO degenerate system which exhibits high multiplicity. However, by including the effect of electron correlation, Non-Disjointed type molecules thus obtained may be sometimes more stable in the singlet state than in the other multiplet states. Therefore it would be important to design Non-Disjointed type molecules with a large mixing between the degenerate NBMOs even at Hartree-Fock level. In this work, they defined an index to estimate the mixing between the degenerate NBMOs and applied it to various organic molecules which are well known as Ferromagnetic organic polymers.

1.2 Molecular Dynamics and Monte Carlo Approach

Y. Abe, K. Tashiro *et al.* (3664, E884) performed molecular dynamics simulations to clarify the ferroelectric phase transition in vinylidene fluoride-trifluoroethylene (VDF-TrFE) copolymers. The MD unit cells of VDF 50 and 70 mol% copolymer systems were constructed by packing the 16 chains consisted of random sequences of VDF and TrFE monomer units. The results showed that the average phase transitional temperature of the VDF 70 mol% system was higher than that of VDF 50 mol% system. The mean square displacement of the carbon atoms in the c-axis direction was larger than that in the directions of the a and b axes in both the phases of the low temperature phase and the high temperature phase. It was found that the sequences related to TrFE segments tend to keep the trans conformation in the molecular chains even above the transition point.

T. Koda, Y. Morito *et al.* (3716, E892) performed a Monte Carlo simulation to discuss the polarization reversal of ferroelectric crystal of poly(vinylidene fluoride) (PVDF). Applied electric field can reverse the direction of spontaneous polarization of PVDF. Starting with a poled state against applied electric field, the simulation showed microscopic behavior of growing domains of flipped chains. It was indicated that a certain size is needed for a domain to grow stably. Their results showed that the strength of electric field affects this domain size of stable growth.

2 POLYMER CONFORMATION

2.1 Microscopic Approach

K. Ueda, A. Imamura *et al.* (3688, E888) studied the solution conformation of the sulfated polysaccharide of carrageenan. Solvent water plays an important role on the solution conformation of biopolymers, such as polysaccharides and proteins. However, it is generally very difficult to obtain a free energy of biopolymers which is calculated by taking into account the solvation effect exactly owing to their large freedom of conformation. In their study, molecular dynamics calculation with umbrella sampling was applied in order to obtain the two dimensional free energy surface for (ϕ, ψ) dihedral angles of glycosidic linkage of the dimer unit of carrageenan.

H. Shimizu, K. Uehara *et al.* (3692, E888) calculated the free energy of the di-block copolymer by applying the multi-canonical molecular dynamics method. Di-block copolymer has been considered as a simple model of biopolymers and been investigated for the study of the folding problem. Multi-canonical method has great advantages of avoiding a system to stay in local minimum states and being able to sample in a wide area of the phase space. They discussed the structural (phase) transition for such a particular model from the thermodynamic point of view as well as free energy which determines most stable states.

Y. Tamai, H. Tanaka (3698, E889) performed molecular dynamics simulations on hydrogels of poly (vinyl alcohol) and pure water at 135–400 K in order to investigate the effects of water on the dynamics of polymer chains and effects of suppression of chain dynamics caused by the glass transition on the structure of water. A distinct break was observed at around 200–250 K in the specific volume, the potential energy of water, and the orientational autocorrelation function of bond vector of main chains, which can be identified as a glass transition. Perfectness of hydrogen bond structure was examined by the fraction of water molecules which form four hydrogen bond, P(4). Above glass transition temperature *Tg*, the value of p(4) of water in hydrogels were approximately the same as that in pure water. On the other hand, structurization of water was hindered around hydrophilic groups of polymer chains below *Tg*.

2.2 Macroscopic Approach

H. Noguchi, K. Yoshikawa (3684, E887) performed a Monte Carlo simulation on the folding transition of a single stiff polymer chain by using a beads-stick model. The results showed that the coil-globule transition of a stiff chain is first-order phase transition. Among the products of the folding from the single chains, torroidal structure was found to be the most stable. Rod structure was also generated as a metastable state. These morphologies resemble the experimental structures observed with electron microscopy for the products of collapse from single duplex DNA chains.

M. Monzen, M. Doi (3694, E889) investigated the equilibrium structure of linear homopolymers grafted periodically on a solid surface. Calculations were carried out using both Monte Carlo (MC) simulation and Self-Consistent Field (SCF) theory for several solvent conditions. Good agreement was found between these two methods. In the case of low graft density, "mushroom" like conformation of the grafted polymers was observed by both methods (MC and SCF). In the case of very high graft density, "brush" like structure appeared. In a good solvent, "swollen brush" was observed. In a poor solvent, "melt brush" was observed since solvent molecules cannot penetrate into the brush. Furthermore, they proposed a new technique to make a initial condition of MC simulation using "self-consistent field" of SCF theory.

K. Matuura, M. Doi (3704, E890) studied the gelation process of telechelic polymers which have two reaction sites at both ends of the chain by using the Brownian Dynamics. When the distance of the reaction sites was below certain value, they always connect irreversible. It was found that the final state is dependent on the initial density of polymer and the solvent quality and that there is a critical density for gelation.

N. Takahashi (3730, E895) proposed a new simulation method to predict the three-dimensional structure of protein. Their method "homology reconstruction" is based on a "local structure database". The database was made from the results of a molecular dynamics simulation. The basic concept and an example of application were shown. A description of time evolution of the chain on a locally defined coordinate (bond angles) gives a repeating of the local variables. A portion of the MD orbit of each bond angle which has homology to the other part of the MD orbit is connected to the MD orbit. The connected parts are then adjusted and the global time evolution was predicted. This method was applied to the conformation of n-butane.

3 MOLECULAR DESIGN OF POLYMER

M. Sisido (3666, E884) developed a software (PROCON) for design of artificial prosthetic group and substrates through molecular mechanics calculation. This program was extended to design ferrocenelinked FAD prosthetic molecules that may be properly bound to D-aminoacid oxidase (DAO) and may mediate electrons between electrode and FAD moiety. The FAD part of the artificial prosthetic group was positioned at the FAD binding site of DAO and the conformational energy calculations were carried out by using the PROCON program to find the most stable orientation of the ferrocenyl group.

M. Oka, T. Hayashi (3668, E884) carried out theoretical conformational analysis by using ECEPP and conformational optimization procedure for the super helical structures constructed by β-strands. Conformational optimization procedure was performed under the condition having conformational constraint at the loop portion. Calculated results indicated that relative stability of the super helical structures constructed by β-strands are significantly changed by introducing such constraint. Some of them are very interesting for the backbone structures of β-type artificial proteins.

T. Matsuoka, S. Yamamoto *et al.* (3726, E894) applied generic algorithm to design microstructures of polymer mixtures by combining with a finite element stress analysis. As a working example, this method was applied to find microstructures of binary mixtures that do not shrink transversely when they are stretched. They succeed to design a new network structure from the results of the generic computing for mixtures of which Poisson's ratio is negative.

Polymer Dynamics and Rheology

NORIO NEMOTO

Department of Molecular and Material Sciences, IGSES, Kyushu University, Hakozaki, Fukuoka 812-8581, Japan

This article reviews papers presented in a special session "New Development of Polymer Alloy" and papers in a session "Polymer Dynamics and Rheology" in the SPSJ 45th fall symposium.

KEYWORDS: Phase separation process, Polymer melt, Domain structure, Reactive processing, Dynamic viscoelasticity, Block copolymer, Polymer blend, Dispersion, Gel and Local motion.

POLYMER ALLOY

In 1981, The Society of Polymer Science, Japan, published a monograph titled "Polymer Alloy: Fundamentals and Applications",[1] which was quite successfull in systematic reorganization of various ideas and concepts being independently developed in respective fields of multicomponent systems such as polymer blends, polymer composites, block and graft copolymers, and promoted technological developments in polymer industry. We can see many fruitful results in the second edition[2] published in 1993. Though incipent enthusiasm looks to have calmed down, papers presented in the special session show that basic research on polymer alloy is continuously expanding to reach to the scientific level of metallic alloys.

1 Polymer Blend

There is surely a limit to the improved mechanical properties or new functional properties obtainable by simple blending of two compatible or incompatible polymers, even if it is low cost commercially. As dynamic vulcanization gave a break-through to improvement of elastic properties of thermoplastic elastomers, interconnection of imcompatible polymer chains by chemical reaction is useful. For example, high impact polystyrene and ABS resins constitute an important class of industrial thermoplastics. T. Inoue (E709) pointed out in the invited lecture that, in addition to these alloys by "wet processing" two families of polymer alloys by "dry processing" were going to be developed. Chemical reaction usually occurs on the interface to yield block or graft copolymers for immiscible polymer–polymer systems, and copolymer formation drastically affects interfacial thickness, morphology, and bulk properties. Cure reaction in single-phase mixtures induces phase transitions, which mostly proceeds by a spinodal decomposition mechanism. One can control the morphology in a wide range of 10 nm–10 μm using reactive processing techniques.

T. Sato, T. Shiomi *et al.* (E708) discussed miscibility and immiscibility of random copolymer blends using the Flory-Huggins theory for the equation of state. For methacrylate random copolymer systems, the temperature dependence of the interaction parameter χ is represented as a U-shaped curve reproduced by the observed UCST-type phase diagram. The χ was also calculated for poly(vinyl chloride-ran-vinyl acetate)/poly(n-butyl methacrylate-ran-isobutyl methacrylate) blends from experiments for their ternary solutions in cyclohexanone. The immiscibility window for the blends was qualitatively explained by changes in χ values from negative → positive → negative with copolymer composition. Monotonic increase in χ with temperature may indicate that the blends are miscible regardless of the copolymer composition below a certain temperature. M. Hayashi, H. Jinnai *et al.* (E709) studied the phase separation process induced by a two-step temperature jump for a deuterated polybutadiene/polyisoprene blend with the LCST type phase diagram and a spinodal temperature of 36°C. The first T-jump was made from room temperature to 42°C and during the later stage spinodal decomposition occured, the second T-jump was performed from 42 to 70°C. Light scattering profiles showed not only a peak due to larger domains but also, in the higher q-regions, another peak due to newly induced concentration fluctuations inside the previously formed domain by the first T-jump. When one component of polymer blend can crystallize, phase separation phenomena may be affected due to competition between crystallization and liquid–liquid phase separation. A study on tetramethyl-bisphenol-A polycarbonate/polystyrene blend (J. Kim, J. Joi *et al.*, E713) shows that the morphology is strongly dependent on the relative ratio between crystallization and separation rates which resulted from molecular weight difference of the PSs used for the study. For blends of poly(3-hydroxybutylate) (PHB) with poly(vinylidene chloride-co-vinylchloride) (PVDC-VC), J. Lee, T. Nishi *et al.* (E713) found that melting point T_m of PHB decreased with increasing PVDC-VC content above 70%, but showed no melting point depression below 70%. Isothermal spherulitic growth rate measurements indicates that PHB/P VDC-VC blends form homogeneous mixtures in the range of 0–30% PHB, while a mixture (30:70) coexists with an almost pure PHB phase at higher PHB content.

Several papers dealt with compatibilization of immiscible polymer pairs for structure control and toughening. For fine dispersion of RTV-silicone elastomer particles in a bisphenol-A-type epoxy resin, M. Ochi, A. Koyama *et al.* (E714) proposed use of silicone-methyl methacrylate graft copolymer, and showed that the graft copolymer with optimal structure as an effective compatibilizer was more effectively concentrated at the interface between silicone dispersed phase and epoxy resin matrix. Fracture toughness of the modified resin increased with a decrease in the diameter of silicone particles. M. Okamoto and T. Kotaka (E714) studied phase structure and viscoelastic properties of poly(ethylene naphthalene 2,6-dicarboxylate) (PEN)/poly(ethylene terephthalate) (PET) blends with or without PEN-PET random copolymer as compatibilizer. Palierne emulsion model was applied to estimate the interfacial tension Γ from the plateau of the storage modulus G'.

Incorporation of the random copolymer suppressed the domain growth and resulted in a decrease of Γ. In the intermediate stage, the domain growth was retarded by transesterification between the two polyesters through the domain interphase, and the whole system was gradually homogenized due to the miscibility enhancement by the produced PEN-PET multiblock copolymer species. S. Horiuchi, T. Kitano *et al.* (E715) studied compatibilizing effect of SEBS functionalized with maleic anhydride through a chemical reaction induced phase formation in blends of polyamide 6 and polycarbonate. In the PA6 rich blends, interfacial reaction between PA6 and SEBSgMA induces an encapsulation of SEBS onto the PC domains, whereas unfuctionalized SEBS does not give such a phase formation and attaches to the PC domains. Poly(ethylene phthalate) (PEP) is a useful modifier for toughening of bisphenol-A type cyanate resin (BACE). Mixing of 20 wt% PEP gives rise to an increase in fracture toughness by 120% with no reduction in flexural properties, but results in an increase in the extent of moisture absorption. S. Katsurayama, M. Tomoi *et al.* (E715) used poly(ethylene phthalate-co-*p*-phenylenaphthalate) (PEPP) having *p*-hydroxylphenyl units as end groups as modifier and showed that the PEPP-modified resin exhibited lower moisture absorption than the PEP-modified resins. An attempt to compatibilize a novel high-temperature-resistant polymer alloy of polysulfone/polyamide was made from introduction of carboxylic acid functions to the aromatic ring and grafting of PA onto the modified PSU (A. Ribbe, T. Hashimoto *et al.*, E716). Photochemical reaction also looks useful for morphology control (Q. Trang-Cong, O. Urakawa *et al.*, E716).

M. Matsushita, H. Takahashi *et al.* (E717) reported technological developments for blending thermosetting polyurethane (RIM-PU) and thermoplastic resins (PP) with reactive extrusion. Blends with PU content of 0–30% were heat-treated at 200–220°C, and their elongational and impact properties were improved due to plasticization and dispersion of RIM-PU which lead to an increase in the capacity of deformation energy absorption by microvoids and microcrazes that were progressed from the interface of RIM-PU and PP. They also attempted to obtain new raw materials of polyurethane rigid form by powderization and platicization with reactive extrusion (E716), and also studied curing behavior and physical properties of EPDM rubber reclaimed by reactive extrusion (E717).

2 Block Copolymer

A series of experiments on the ordering process were performed by T. Hashimoto's group (E710, E711) using polystyrene-block-polyisoprene diblock copolymers (SI) near the order–disorder transition temperature T_{ODT}. The SI diblock cxopolymer with lamella microdomain structure was quenched from the disordered state to the ordered state very close to T_{ODT}, and the ordering process was examined by time-resolved small-angle and ultra small-angle X-ray scattering diffractometer ($q = 0.0002$ Å^{-1}). The time evolution of SAXS profiles shows that there is an incubation period in which the profiles do not change before the ordering starts. TEM pictures and USAXS data show that the ordered lamellar state and the disordered state coexist during ordering and the shape of the lamellar grain observed in the disordered phase is very anisotropic and elongated in the lamellar normal direction.

These results indicate that this ordering process is a nucleation and growth process. The existence of the incubation period was also found for the SI diblock copolymer with cylindrical microdomain structure during ordering, being a proof that the ordering process is not a spinodal decomposition type but a nucleation and growth type. Pressure effect on order–disorder transition was studied using a diblock copolymer of deuterated polybutadiene (DPB) and protonated polyisoprene (HPI). Changes in SANS scattering profiles with increasing temperature were characterized by a single peak typical for the disordered state at low temperature to the appearance of the second-order peak aasociated with the microphase separation. T_{ODT} estimated from the temperature at which the second-order peak appeared was found a linear function of pressure, impling that pressure enhances the miscibility. This result is in contrast to the observation of PS-PI diblock copolymer which exhibits the UCST type of phase separation.

H. Umeda, S. Nomura *et al.* (E712) performed time-resolved SAXS study on ordering of microphase separated structures using polystyrene-block-polyethylene-butylene-block polystyrene) (SEBS) triblock copolymer. The sample formed a non-equilibrium morphology of lamella when cast from its toluene solution where toluene is a selective solvent, being good for PS but poor for PEB, and cylindrical microdomain structure was formed when fully annealed at temperature above the glass transition temperature of PS. Time profiles of SAXS data gave that the first-order peak position shifted to a wider angular region with increasing annealing time, but higher-order peaks for lamellar microdomains decreased without peak shifts. Crystallization and melting behaviors of poly(ε-caprolactone)-block-polybutadiene diblock copolymer were studied from synchrotron SAXS measurements (S. Nojima, S. Sasaki *et al.*, E713). They report that the melting behavior is quite different from the crystallization behavior for this block copolymer, in such a way that angular positions of the two intensity peaks to be related to microdomain structure and lamellar morphology do not change during crystallization, whereas these peaks are intimately correlated to each other in the case of melting to result in the complicated time-resolved SAXS curves.

POLYMER DYNAMICS AND RHEOLOGY

1 Polymer Blend and Block Copolymer

This section is complementary to summaries of studies on structure control and structure formation process in polymer alloy given in the previous sections, and is mainly focused on viscoelasticity of polymer blends and block copolymers as well as the effect of external mechanical force on their structures. It is well-known that external force affects phase separation as well as phase transition phenomena of polymer blends. S. Kitade, I. Noda (3320, E865) measured viscoelasticity of immiscible polymer blends of polydimethylsiloxane/polyisoprene under steady and oscillatory shear flows in order to clarify relations between domain morphologies under flow and their viscoelatic properties. Under steady shear flow, the shear stress σ and the first normal stress difference N_1 are both inversely proportional to shear rate $\dot{\gamma}$, and roughly uniform size of domains with diameter D decreases linearly with $\dot{\gamma}$. Their viscoelastic behavior can be qualitatively explained by a theory of Doi and Ohta.[3] Under oscillatory shear flow, they observed shoulders in the storage and the loss shear moduli, G' and G'', vs. ω curves, which can be interpreted by the linear theory of Palierne.[4] It is to be noted that the higher frequency components were not observed for this system in contrast to suspension system. 3.3% dioctylphthalate solutions of polystrene/polybutadiene blends were sheared at $\dot{\gamma} = 4.0\,s^{-1}$ so as to form phase-separated structure, and their structural changes with time after cessation of flow was investigated by light scattering measurements and also by direct observation with optical microscopy (K. Matsuzaki, T. Hashimoto (3336, E866). For the 50:50 mixture of the crtical composition, microscopic images and light scattering profiles demonstrate that string-like structure formed at $\gamma = 4.0\,s^{-1}$ broke into series of spherical form, due to Tomotika's instability. When shear rate was decreased from $\dot{\gamma} = 4.0\,s^{-1}$ to $0.1\,s^{-1}$, the string-like structure broke into bicontinuous structure without Tomotika's instability. For the 80:20 mixture, similar structural change was observed after cessation of flow, but it took much longer time for formation of a spherical form. Shear flow enhances concentration fluctuation, thus leading to shear-induced phase separation for semidilute homopolymer solutions. Extensive studies on semidilute solutions of very high molecular weight polystyrene and polyethylene were made by T. Hashimoto's group (3374–3380, E872, 873) using various techniques such as light scattering, viscoelasticity, flow dichroism, and birefringence. Nonlinear stress relaxation behavior was studied for LDPE/PP and LDPE/PS blends in both of which the LDPE component was dispersed as sphere in the matrix (H. Kashihara, T. Masuda *et al.*, 3334, E865). Relaxation modulus $G(t, \gamma)$ was separated into the linear relaxation modulus $G(t)$ and strain dependent damping function $h(\gamma)$ in the time region shorter than 20s. The $h(\gamma)$ is found to be close to that of the continuous phase. At longer times than 20s, $G(t, \gamma)$ for various γ converges to form a single curve. There exists an extra relaxation mode with a relaxation time much longer than the reptation time, which cannot be observed in the linear viscoelastic region. Basic research on tribology of polymer blend was started by T. Horiuchi, M. Takahashi *et al.* (3412, E 878). They measured the specific wear rate on blends of polyamide 6 with maleic anhydride grafted high density and low density polyethylene and polypropylene. Complicated results obtained suggest more extensive study.

T. Hashimoto and his associates continue studies on deformation mechanism of block copolymer. In three papers presented (G. Shin, K. Saijo *et al.*, 3416–3420, E879–880), they report results of dynamic small-angle X-ray scattering experiments on three block copolymers with spherical or lamellar microdomain structures under oscillatory shear strain. For polystyrene-block-poly(ethylene-alt-propylene) diblock copolymer which forms a body-centered cubic lattice, deformation amplitude of the spherical microdomain and that of {110} lattice plane both decay with the number of strain cycle, N, and after 40 cycle the spherical domain and the {110} lattice plane almost cease to deform. This stress-hardening type of process may be related to the slip at the grain boundary. When large oscillatory shear strain ($\gamma = 0.5$ and $\omega = 0.0944\,\mathrm{rad\,s^{-1}}$) is imposed on the same diblock copolymer sample, we can estimate two dynamic lattice strains, one being γ_{orient} for the strain obtainable from the orientation angle of {110} lattice plane and another γ_{simple} the strain described by the simple shear deformation from analysis of two-dimensional SAXS patterns. γ_{orient} is in about the same phase as the macroscopic strain, and γ_{simple} is advanced by 15°. With elevating measuring temperature, the change of γ_{simple} increasingly leads forward the macroscopic strain but γ_{orient} lags behind it. Lamellar-forming PS-alt-PEP diblock copolymer deforms under shear deformation by the biaxial orientation of lamellar microdomains with their normal direction preferentially oriented along either the shearing direction or the velocity gradient direction, which may be supposed to be a folding process of lamellar microdomains at the grain boundaries. The system shows non-linear mechanical response, and the amplitude of stress decreases with increasing strain cycle. The non-linear mechanical response of the system was analyzed in terms of higher Fourier components of the shear stress as a function of the domain orientation, the strain amplitude, and temperature. It is suggested that the shear orientation process may be related to the increase of the volume fraction of grain boundaries with increasing strain cycle.

2 Polymer Gel

The volume phase transition phenomenon of chemical gels is attracting many researchers because of scientific interest as well as practical application. H. Ushiki, J. Rouch *et al.* (3371, E871) studied effects of various metal ions and poly(ethylene oxide) on the volume phase transition temerature T_c of poly(*N*-isopropylacrylamide) gels with anticipation that affinity of these substances with water molecules or clusters might depress T_c. The dependence of T_c on concentration C of added compounds is given by $T_c = (2\times(273.15 + T_{c,o})/(2 - \eta[C]) - 273.15$, where η is a measure of affinity of added compounds with water and is found independent of amount of surface charges of the compounds. They show that this equation can be derived from the extended protein lattice model based on the Ising model. C. Hashimoto and H. Ushiki (3372, E872) also made a kinetic study on shrinking and whitening process at T_c of PNIPA gels from direct observation by a video camera system. The time when turbidity of the gel reaches a maximum is shown to coincide with the time when the area, S, of the gels becomes a minimum, and the time dependence is given, after an incubation period, by the KWW type of the equation (1).

$$S = S_z + (S_0 - S_z)\exp\left[-(t/\tau)^{\beta}\right] \tag{1}$$

where S_0 and S_z are the area at the swollen and the shrinked states, respectively. They suggest that β and τ are quantities characteristic of the collapse process of the skin layer formed during the incubation period and the holding time of the skin layer, repectively, which may emphasize importance of the concept of the skin layer in the process. T. Ikehara and T. Nishi (3397, E876) investigated volume change dynamics of acrylamide gels in poly(vinyl methyl ether) solution with polymer concentration C range of 0.1–5%. The swollen gels in pure water first contract when they are transferred into PVME solutions and they begin to swell after several hundreds of hours. The late reswelling process takes place by penetration of PVME molecules into the gel network, and the period until the reswelling starts is governed by the self diffusion coefficient of PVME roughly estimated as $D_s \sim 10^{-9}\,cm^2s^{-1}$, whereas the initial deswelling process is dominated by the cooperative diffusion coefficient $D_c \sim 10^{-7}$ cm^{2}s^{-1}. They conclude that the dynamics are a superposition of two diffusion processes with different rate-determining factors, D_s and D_c.

Two papers are concerned with inhomogeniety of gels. As a basic research for preparation of rapid response gels, T. Miura and H. Ichijo (3392, E875) studied the formation process of heterogeneous gels resulted from competition between simultaneous liquid–liquid phase separation and the chemical gelation. 30 wt% Solutions of PVME pre-irradiated for various time intervals were quenched into the two phase region and formation of semi-macroscopic heterogeneous gel structures were observed using optical microscopy. Image analysis gave the characteristic wave number q_c^{-1} for respective heterogeneous structures. q_c^{-1} is found to vary drastically as the phase separation temperature is varied only by 0.5°C. Preparation of the rapid response gel appears impossible with this method at present, but porous gel can be easily prepared under conditions examined. The gel formation process of agarose is studied by S. Nakamura, K. Morisawa *et al.* (3394, E875) with two-dimensional light scattering method. Total intensity suddenly increased as the gel was formed and asymptotically approached to a constant value. They conclude from scattering pattern and the correlation length that fine particles are formed during the late stage of the gel formation process.

3 Local Motion

Local motions of polymer chains in solution, solid, and glass are quite complicated and there remain a lot of unsolved problems. Two groups used the fluorescence anisotropy decay method to obtain informations on local molecular motion in dilute polymer solution. S. Amano, M. Yamamoto *et al.* (3502, E893) estimated the orientational relaxation time of poly(oxyethylene as about 0.1 ns, which is one order shorter compared to corresponding values of other chains with side chains. Y. Katsumoto, H. Ushiki *et al.* (3366, E871) examined polystyrene solutions from the dilute to the semidilute regime. They found that fluorescence decay curve could be fitted by the KWW function in the dilute regime and by the hyperbolic function in the semidilute regime. They show that the results are in good agreement with their theory constructed on the basis that polymer main chains move intermitently. T. Shimomura, R. Hayakawa, *et al.* (3364, E870) developed a new apparatus for the frequency-domain electric birefringence (FEB) in a wide frequency range form 0.1 to 50 MHz with comparable sensitive to a conventional dielectric relaxation spectroscopy. They applied this apparatus to the dilute and non-dilute solutions of poly (3-hexylthiophene) for a study of intra-molecular carrier dynamics of conjugated conducting polymer. There exists a high-frequency relaxation mode above 1 MHz due to the diffusion of mobile carriers within a local region between neighbouring defects on a polymer chain. With increasing the polymer concentration, the relaxation frequency shifts to the high frequency side, which suggests that the conjugation length becomes longer by association of polymers.

Molecular motion of polymer chains tethered on the surface of other polymers is affected by the segmental motion as well as the structure of the latter. ESR measurements show that molecular mobility of poly(methyl methacrylate) copolymer chain tethered on the surface of high density PE is higher than that of PMMA homopolymer, whereas the mobility of poly(*n*-butyl methacrylate) copolymer chain is lower than that of PnBMA homopolymer (M. Kozakai, M. Yamamoto *et al.* (3496, E892) This peculiar result may be ascribed to the fact the PMMA chain has a low segmental concentration.

Dielectric measurements were performed to study the α-and β-relaxation in miscible blends of poly(vinyl methylether) and poly(2-chlorostyrene) (O. Urakawa, Q. Trang-Cong, *et al.*, 3340, E866). Two α-relaxation peaks were observed in the dielectric tan δ for all blends and attributed to each component relaxation which arised from local composition fluctuation. For the β-relaxation of PVME components in the blends, the relaxation time and its activation energy remain unchanged with the blend composition. This indicates that the side chain motion of PVME occurs independently and is unaffected by the change of environment.

Polymer electrolytes have potential applicability for solid electrolytes due to the unique characteristics such as flexibility, adhesivity and processibility into the membranes. A. Nishimoto, M. Watanabe *et al.* (3506, 3508, E894) have chosen three networks composed of poly(ethylene oxide) (PEO) with and without dendric side chains as ion-conducting polymer solids and studied relations between the mechanism of ion conduction and fast side chain relaxation. They found that, when ionic conductivity σ was compared at their respective glass transition temperature, (1) σ took a maximum with increasing the dendric side chain length; (2) σ of the network with dendric side chains was larger by one order of magnitude than σ of the network of linear PEO. Positron annihilation spectroscopy revealed that the latter result was related to an increase in local free volume due to introduction of dendric side chains.

Recently Sokolov *et al.*[5] reported that fragility of glass-forming material, defined from temperature dependence of viscosity, was correlated to two ratios, R_1 and R_2. R_1 is an intensity ratio of the "fast" process in a picosecond order to the Boson peak at the glass transition temperature T_g and R_2 is a ratio of minimum to maximum of heat capacity divided by T^3 far below T_g. It is well-known that the fragility is a property of the α-process while R_1 is a property in very high frequency region and R_2 of a very low temperature nature. This lead Kanaya to raise an issue, "Why can those properties be correlated?" (3414, E879). He roughly estimated the length scale of cooperatively rearranging region (CRR) for the α-process as 10–30 Å and the length of the Boson peak as 10–50 Å. He suggests that correlated molecular motions in glass are allowed only in this restricted region and may give the correlation mentioned above. Inoue and Osaki (3424, 3426, E880, 881) proposed two orientation models for amorphous polymers in the glassy state to describe the strain-induced birefringence and visocelasticity around the glass transition zone from the molecular point of view. Using the models, they calculated the strain dependence of two characteristic orientation functions, P_R and P_G, which corresponds to the orientation of the chord vector (chain direction) of the structure units and the tilting of the structure units toward the stretch direction by rotating around the chain axis. They already analyzed dynamic birefringence and dynamic viscoelasticity of many vinyl polymers with various side chain groups with the modified stress-optical rule to obtain the two components functions (R for the rubber and G for the glass component) for the birefringence and stress. Making use of those data, the relation between P_R and P_G were studied. It is found that $P_G \sim 2P_R$ at small strain and P_G tends to increase with increasing the size of the side chain.

4 DISPERSION

Suspensions of monodisperse spherical silica particles in organic solvent such as ethylene glycol (EG) may be considered as an ideal system for a study of Brownian dynamics under the repulsive potential due to collision of rigid bodies. Since EG is not only a visous medium but also prevent fatal effect due to electrode polarization, accurate dielectric measurements become feasible. T. Moriwaki, T. Shikata *et al.* (3360, E870) found two distinctive relaxation processes for all samples examined. The relaxation time in the slow process is proportional to the square of the particle diameter as found for aqueous suspension of polystyrene latex and obeys the prediction of Schwarz theory[6] which states that the slow mode is originated from fluctuation of the distribution of counterions on the particle surface. The fast relaxation process with small amplitude is essentially independent of the particle size and fluctuation of the counterion distribution in the radial direction of the particle is the origin for the fast mode. Nonlinear rheology was examined for a suspension of same silica particle (radius = 40 nm, volume fraction = 0.34) in EG/glycerol mixture (H. Watanabe, Y. Morishima *et al.*, 3402, E877). Brownian motion of these particles was detected as slow, linear viscoelastic relaxation. The stress relaxation modulus $G(\gamma, t)$ showed damping behavior for $\gamma > 0.2$ and the damping function $h(\gamma)$ is found different from that obtained for the entangled polymer system. The viscosity growth function and the steady state viscosity exhibited shear-thinning for small $\dot{\gamma}$, which was well described by a BKZ type constitutive equation, but shear-thickening for larger $\dot{\gamma}$. The latter is discussed in relation to shear effect on the spatial distribution and motion of the suspended particles.

Linear and nonlinear viscoelastic relaxations of polystyrene-block-polyisoprene diblock copolymer micelles (with S cores and I corona) were extensively discussed by H. Watanabe, T. Sato *et al.* (3404–3408, E877, 878). In a nonentangling and also an entangling homopolyisoprene (hI) matrix, the micelles exhibited fast and slow relaxation processes. The fast process was attributed to relaxation of individual corona I blocks, and a nearly universal relationship was obtained for reduced modului $G_r^* = [M_{bI}/C_{bI}RT]G_{SI}^*$ and reduced frequency $\omega\tau^*$, where G_{SI}^* was the contribution of the SI micelles to G^*, M_{bI} and C_{bI} were the molecular weight and concentration for the I block, and τ^* was the relaxation time that increased exponentially with C_{bI} for large C_{bI}. These features were similar to those observed for star chains. The relaxation time of the slow process was found close to the diffusion time of the micelles determined from FRS measurements in the nonentangling hI matrix, whereas the process was much faster than that expected for the simple Einstein-Stokes diffusion mechanism in the entangling hI matrix. Nonlinear relaxation moduli $G(\gamma, t)$ of the SI micelles in the nonentangling hI matrix exhibited two-step relaxation and were separated into contributions of the fast and slow processes, $G_f(\gamma, t)$ and $G_s(\gamma, t)$. Damping funtion $h_f(\gamma)$ was only modestly strain-dependent like that of homopolymer chains, while $h_s(\gamma)$ was strongly γ-dependent as observed for silica suspension. Under steady flow, the SI micelles exhibited mild shear-thinning that could be described by a BKZ constitutive equation, which suggests that the thickening mechanism of the suspensions, collision and dynamic clustering of particles, was surpressed for the micelles by the presence of the corona. The nonlinear damping function of the slow process was more weakly strain-dependent in the entangling hI matrix, again demonstrating the difference in the slow relaxation mechanism in these matrices.

Dynamics of threadlike micelles such as CTAB and CDMAO was investigated by two groups. Ultrasonically induced birefringence experiments (K. Yasuda, H. Nomura, 3353, E869) showed that the wave form of transient birefringence after cessation of ultra sonic fields was like a damping oscillation whose period and damping time were 0.25 and 0.11 s for 50 mM and 0.1 and 0.09 s for 100 mM, respectively. T. Shikata, Y. Morishima *et al.* (3356–3358, E869) estimated the orientational relaxation time of a fluorescent probe in the micelles and found that the molecular motion was unaffected by added salt. They succeeded in measuring the lateral diffusion coefficient D_{lat} as about $10^{-5}\,\mathrm{cm^2 s^{-1}}$. Results of dynamic birefringence measurements are also reported.

REFERENCES

1. "*Polymer Alloy: Fundamentals and Applications*", ed. by the Society of Polymer Science, Japan, Tokyo Kagaku Dojin, Tokyo, 1981.
2. "*Polymer Alloy: Fundamentals and Applications*", 2nd edn. ed. by the Society of Polymer Science, Japan, Tokyo Kagaku Dojin, Tokyo, 1993.
3. M. Doi and T. Ohta, *J. Chem. Phys.*, 1991, **95**, p. 1242.
4. J. F. Palierne, *Rheol. Acta*, 1990, **29**, p. 204.
5. P. Sokolov, E. Rossler, A. Kisulik and D. Quitman, *Phys. Rev. Lett.*, 1993, **13**, p. 2062.
6. G. Scharz, *J. Phys. Chem.*, 1962, **66**, p. 2636.

Free-Radical Polymerization

TAMAKI NAKANO

Department of Applied Chemistry, Graduate School of Engineering, Nagoya University, Furo-cho, Chikusa-ku, Nagoya 464-0814, Japan

KEYWORDS: Living Polymerization, Block Copolymer, Cptodative Monomer, Chain Transfer, Branched Structure, Stereochemistry, Topochemical Polymerization.

A special session, "Frontiers in Radical Polymerization", was held at the fall meeting of the Society of Polymer Science, Japan, in 1997. Papers dealing with free-radical polymerization were also presented at the poster session on "Polymer Synthesis". In this article, selected topics presented at the two sessions are reviewed. Several papers dealing with living free-radical polymerization which uses stable nitroxyl radical species[1] were presented.

T. Fukuda and coworkers (Kyoto University) achieved living polymerization of styrene derivatives bearing a sugar like moiety (**1**) using di-*t*-butylnitroxyl-based initiator (**2**) (1526, E630). The polymerization of **1a** proceeded in a living manner but the Mn of the products increased to ca. 6000 probably due to chain transfer to the hydroxyl groups in the sugar moiety. When **1b**, the acetylated form, was used, chain transfer was suppressed and higher molecular weight was attained. The polymer having acetylated sugar group thus obtained had narrow molecular weight

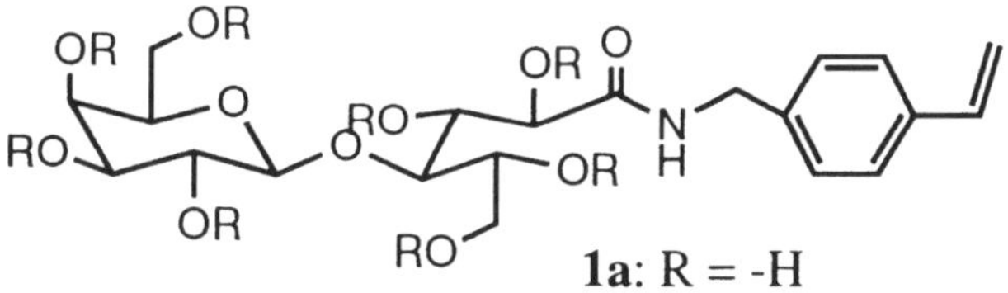

1a: R = -H
1b: R = -Ac

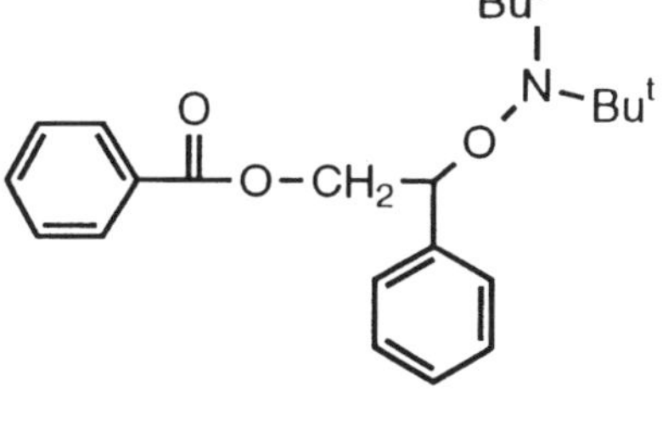

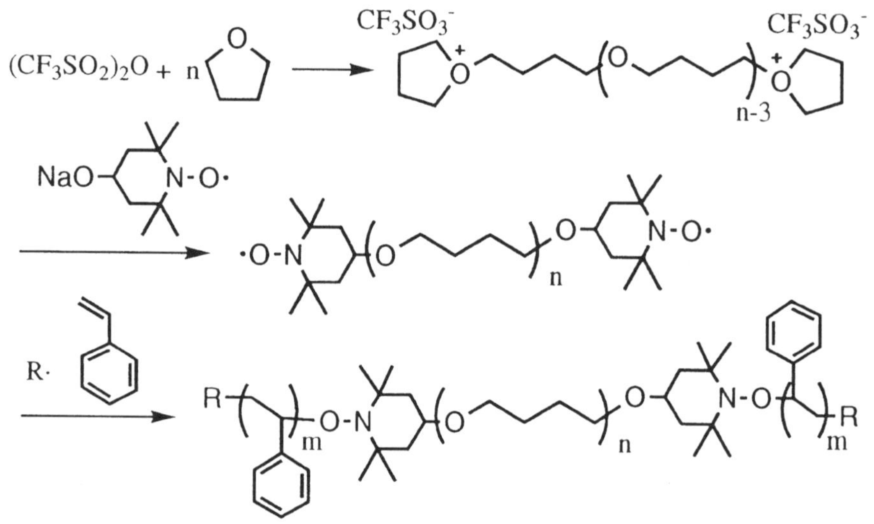

Scheme 1

distribution and was deacetylated using hydrazine. Fukuda's group also succeeded in synthesizing a block copolymer of styrene and *p*-*t*-butoxystyrene which was converted to the block copolymer of styrene and *p*-vinylphenol (1524, E630): the block copolymer exhibited lamella and cylindrical microdomain morphologies depending on the copolymer composition.

E. Yoshida and coworkers (Kyoto Institute of Technology) prepared a triblock copolymer consisting of polystyrene and polytetrahydrofuran segments (Scheme 1) (1530, E631). Tetrahydrofuran (THF) was polymerized by trifluoromethanesulfonic anhydride to give a telechelic living poly(THF). This living polymer was coupled with sodium salt of 4-hydroxy-2,2,6,6-tetramethylpiperidine-1-oxyl to give poly(THF) having TEMPO moieties at the chain ends. This species promoted living free radical polymerization of styrene to afford a novel triblock copolymer. TEM observation indicated microphase segregation on the surface of a film obtained from the block polymer.

A novel method of free-radical polymerization using Ni(0) and Ni(II) complexes was presented by M. Sawamoto and coworkers (Kyoto University) (1506, E627). In the presence of $Al(OPr^i)_3$, combinations of alkyl bromides with $Ni(PPh_3)_4$ or $NiBr_2(PBu^n_3)_2$ promoted living polymerization of MMA to give polymers with narrow molecular weight distribution. Block and random copolymers of MMA with acrylates were also synthesized in a living manner. Although the living polymerization using Ni(0) complex requires the presence of $Al(OPr^i)_3$ similarly to the living polymerization using Ru(II) species[2] which was developed by the same research group, the polymerization using the divalent Ni complex proceeds in a living manner even in the absence of the Al complex. Also, Sawamoto's group extended their living free-radical polymerization method using $CH_3CH(Ph)Br/RuCl_2(PPh_3)_3/Al(OPr^i)_3$ initiator system[2] to the synthesis of a novel "block-random" copolymer from styrene and MMA which consists of three segments each of which is a random-copolymer with different monomeric unit ratios of styrene/MMA (1536, E632). Prior to the block-random synthesis, random copolymerization of styrene and MMA was tested and it was clarified that the polymerization proceeds in a nearly completely random and living manner regardless of the ratio of the two monomers in feed. The block-random copolymer was obtained by initially polymerizing a mixture of styrene and MMA in a 75:25 ratio and by sequentially adding two portions of MMA at different monomer conversions (Scheme 2): the polymer obtained has a styrene unit-rich and a MMA unit-rich segments which are separated by a segment with a comparable composition of MMA and styrene units.

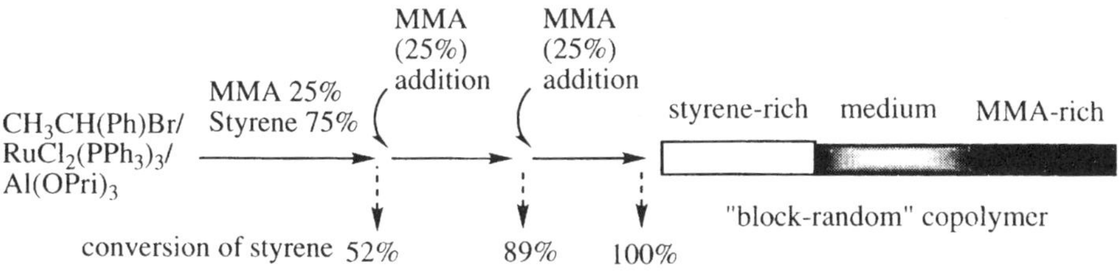

Scheme 2

Selenide[3] and telluride compounds were found to promote living free-radical polymerization of styrene and its derivatives by S. Kondo (deceased August 1997) and coworkers (Nagoya Institute of Technology) (1498, E626; 1117, E904; 1522, E630; 1119, E905). When styrene is polymerized in the presence of BPSE under irradiation by a high-pressure mercury lamp, the Mn of the products increased with monomer conversion, suggesting a living propagation.

As well as BPSE, DDSE, a diselenide compound, DDTE, a telluride compound, and XBSE, a bifunctional version of BPSE, led to living polymerization of styrene. BPSE was also effective in promoting living polymerization of *p*-methyl, *p*-bromo, *p*-chloromethyl, and *p*-hydroxymethyl derivatives of styrene. The mechanism of polymerization seems to be based on homolysis of C—Se bonding by irradiation, attack of the C radical to monomer, and coupling of the C radical and Se radical to give a polymer chain having C_6H_5Se-group at the ω-end (Scheme 3). The Se containing polymer can initiate polymerization of other monomers and block copolymerization of styrene and *p*-chloromethylstyrene was demonstrated.

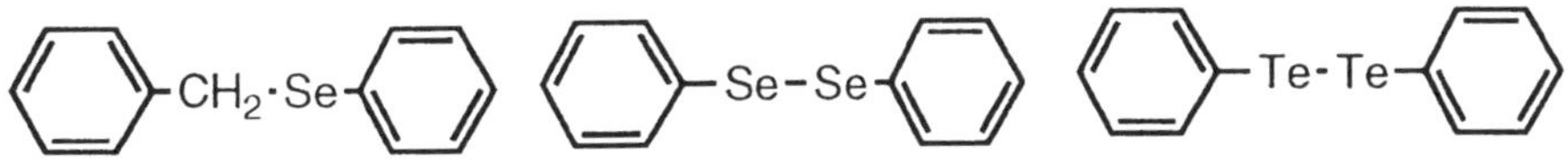

BPSE **DDSE** **DDTE**

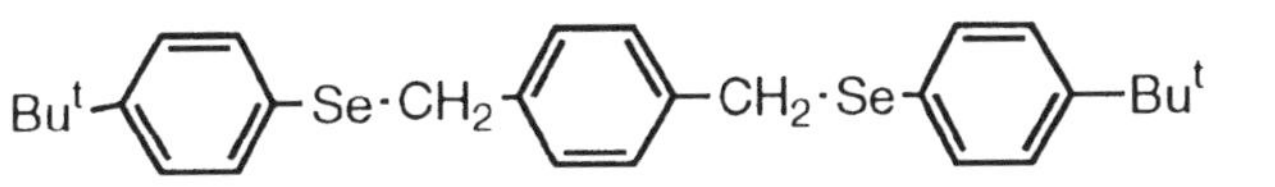

XBSE

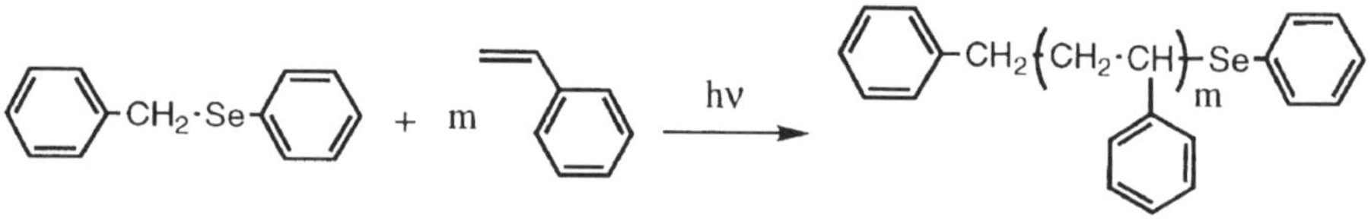

Scheme 3

The polystyrene having a Se atom at the ω-end can be reduced by n-Bu_3SnH and converted to the ω-end unsaturated form using H_2O_2. The ω-end unsaturated polymers were successfully converted to a polymer having an epoxide group or a hydroxyl group at the ω-end by epoxidation or hydroboration, respectively (Scheme 4). Thus, the Se mediated polymerization was indicated to be an effective method of synthesizing a polymer with controlled molecular weight and end group.

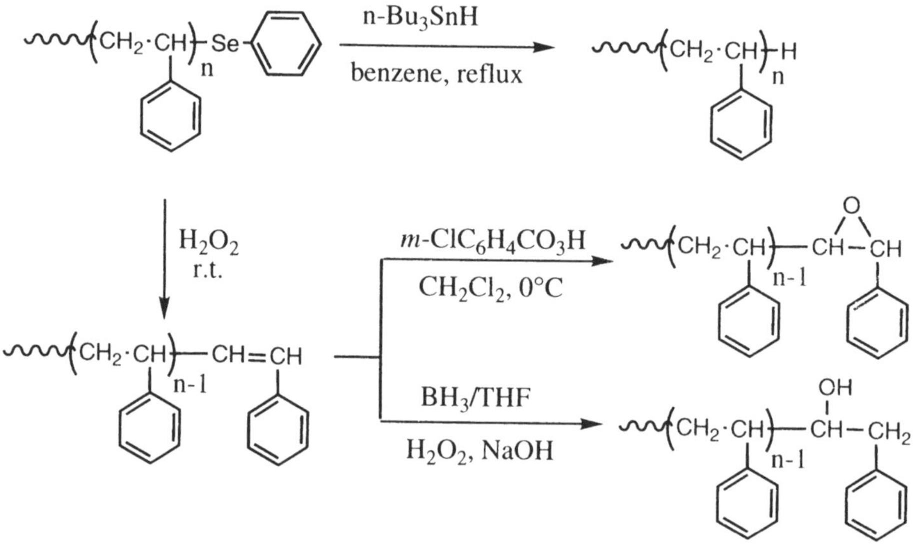

Scheme 4

A vinyl monomer having a electron-withdrawing and a electron-donating groups attached to the same carbon atom is called "captodative" monomer.[4] H. Tanaka's group (Tokushima University) carried out the polymerization of captodative monomers and found intriguing polymerization behaviors which are not seen for the polymerization of monomers having only either of a electron-withdrawing or a electron-donating group (1552, E635). In the polymerization of MAA and EAA, the Mn of the products increased with an increase in monomer conversion ratio similarly to a living system although the reason for this observation was not clear. Viscosity measurement and NMR study of poly(MAA) suggested that the polymer chains associate in solution. The association between polymer chains seems to be based on the dipole-dipole interaction between the captive groups and the dative groups. The poly(MAA) exhibited a large non-linear optical effects.

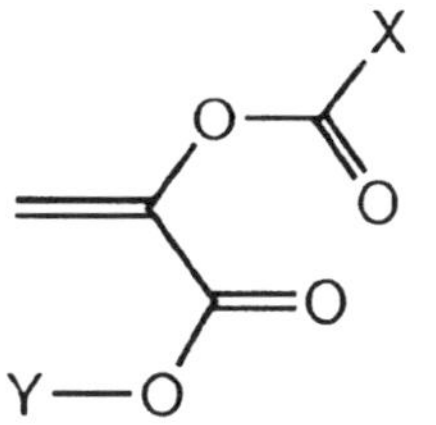

MAA: X = -CH_3, Y = -CH_3
EAA: X = CH_3, Y = C_2H_5

Polymers with branched structures including dendrimers are attracting attention since such polymer as are expected to show novel properties and functions which are impossible for linear polymers. B. Yamada's group (Osaka City University) presented a novel, convenient method of hyperbranch synthesis through free-radical mechanism (1542, E633). The method is based on a reaction which involves a chain-transfer agent which releases a free radical leaving vinylidene group on addition of a growing polymer radical (Scheme 5). Yamada and coworkers synthesized **3–5** as chain transfer agents and used them for MMA and styrene polymerizations. Polymerization of MMA in the presence of **3** gives **6** whose vinylidene group is regenerated through β-scission even when PMMA radical attacks. When styrene polymerization is carried out in the presence of **6**, two polystyrene radials add to the vinylidene group to give three-armed molecule, **7** (Scheme 6). In a similar manner, **4** can give a molecule carrying six polymer chains. Copolymerization of MMA with a small amount of **5** (2.9 mol% in the feed) gives a soluble polymer whose constitutional units in addition to MMA units have the structure **8** which can add two polystyrene radicals to generate a branching point.

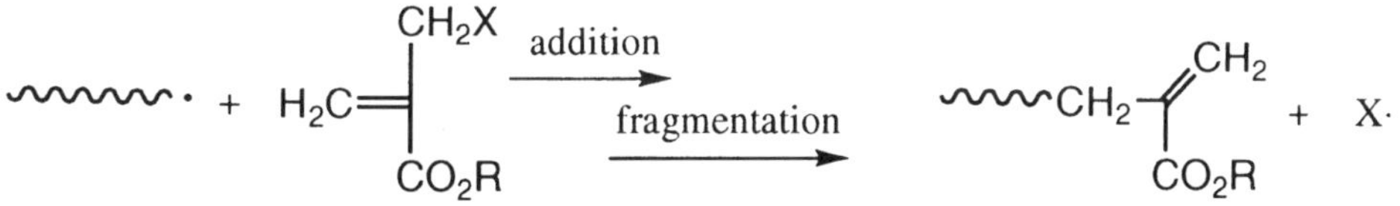

Scheme 5

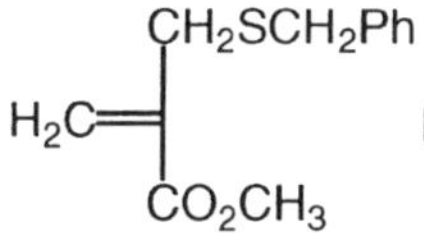

3

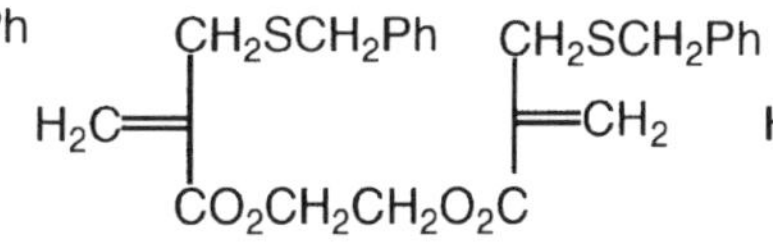

4

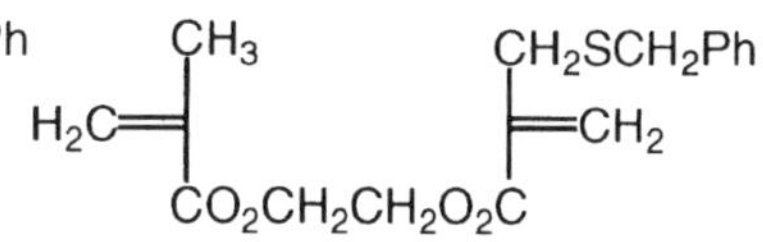

5

T. Nakano, Y. Okamoto, and coworkers (Nagoya University) studied the possibility of stereocontrol of free-radical polymerization using the Co(II) complexes (1500, E626). The research group carried out radical polymerization of triphenylmethyl methacrylate (**9**) using divalent cobalt complexes including **10** and analyzed the stereochemistry of the polymerization. Triad isotacticity of the poly-**9**

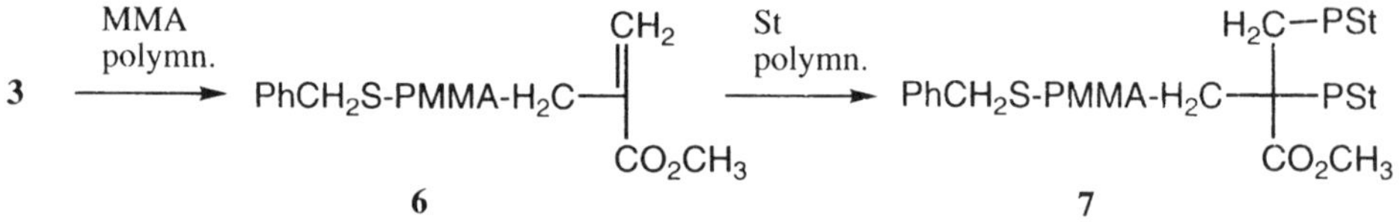

Scheme 6

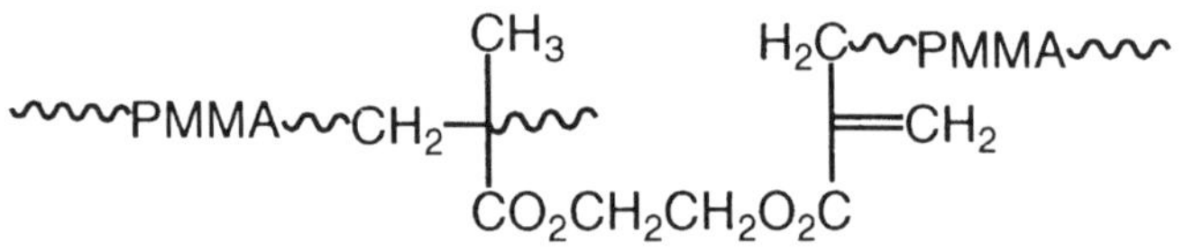

8

obtained in the presence of **10** was found to be lower (ca. 52%) than that of a control polymer (72%) although the presence of **10** also decreased the molecular weight of the polymer. The stereoeffect may be based on the interaction between growing polymer radical and the Co(II) radical species. The cobalt complex **10** was also effective in regulating the regiochemistry of sorbate polymerization. Radical polymerization of methyl sorbate gave a mixture of a higher-molecular-weight component with mainly 1,4-structure and a lower-molecular-weight component with a lower regioregularity. When the polymerization was carried out in the presence of **10**, the formation of the lower-molecular-weight component was effectively suppressed.

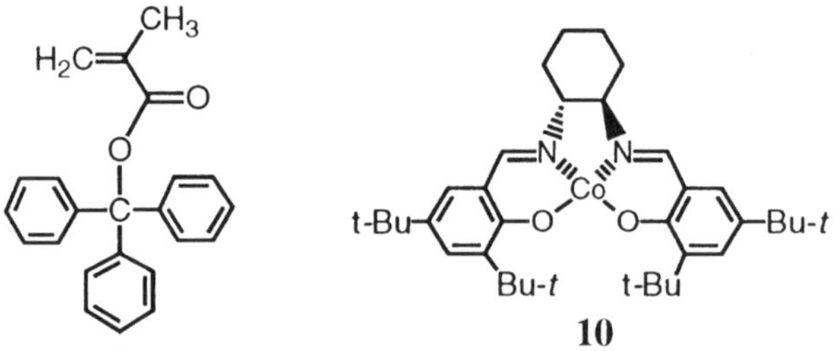

9 **10**

A. Matsumoto and coworkers (Osaka City University) investigated the solid-state polymerization of muconic acid derivatives (1512, E628; 1514, E628). Diethyl *cis, cis*-muconate gives a polymer with a meso-diisotactic-trans-2,5-structure by crystalline state radial polymerization (topochemical polymerization) (Scheme 7).[5]

Although polymerization of several esters was tested, only ethyl(-d_5) was found to give the stereotactic polymer. 2-Fluoroethyl ester also led to a polymer in addition to isomerized monomer ((E,E)-isomer). Matsumoto assumed that the solid state polymerization of 2-fluoroethyl ester involves isomerization of the monomer which competes with polymerization. Polymerization of amides of *cis, cis*-muconic acid

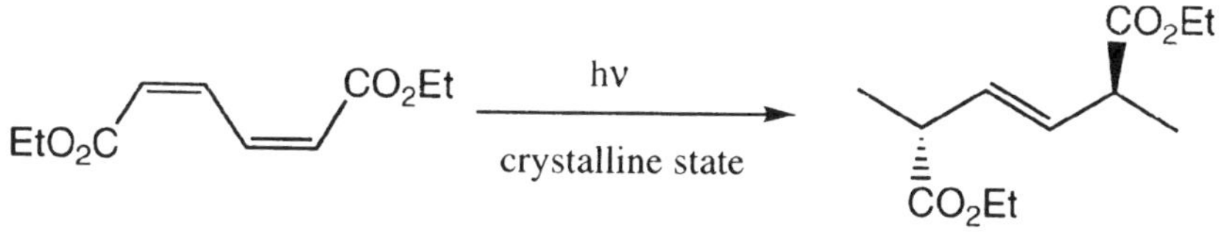

Scheme 7

(RMAM) was also studied but the monomers only underwent isomerization or led to no reaction. Since no (E,Z)-isomer was found in the products, the isomerization should be based on a one-step reaction involving diradical species generated by irradiation of monomers. Among several ammonium salts of *cis,cis*-muconic acid (RAMU), benzyl and *p*-chlorobenzyl ammonium salts gave trans-2,5-polymers and *n*-butyl and isopropyl derivative only gave isomerized (E,E)-monomer while other derivatives including several alkyl ammonium salts resulted in no reaction. The polyammonium salts were converted to poly(muconic acid) by hydrolysis or thermolysis: the polyacid could be led to various derivatives via polymer reaction.

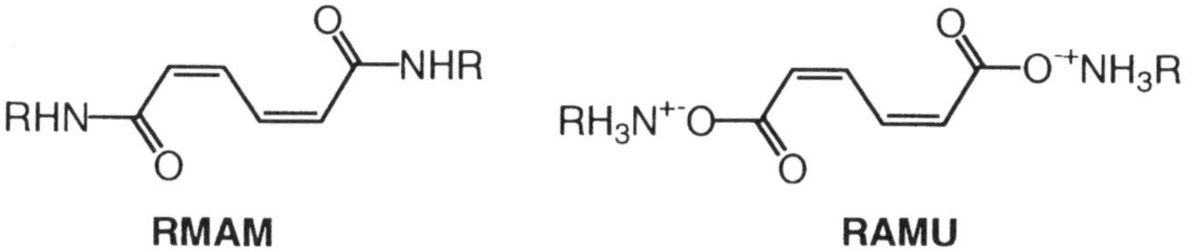

Matsumoto's group attempted molecular weight control in the polymerization of the diethyl ester by preparing monomer crystals with different sizes. The monomer crystals were made by recrystallization from ethanol (crystal size $> 10^{-4}$ m), freeze-drying of a benzene solution (crystal size 10^{-5} m), milling (crystal size 10^{-5} m), and reprecipitation in a mixture of ethanol and water (crystal size $< 10^{-5}$ m). Polymerization of these crystals gave polymers with $[\eta]$ of $13.4 \times 10^{-2}\,cm^3/g$, $6.6 \times 10^{-2}\,cm^3/g$, $2.0 \times 10^{-2}\,cm^3/g$, and $0.6 \times 10^{-2}\,cm^3/g$, respectively, suggesting that a larger crystal results in a polymer with higher molecular weight.

REFERENCES

1. M.K. Georges, R.P.N. Veregin, P.M. Kazmaier and G.K. Hamer, *Macromolecules*, 1993, **26**, p. 2987.
2. H. Uegaki, Y. Kotani, M. Kamigaito and M. Sawamoto, *Macromolecules*, 1997, **30**, p. 2249.
3. H. Ochiai, S. Kondo, H. Kunisada and Y. Yuki, *Polym. Prepr. Jpn.*, 1996, **45**, p. 134.
4. H. Tanaka and S. Yoshida, *Macromolecules*, 1995, **28**, p. 8117.
5. A. Matsumoto, T. Matsumura and S. Aoki, *Macromolecules*, 1996, **29**, p. 423.

Ionic Chain Polymerization: Anionic, Cationic, and Coordination Polymerizations of Vinyl Monomers and Related Compounds

TAMOTSU HASHIMOTO

Department of Materials Science and Engineering, Faculty of Engineering, Fukui University, Bunkyo, Fukui 910-0017, Japan

This review concerns anionic, cationic, and coordination polymerizations of vinyl and related monomers and new polymer synthesis by these mechanisms. The article presents highlights selected from the papers presented at the 46th Annual Meeting and Symposium of the Society of Polymer Science, Japan (SPSJ) which were held in 1997.

KEYWORDS: Ionic polymerization, Chain polymerization, Vinyl polymerization, Anionic polymerization, Cationic polymerization, Coordination polymerization, Metathesis polymerization, Metallocene-catalyzed polymerization, Living polymerization, New polymer synthesis

1 ANIONIC POLYMERIZATION

1.1 Living Anionic Polymerization of 1,3-Cyclohexadiene

Polyolefins having cyclic repeating units in their main chains are expected to possess good thermal stability, chemical stability, and mechanical strength.[1] I. Natori and K. Imaizumi, researchers of Asahi Chemical Industry, reported the first successful example of living anionic polymerization of 1,3-cyclohexadiene (**1**) by using the *n*-butyllithium (*n*-BuLi)/N,N,N',N'-Tetramethylethylenediamine (TMEDA) initiating system (1145, E929). When 1,3-cyclohexadiene was polymerized in cyclohexane solvent with TMEDA/*n*-BuLi molar ratio being unity or above, the number-average molecular weights ($\bar{M}n$) of the polymers obtained increased in proportion to the monomer conversion and their molecular weight distributions (MWD) were very narrow ($\bar{M}w/\bar{M}n = \sim 1.1$; $\bar{M}w$: weight-average molecular weight) [Equation (1)]. The number-average degrees of polymerization ($\overline{DPn}$) of the polymers were in good agreement with the monomer to *n*-BuLi feed ratio, indicating that each *n*-BuLi molecule forms one polymer chain. Under the conditions where these living polymers generate, the ratio of 1,2-addition and 1,4-addition structural units of the polymer chains (**2** and **3**, respectively) is about 50/50. The use of a lower amount of TMEDA (TMEDA/*n*-BuLi molar ratio below unity) and of other amine compounds resulted in non-living polymers and the ratio of the amounts of 1,2- and 1,4-addition units was also changed.

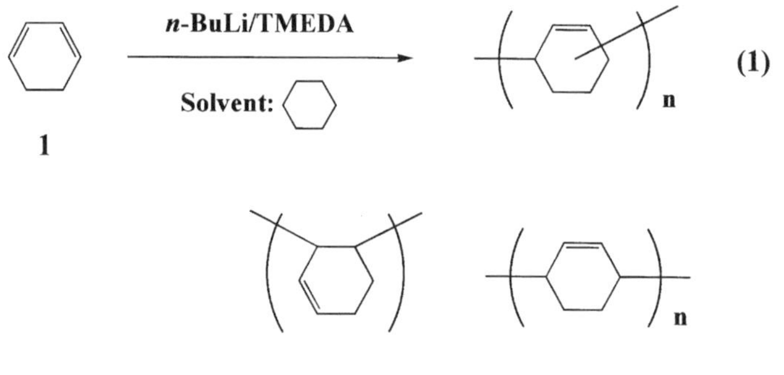

Scheme 1

1.2 Stereospecific Anionic Polymerization of α-Substituted Acrylates

Y. Okamoto and his coworkers are continuing their search for stereospecific anionic polymerization of α-substituted acrylates[2] and found that α-(*N-tert*-butylaminomethyl)acrylate (**4**), a new acrylate monomer having unprotected secondary amino group in the α-position, can undergo stereospecific polymerization leading to highly isotactic polymers (1167, E933). For example, polymerization of **4** with lithium diphenylamide/TMEDA complex as an initiating system in toluene as solvent at −78°C afforded polymer rich in isotacticity (triad tacticities; mm:mr:rr = 83:17:0). In contrast, the polymerization in tetrahydrofuran solvent under the otherwise similar conditions resulted in moderately syndiotactic enchainments (triad tacticities; mm:mr:rr = 15:37:48).

The Nagoya University group also studied polymerizations of other α-substituted acrylates including α-(alkoxymethyl)acrylates **5** (1169, E933) and **6** (1171, E934). Among them, monomer **5** is an acrylate of optically active substituent. Anionic polymerizations of (R)-**5** and (S)-**5** with *n*-BuLi initiator in toluene solvent gave isotactic polymers exhibiting higher specific rotation than the monomers. CD spectra of these polymers also showed a spectral patterns opposite to those of the corresponding monomers, indicating that the chiralities of poly[(R)-**5**] and poly[(S)-**5**] are different from those of monomers (R)-**5** and (S)-**5**.

1.3 Anionic Cyclopolymerization of α-Substituted Acrylates

According to M. Urushisaki and T. Kodaira, anionic cyclopolymerization of α-(allyloxymethyl)acrylates (**7**) led to five-membered cyclic repeating units in the linear polymer chains which were produced (1079, E898). This is particularly interesting because the formation of five-membered ring via anionic cyclopolymerization of 1,6-dienes demonstrates that head-to-head and tail-to-tail addition linkages are gener-

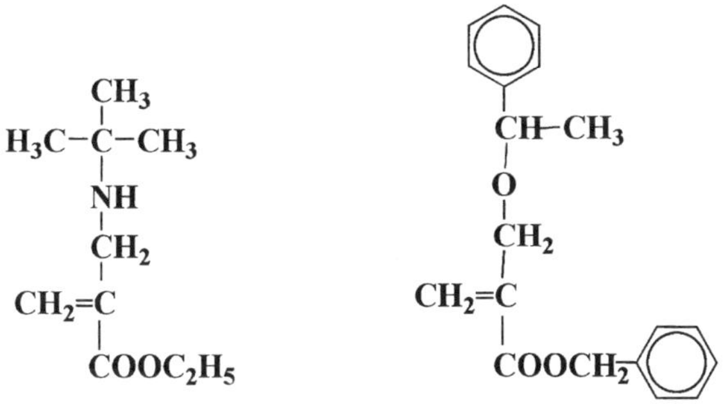

4 **5**

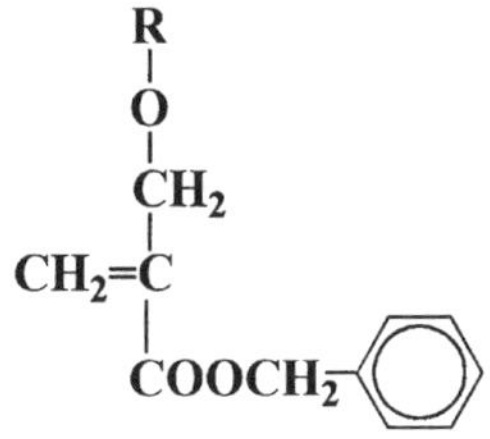

6

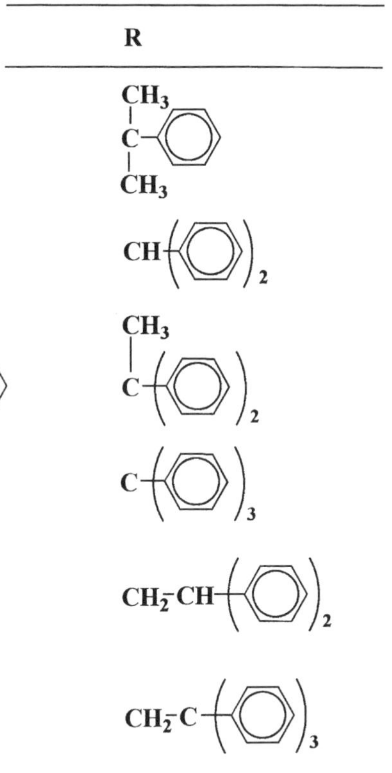

Scheme 2

ated by an anionic mechanism.[3] The degrees of cyclization of the polymers obtained by *tert*-BuMgCl-initiated bulk polymerizations of **7** with $R = CH_3$ and **7** with $R = C(CH_3)_3$ at $-78°C$ were 80% and 87%, respectively, and the residual pendant unsaturations were all allyloxy groups. The Fukui University group pointed out that monomer conformations favorable to five-membered ring formation play important role in the unusual anionic head-to-head and tail-to-tail additions.

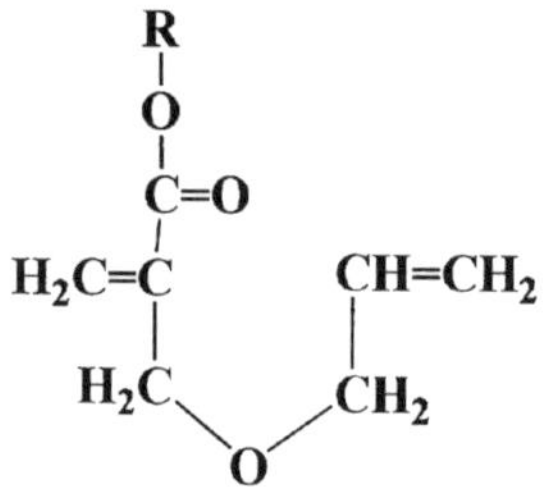

7

R
CH_3
CH_2CH_3
$C(CH_3)_3$

Scheme 3

1.4 Anionic Polymerization of Enynes

I. Tomita and T. Endo at Tokyo Institute of Technology have already developed controlled polymerizations of allene derivatives and synthesized a variety of reactive polymers having unsaturated double bond in repeating units[4] (cf., **3.1** below). The research group has now extended their research to polymerization of enyne monomers which may also form novel reactive polymers bearing unsaturated functional groups. With the *n*-BuLi/TMEDA complex as initiator, anionic polymerization of 4-phenyl-1-butene-3-yne (**8**) proceeded in quantitative yield in tetrahydrofuran

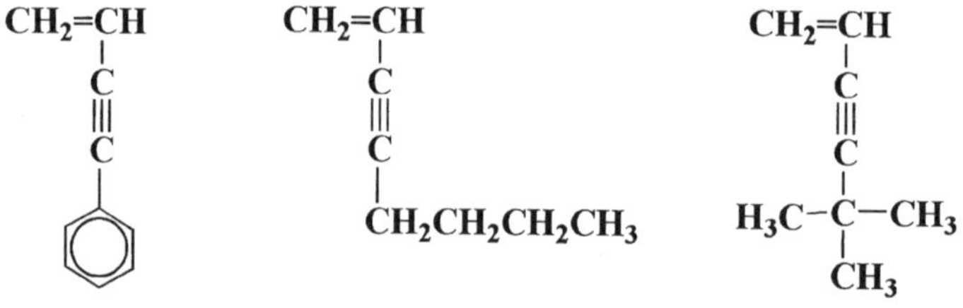

8 **9** **10**

Scheme 4

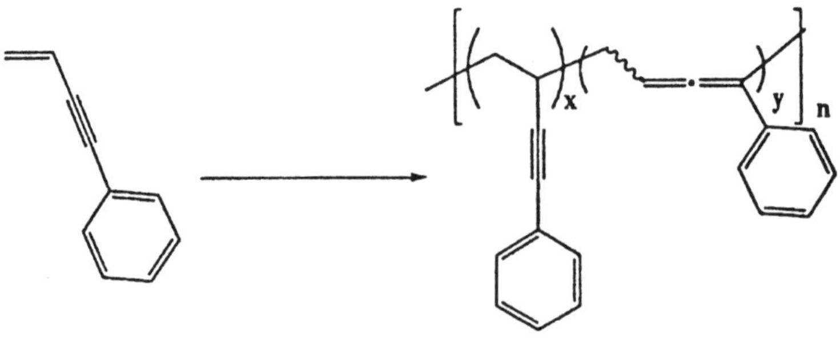

(2)

Scheme 5

solvent at −78°C (1183, E936). The polymers obtained have relatively narrow MWDs ($\bar{M}w/\bar{M}n = \sim 1.1$) and comprise 90% 1,2-addition units and 10% 1,4-addition units [Equation (2)]. In contrast, anionic polymerizations of aliphatic substituted enynes **9** and **10** using the *n*-BuLi/*tert*-BuOK mixed catalyst yielded 1,4-addition polymers selectively. Coordination polymerization (1185, E936) and radical polymerization (1195, E938) of similar enyne monomers were also reported.

2 CATIONIC POLYMERIZATION

2.1 Cationic Polymerization in Aqueous Media

Unlike radical polymerization, cationic polymerization usually requires a highly purified reaction system, since basic impurities such as water and amines cause side reactions of the growing carbocation. M. Kamigaito and M. Sawamoto at Kyoto University reported that cationic polymerization of *p*-methoxystyrene can proceed even in aqueous media with the *p*-methoxystyrene-HCl adduct/lanthanoid triflates [$Ln(OSO_3CF_3)_3$ Ln = Yb, etc.] initiating system at 30°C to give long-lived polymer (1069, E896) [Equation (3)]. Interestingly, addition of emulsifier such as $CH_3(CH_2)_{11}N^+Cl^-$ accelerated the reactions and produce narrower MWDs polymer. The versatility of *p*-methoxystyrene-CF_3COOH adduct as initiator was also demonstrated by applying it to emulsifier-assisted aqueous polymerizations. The key to these successful aqueous living-like polymerizations is apparently the use of the styrenic carbocation intermediates stabilized by the highly nucleophilic counter anion[5] (Cl^- and CF_3COO^-) and of water-tolerant Lewis acid activators [$Ln(OSO_3CF_3)_3$].

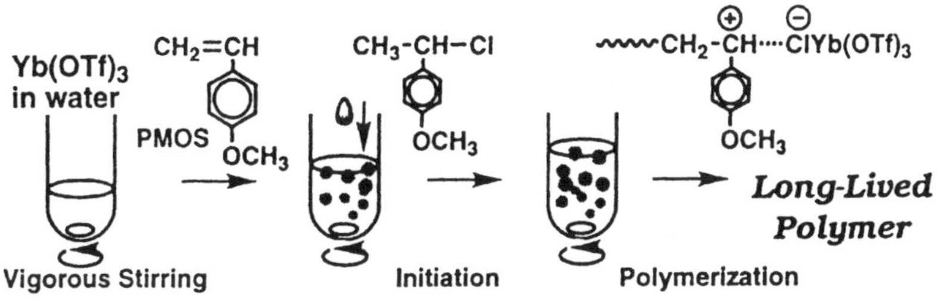

(3)

Scheme 6

2.2 New Method of Star-Shaped Polymer Synthesis

S. Kanaoka and T. Higashimura presented a new method of synthesizing star-shaped polymers by living cationic polymerization (1067, E896). Short living poly[isobutyl vinyl ether (VE)] linear chains ($\overline{DPn} = 10$) (**11**) were first reacted with small amount of divinyl ether **12** and the resulting soluble microgel core (**13**) initiated living polymerization of isobutyl VE to give star polymers (**14**) [$\bar{M}w = 115600$; $\overline{DPn}$ (arm) = 200] [Equation (4)]. According to the group of the University of Shiga Prefecture, this “core-first” method provides a higher-molecular-weight star polymer than the conventional method[6] by simple linking reaction of living linear chains with **12** and may be more suitable to obtain star-shaped polymers having long arms in high yield.

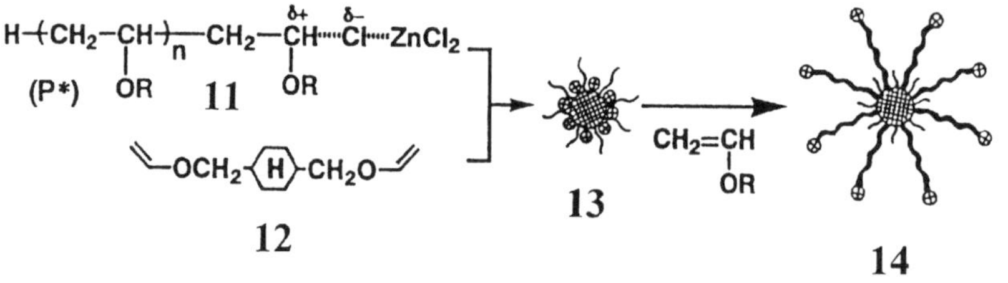

(4)

Scheme 7

2.3 Approach to Stereoregulation

M. Sawamoto and his group employed bulky phenoxy-substituded titanium chloride[7] (**15**) as a Lewis acid activator along with $CH_3CH(O\textit{i}Bu)$-Cl (initiator) and 2,6-di-*tert*-butyl-4-methylpyridine (supposedly proton trap) to induce isotactic-specific cationic polymerizations of various alkyl VEs in *n*-hexane solvent at −78°C (1071, E897). Examples of isotactic-rich poly(VE)s include: Poly(isobutyl VE) 90% meso, poly-(isopropyl VE) 88% meso, poly(*n*-butyl VE) 76% meso, and poly(*tert*-butyl VE) 69% meso. Thus, the isotacticities were higher for VEs whose pendants are branched near the ether oxygen (isobutyl and isopropyl) than for VEs with linear and too bulky substituents (*n*-butyl and *tert*-butyl, respectively).

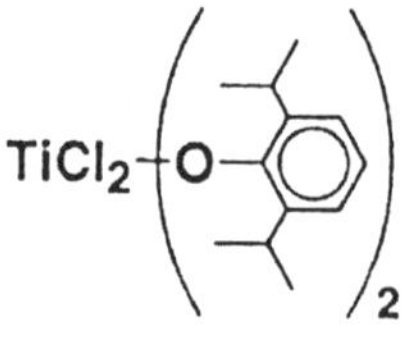

15

Scheme 8

In another contribution S. Aoshima and E. Kobayashi, Science University of Tokyo, utilized optically active basic additives [like (S)-methyl 2-methoxypropionate (MMP)] to effect possible stereoregular living cationic polymerization of VE (1065, E896). When isobutyl VE was polymerized with the $CH_3CH(O\textit{i}Bu)$-$OCOCH_3$/$EtAlCl_2$ system[8] in the presence of (S)-MMP in *n*-hexane solvent at 0°C, the reaction led to living polymers with moderate isotacticity (ca. 65% meso). With racemic MMP under similar conditions, living polymers were also formed but their isotacticities were slightly lower than those with (S)-MMP.

2.4 Synthesis of Water-Soluble Fullerene Derivatives by Living Cationic Polymerization

M. Minoda and Miyazono at Kyoto University applied living cationic polymerization technique[9] to the synthesis of new fullerene derivatives with solubility in water (1615, E1074). For instance, living poly(VE) with malonate pendants ($\bar{M}n$ = ca.1700) was first prepared by living cationic polymerization of $CH_2{=}CH[OCH_2CH_2CH(COOCH_2CH_3)_2]$ using the $CH_3CH[OCH_2CH_2CH(COOCH_2CH_3)_2]{-}Cl/ZnI_2$ initiating system and then used for the subsequent coupling reaction with mono-octynylfulleride anions via 1,2-addition manner to give fullerene-terminated polymers as dark brown gummy solid (>70% yield) (**16**). Alkaline hydrolysis of the pendant malonate ester groups of the products resulted in water-soluble fullerene-capped polymers.

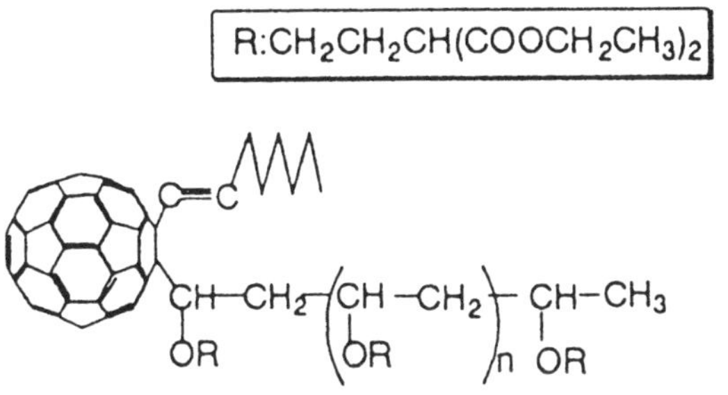

16

Scheme 9

3 COORDINATION POLYMERIZATION

3.1 Living Coordination Polymerization of Allenes

The research by Endo's group led to a further extension of the scope of allen monomers with pendant functional groups for living coordination polymerization (Scheme 9). The monomers include such functional groups as carboxylic acid esters (**17–19**) (1225, E967), amides (**20–22**) (1227, E967), sulfides (**23** and **24**) (1237, E969), naphthalene units (**25–28**) (1239, E969), and long oxyethylene chains (macromonomer **29**) (1229, E967). Similar to other substituted allene monomers, previously reported,[10] these monomers can be polymerized into living polymers with allylnickel catalyst, mostly in the presence of PPh_3.

3.2 New Catalyst for Living Metathesis Polymerization of Substituted Acetylenes

T. Masuda and his associates have already developed a series of $MoOCl_4$-based three- or two-component catalysts (like $MoOCl_4$-n-Bu_4Sn-EtOH, etc.[11] and

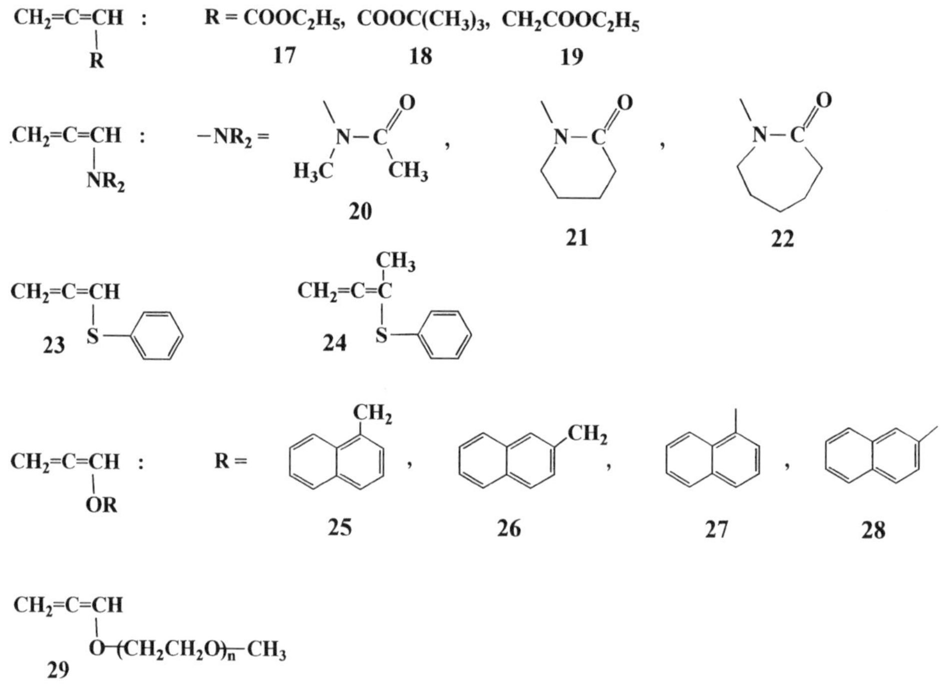

Scheme 10

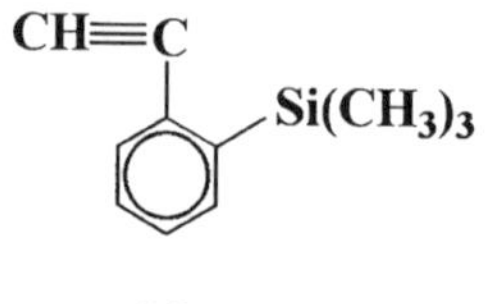

30

Scheme 11

$MoOCl_4$-*n*-BuLi[12]) for living metathesis polymerization of substituted acetylenes. However, the main component in the catalyst systems has been limited so far to Mo metal. The Kyoto University group described in their this year's report that $WOCl_4$-based catalyst can also effect living polymerization of acetylenic monomers such as *o*-trimethylsilyl-phenylacetylene (**30**) (1295, E1002). With the $WOCl_4$-*n*-Bu_4Sn-*tert*-BuOH (1:1:1 molar ratio) system, for example, monomer **30** gave living polymers of very narrow MWDs with $\bar{M}w/\bar{M}n$ below 1.1. The bulkiness of third components is apparently important to achieve living nature; the use of less bulky EtOH and MeOH broadened the polymer MWDs ($\bar{M}w/\bar{M}n = 1.17$–1.21).

3.3 Metallocene-Catalyzed Living Polymerization

T. Shiono and his coworkers at Tokyo Institute of Technology found that living polymerization of propylene can proceed with [*tert*-$BuNSiMe_2Flu$]$TiMe_2$ complex in conjunction with $B(C_6F_5)_3$ as cocatalyst and $Al(Oct)_3$ as scavenger in toluene solvent at −50°C (1601, E643). The $\bar{M}n$ of the polymers obtained increased in proportion to polymer yield and the polymer MWDs were narrow ($\bar{M}w/\bar{M}n$ = 1.15–1.40). Raising the reaction temperature (0°C) and the use of $Ph_3CB(C_6F_5)_4$ in place of $B(C_6F_5)_3$, however, resulted in deactivation of the living growing ends. The similar [*tert*-BuNSiMe$_2$Flu]TiMe$_2$-based catalyst system was reported to afford syndiotactic-rich poly(propylene) (triad tacticities; rr = 0.55–0.64).[13]

REFERENCES

1. I. Natori, *Macromolecules*, 1997, **30**, p. 3696.
2. (a) S. Habaue, H. Yamada and Y. Okamoto, *Macromolecules*, 1996, **29**, p. 3326.
   (b) S. Habaue, H. Yamada, T. Uno and Y. Okamoto, *J. Polym. Sci., Part A: Polym. Chem.*, 1997, **35**, p. 721.
   (c) S. Habaue, T. Uno and Y. Okamoto, *Macromolecules*, 1997, **30**, p. 3125.
   (d) S. Habaue, T. Uno, H. Baraki and Y. Okamoto, *Polym. J.*, 1997, **29**, p. 983.
3. (a) T. Kodaira and H. Tanahashi, *Macromolecules*, 1989, **22**, p. 4643.
   (b) T. Kodaira, M. Urushisaki, M. Usugaya, K. Ohora and M. Okuyama, *Macromolecules*, 1994, **27**, p. 1320.
4. A recent review: T. Endo and I. Tomita, *Prog. Polym. Sci.*, 1997, **22**, p. 565.
5. T. Higashimura, Y. Ishihama and M. Sawamoto, *Macromolecules*, 1993, **26**, p. 744.
6. S. Kanaoka, M. Sawamoto and T. Higashimura, *Macromolecules*, 1991, **24**, p. 2309.
7. M. Kamigaito, M. Sawamoto and T. Higashimura, *Macromolecules*, 1995, **28**, p. 5671.
8. (a) S. Aoshima and T. Higashimura, *Macromolecules*, 1989, **22**, p. 1009.
   (b) S. Aoshima, Y. Ito and E. Kobayashi, *Polym. J.*, 1993, **25**, p. 1161.
9. H. Okamura, M. Minoda, K. Komatsu and T. Miyamoto, *Macromol. Chem. Phys.*, 1997, **198**, p. 777.
10. (a) I. Tomita, Y. Kondo, K. Takagi and T. Endo, *Macromolecules*, 1994, **27**, p. 4413.
    (b) I. Tomita, Y. Kondo, K. Takagi and T. Endo, *Acta Polymer.*, 1995, **46**, p. 432.
    (c) I. Tomita, T. Abe, K. Takagi and T. Endo, *J. Polym. Sci., Part A: Polym. Chem.*, 1995, **33**, p. 2487.
    (d) K. Takagi, I. Tomita and T. Endo, *Macromolecules*, 1997, **30**, p. 7386.
11. (a) T. Masuda, T. Yoshimura and T. Higashimura, *Macromolecules*, 1989, **22**, p. 3804.
    (b) S. Hayano and T. Masuda, *Macromol. Chem. Phys.*, 1997, **198**, p. 3041.
12. A recent review: S. Hayano, H. Kaneshiro and T. Masuda, *Kobunshi Ronbunshu*, 1997, **54**, p. 587.
13. H. Hagihara, T. Shiono and T. Ikeda, *Macromolecules*, 1997, **30**, p. 4783.

Electroactive Polymers

KATSUFUMI TANAKA

Department of Polymer Science and Engineering, Kyoto Institute of Technology, Matsugasaki, Kyoto 606-8585, Japan

In this paper, we will review four papers related to the electroactive polymers to which attention was drawn at the 1997 meetings of The Society of Polymer Science, Japan in view of potential applications in rechargeable batteries and other potential applications in electro-optic devices.

KEYWORDS: Rechargeable Batteries, Polyacenic Semiconductive Materials, Laser Ablation, Poly(dithiodianiline), Charge Capacity, Aluminate Polymer Complexes, Oligothiophenes, Optical Waveguide Modulator.

POTENTIAL APPLICATIONS IN RECHARGEABLE BATTERIES

Preparation of Polyacenic Semiconductor by Excimer Laser Ablation

Pyrolysis of polymers such as phenol formaldehyde resin was found to give "polyacenic semiconductive (PAS) materials" which are stable in air. The PAS materials showed a wide range of electrical conductivity by controlling the pyrolytic temperature. The conductivity of the PAS materials can be varied by up to 11 orders of magnitude upon doping with either an electronic acceptor or a donor. Furthermore, ion entry and accommodation is also facilitated in the PAS materials by mean distances between carbon ring layers in excess of 0.40 nm which is much larger than the lattice spacing of 0.335 nm in graphite. Such distances are held responsible for the higher structural stability during the charge–discharge cycles, as compared to graphite. The PAS materials can be doped up to the C_2Li stage, which is three times as large as that of graphite. These features of the PAS materials have been utilized for the fabrication of the electrodes for commercially available rechargeable batteries.[1] However, difficulties in preparation of thin films of the PAS materials limit their potential for electric and electronic devices because the polyacenes are infusible and insoluble. There is an urgent requirement, to develop a method for preparing the PAS as thin films.

Recently, much attention has been given to deposition of polymer films using laser ablation. Deposition of polymers by laser ablation definitely constitutes a promising new technology for the preparation of thin films of hard to process materials.[2] S. Yata *et al.* (1885, E681) reported that a new PAS material prepared by ablation of a phenol formaldehyde resin with 308 nm (XeCl) excimer laser beams. They prepared the PAS thin films on a glass substrate under evacuation below 10^{-3} Torr. The thin films deposited at a substrate temperature of 20°C were homogeneous dark brown thin films with a thickness of about 1 μm. The electric conductivity of the PAS thin films was about 10^{-8} S/cm at room temperature and X-ray structural analysis showed that it is essentially amorphous. Elemental analysis showed a considerably large content of hydrogen (H/C = 0.51) compared with a pyrolytic PAS material with comparable electric conductivity. Further, the electrical conductivity increased remarkably with an increase in the substrate temperature during the deposition process. In particular, the conductivity of the PAS thin films deposited at a substrate temperature of 300°C was as high as 10^{-2} S/cm, which is comparable to that of bulk PAS materials prepared by pyrolytic treatment at a temperature of 775°C. These results showed that a high electric conductivity can be obtained at a substrate temperature much lower than the temperature necessary for preparation of the PAS materials by pyrolytic treatment alone.

Electrochemistry of Poly(2,2′-dithiodianiline) and their Application in Lithium Batteries

Organodisulfides have recently been introduced as a new candidate for high energy cathodes in lithium polymer secondary batteries. A series of compounds having -SH group within the molecules are being considered as energy storage materials, whereby energy exchange occurs based on a reversible polymerization-depolymerization process (2SH $\longleftrightarrow$ S—S). However, the efficiency of the cleavage and recombination (or charge retention) of S—S bonds was low for the organodisulfides so far proposed. The efficiency strongly depends on their structure and conformation. As shown in Figure 1, the recombination efficiency can be improved if the material has a confined polymer structure or conformation which is interconnected with S—S bonds. In this case, the cleavage and recombination of S—S bonds is expected to be facile. K. Naoi *et al.* (1887, E682) presented a new class of higher energy cathode material, poly(2,2′-dithiodianiline) (poly(DTDA)) which is based on polyaniline chains having disulfide bonds sandwiched by them. Poly(DTDA) is expected to show higher electrochemical activity and higher electrical conductivity by virtue of its intermolecular or intramolecular electrocatalytic effect as well as the conducting nature of the material.[3] The poly(DTDA) has some advantages because of its high

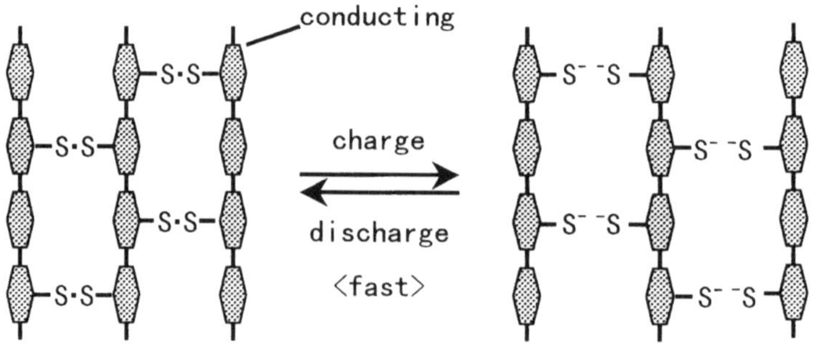

Figure 1 Concept of the redox of poly(dithiodianiline).

theoretical energy density, faster kinetics, and higher electrical conductivity than an organosulfur cathode when used in lithium batteries. They polymerized DTDA electrochemically to form an electroactive thin film. The structure of the poly-(DTDA) was similar to that of polyaniline, in addition the S—S bond was preserved after electropolymerization of DTDA. From the results of the cyclic voltammetry and the *in-situ* surface-enhanced Raman spectroscopy (*in-situ* SERS), poly(DTDA) showed a combined redox processes of the polyaniline and the S—S moiety both of which have a good contribution to the energy storage. The discharge test of Li/poly(DTDA) cell showed flat curve with a charge capacity of 270 Ah/Kg-cathode which is in excess of theoretical charge capacity of 150 Ah/Kg-cathode for polyaniline alone.

Rechargeable Lithium Battery Composed of Aluminate Polymer Complexes as Single-ionic Solid Electrolytes

Solid polymer electrolytes of [alkali metal salt/polymer] hybrids have been extensively studied. When used in a rechargeable batteries, two ionic species, i.e., lithium ions and their counteranions, migrate between two electrodes during charging and discharging processes. In such "bi-ionic" conductors, the migration of anions toward the cathode causes polarization, resulting in a serious decay of dc conductivity or the time-dependent increase of cell impedance. On the other hand, the migration of lithium ions via fixed anionic sites is the major event in a "single-ionic" conductor with minimized polarization. To realize the single-ionic nature, side-chain anionic polymers carrying lithium ions as counterparts have been proposed as a plausible model. Shigehara *et al.* synthesized aluminate polymer complexes as single-ionic solid electrolytes, which have oligo(oxyethylene)aluminate chain backbones attached with two side chains of *end*-methoxy[oligo(oxyethylene)].[4] They reported (1889, E682) the ionic conductivities of the main-chain anionic polymers with lithium cations as shown in Figure 2. The ac conductivity of such aluminate polymer complexes was about $10^{-6}-10^{-7}$ S/cm at room temperature. As the constant current was observed for [Li/aluminate polymer complex/Li] cells under a dc electric field, the single-ionic conduction was confirmed. Thin film lithium secondary battery was fabricated into $5.5 \times 4.5 \times 0.03$ (thick) cm^3 cells from TiS_2 (cathode), aluminate polymer complex (single-ionic solid electrolyte) and lithium foil (anode). The area of the electrodes of the battery was 10 cm^2. The battery showed a minimal decay of the

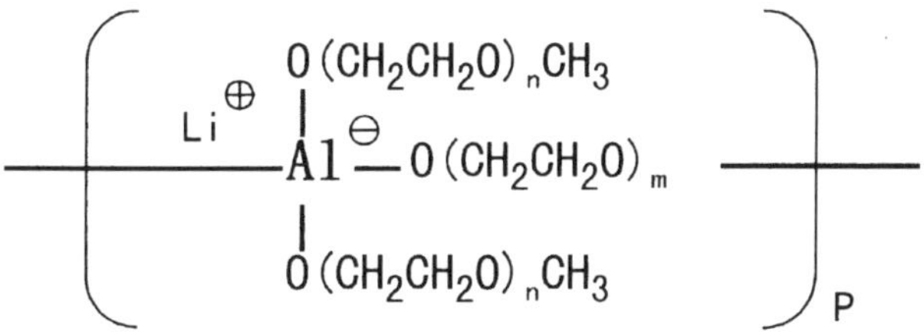

Figure 2 Chemical structure of aluminate polymer complex.

operating voltage and the charge capacity of the first cycle of about 3.3 mAh/Cell, while a typical bi-ionic conductor of 5% $LiClO_4$-doped aluminate polymer complex hybrid system showed a rapid decay of operating voltage and the charge capacity of the first cycle of about 0.13 mAh/Cell.

POTENTIAL APPLICATIONS OF π-CONJUGATED OLIGOTHIOPHENES IN ELECTRO-OPTIC DEVICES

Optical Waveguide Modulator of a Field-Effect Transistor Type using Thiophene Oligomer

π-Conjugated materials have attracted much attention because of their unique optical properties. Some conducting polymers have shown good semiconducting properties and have been applied to the field-effect transistor (FET). The charge carriers of the FET devices have been assumed to be the polaron-like states produced in the band gap. The optical characterization of the charge carriers was performed by modulated optical transmission only through the metal/insulator/semiconductor (MIS) structure in the presence of a modulated gate voltage. The appearance of the absorptions due to the polaron-like states in the midgap was observed. The optical modulation is thought to be one of the candidates for the mechanism applicable to an electro-optical modulator. It is necessary for obtaining a large modulation signals to fabricate an optical waveguide. However, the MIS sandwich-type electrode structure is not suitable for use as an optical waveguide. Recently, an optical waveguide modulator having a field-effect transistor type electrode using a thiophene oligomer, α-sexithienyl (6T) was demonstrated,[5] and much attention has been given to the optical waveguide.

T. Kurata *et al.* (1895, E683) presented the optical waveguide modulator using 6T and discussed the modulation mechanism in connection with the FET operation. The chemical structure of 6T and the fabricated device structure are shown in Figure 3 and Figure 4, respectively. A highly doped silicon wafer with a thick silicon dioxide layer (1.5 μm) was used as the substrate. The silicone dioxide layer functions both as a gate insulator of FET and as a cladding layer of the waveguide. A pair of Au/Cr electrodes evaporated on the silicon dioxide layer was used for source and drain electrodes. The length and the gap of the electrodes were 10 mm and 0.8 mm, respectively. 6T was deposited on the substrate by a molecular beam deposition technique under 2×10^{-7} Torr. Deposition rate was controlled to be 6 nm/min to fabricate the smooth isotropic film. Poly(chloromethylstyrene) (CMS) was spin-coated on the 6T film as the overcoat layer. The channel region between source and drain electrodes is utilized as the slab-type waveguide. This device operates as an

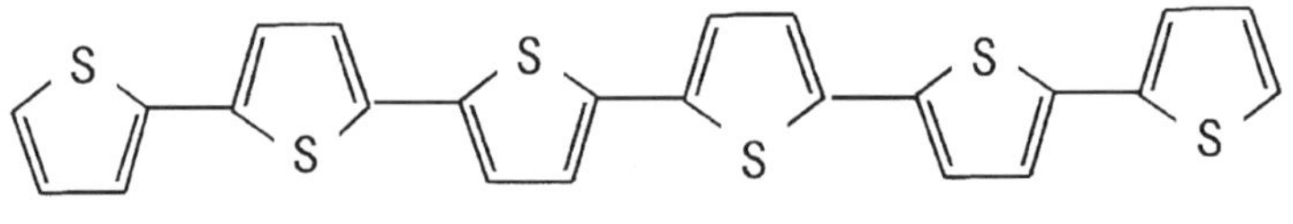

Figure 3 Chemical structure of α-sexithienyl (6T).

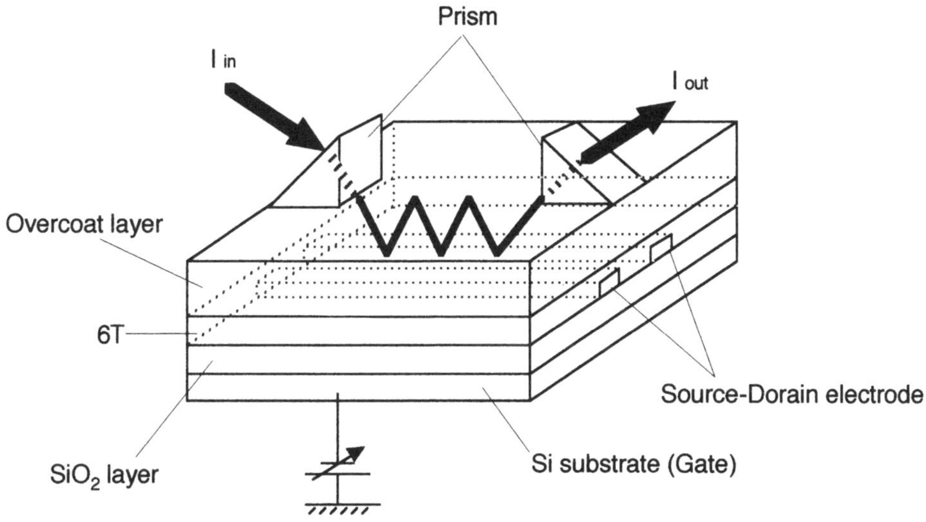

Figure 4 Device structure of the field-effect transistor-type waveguide using 6T.

electro-absorption modulator, decreasing the optical output intensity in response to an applied negative gate bias. The device also functions as a FET transistor, simultaneously.

The FET characteristics of the device without the overcoat layer were analyzed and the field-effect mobility was estimated to be 0.007 cm^2/Vs. The modulated signals for the propagating light with a wavelength of 830 nm were observed at a frequency of 20 Hz of the sinusoidal gate bias with an amplitude of 50 V. The optical modulation ratio, which was defined as the ratio of changes in the output intensity of light induced by the applied gate bias of −100 V (ΔI) to the output intensity of light without the applied gate bias (I), reached 20% below the frequencies of the gate bias of 10 Hz for the propagating light with a wavelength of 830 nm. In the wavelength dependence of the optical modulation ratio, the optical modulation showed the maximum at 830 nm for the propagating light wavelength. The feature of wavelength dependence of the optical modulation ratio almost corresponded to the absorption spectrum of the induced polarons in a solution of 6T. Therefore, the mechanism of the optical modulation was found to be an electro-absorption due to the polarons induced or injected by negative bias. Further, the optical modulation ratio was found to be proportional to the difference between current induced by the applied gate bias of −100 V and the current without the applied gate bias ($\Delta J = J(-100\,V) - J(0\,V)$) in the FET characteristics of the device. It was pointed out that the efficiency of generation of polarons should be taken into account for the understanding of the optical modulation of the waveguide.

REFERENCES

1. S. Yata, Y. Hato, H. Kinoshita, N. Ando, A. Anekawa, T. Hashimoto, M. Yamaguchi, K. Tanaka and T. Yamabe, *Synth. Met.*, 1995, **73**, p. 273.
2. S. Nishio, S. Kato, A. Matsuzaki, H. Sato, H. Kinoshita, S. Yata, K. Tanaka and T. Yamabe, *Synth. Met.*, 1996, **83**, p. 67.
3. K. Naoi, K. Kawase, M. Mori and M. Komiyama, *J. Electrochem. Soc.*, 1997, **144**, L173.
4. K. Onishi, M. Matsumoto, Y. Nakacho and K. Shigehara, *Cem. Mater.*, 1996, **8**, p. 469.
5. T. Kurata, C. Fukada, H. Fuchigami, K. Hamano and S. Tsunoda, *Jpn. J. Appl. Phys.*, 1995, **34**, L1464.

Degradable Polymers

MAAHIRO TSUNOOKA

Department of Applied Chemistry, College of Engineering, Osaka Prefecture University, 1-1 Gakuen-cho, Sakai, Osaka 599-8531, Japan

This review summarizes several topics on biodegardable polymers reported in the polymer symposium in 1997 in Japan. New trends in this area are: (1) Synthesis of copolymers of lactic acid for the modification of their physical properties and biodegradability and (2) Modification of biodegradability of poly(lactic acid) or poly(vinyl alcohol) by blending other polymers.

In this review, synthesis of biodegradable polymers and modification of biodegradability.

KEYWORDS: lactic acid, ε-caprolactum, β-butyrolactone, δ-valorolactone, trimethylene carbonate, depsipeptide, poly(latic acid), polylactide, polycabonate.

1 SYNTHESIS OF BIODEGRADABLE POLYMERS

It is well known that although poly(L-lactic acid) (L-PLA) is biodegradable, they are rigid and very brittle, which is unfavorable for moulding. In order to improve their unfavorable properties and biodegradability, random copolymers of L-lactide (L-LA, DL-LA) with lactones (δ-valerolactone(VL), ε-caprolactone(CL)) were prepared by the use of $AlEt_3/H_2O$ catalysts (H. Shirahama *et al.*, 1665, E1111). Thermal analysis of the resulting polymers by DSC showed the randomness of L-LA/VA copolymers was greater than that of L-LA/CL copolymers. Biodegradation of these copolymers by Proteinase K was carried out. Although P(L-LA) was degraded fairly effectively by the enzyme, P(VL) and P(CL) were not. Degradability of L-LA/CL copolymers bearing higher than 44 mol % if L-LA was pretty high. Although L-LA/VL copolymers (VL $>$40 mol %) were random copolymers and non-crystalline, their degradability was less than that of P(L-LA). For the biodegradation of the copolymers by the enzyme, it was deduced that continuous sequence of L-LA in the copolymers were required.

N. Kawasaki *et al.* (1685, E1114) prepared copolymers of L-LA with ε-caprolactum (CLM) by the use of catalysts (Fe/Al) at 180°C. Resulting copolymers were amorphous and their molecular weights were between 1.0×10^3 and 12×10^3. Some copolymers were degraded by an activated sludge and the degree of decomposition determined by the evolution of CO_2 was 40–60% after 1 month. The degradability of copolymers depended on their polymer composition rather than their molecular weight. In the resulting low-molecular-weight compounds, L-LA, aminocaproic acid and their oligomers were found.

T. Tomoda *et al.* (1675, E1112) prepared copolymers of β-butyrolactone (BL: (R)- and racemic isomers) with CL by the use of the coordinate catalyst ($Sm(O^iPr)_3$-$AlEt_3$/

H_2O) derived from $Sm(O^iPr)_3$ and $AlEt_3/H_2O$. The ring-opening polymerization of (R)-BL using this coordinated catalyst proceeded with retention of the configuration of (R)-BL and the resulting copolymers were random copolymers. The enzymatic degradation of these copolymers by cholesterol esterase showed little substrate specification for (R)-BL units and the copolymers bearing 10–20 mol % (R)-BL were most degradable.

M.S. Audin *et al.* (1671, E1112) synthesized the optically active cyclic carbonate, 1-methyl-trimethylenecarbonate(1-TMC) from 1,3-butanediol((R)- and racemic isomers) and ethyl chloroformate and prepared copolymers of 1-TMC with CL by use of an $AlEt_3/H_2O$ catalyst. Molecular weights of copolymers decreased with increasing content of 1-MTC. The films of copolymers bearing less than 18 mol % of 1-MTC were easily cast. Among the copolymers, those bearing 18 mol % (R)-1-MTC showed the highest degradability by cholesterol esterase.

A. Kanetani *et al.* (1673, E1112) synthesized trimethylene carbonate (TMC) as a cyclic carbonate and prepared its homopolymers and its copolymers with lactones such as CL and VL by the use of an Et_3AL/H_2O catalyst. Their order in biodegradability by lipoprotein lipase was TMC-ran-CL > TMC-ran-VL, TMC-block-CL > TMC-block-VL and the TCL copolymer bearing 50 mol % CL showed highest degradability.

Desipeptide/lactone copolymers were prepared and their biodegradability was investigated. M. Nagasawa *et al.* (1669, E111) synthesized cyclic depsipeptides such as 3-isobutyl-6-methyl-2,5-morpholinedione(PMO) and 3-isobutyl-6-methyl-2,5-morpholinedione(BMO) using L-valine or L-leucine as an amino acid unit. Their copolymers with CL were prepared by ring opening polymerization using tin(II) octylate as a catalyst. Their enzymatic degradation by Proteinase K was investigated. The degradability of copolymer increased with increasing content in the copolymers. K. Umemoto *et al.* (1667, E1111) synthesized cyclic depsipeptides, 3,6-dimethyl-2,5-morpholinedione(L-DMO) and 3-metyl-6-ethyl-2,5-morpholinedione(L-MEMO) and prepared their copolymers with CL. L-MEMO was more easily copolymerized with CL than L-DMO and molecular weights of L-MEMO were higher than those of L-DMO. The crystallinity of L-MEMO copolymers decreased and their glass transition temperature increased with an increasing amount of L-MEMO units. Although they were not hydrolyzed without an enzyme, they were degraded by Proteinase K. The degradability of L-MEMO copolymers was somewhat greater than that of L-DMO copolymers.

2 EVALUATION AND MODIFICATION OF BIODEGRADABILITY

H. Tsuji *et al.* (1677, E1113) investigated the hydrolytic degradation of poly(L-lactide) (PLLA) films in an aqueous 0.01 N NaOH solution at 37°C. The change in molecular weight distribution and surface morphology of PLLA films during the hydrolysis revealed that PLLA film hydrolysis in the solution proceeded mainly via the surface erosion. Hydrolysis of PLLA chains occurred predominately in the amorphous region outside spherulites and between the lamella in the spherulites.

Although PLLA or PDLLA can not be blended homogeneously with poly(ε-caprolactone) (PCL), biodegradable polymers with a wide range of mechanical properties can be obtained by changing their blend-ratio. H. Tsuji *et al.* (1679, E1113) investigated the hydrolysis behavior of phase-separated blend films of PLLA and PCL up to 20 months in phospate buffered solution of pH 7.4 at 37°C. Mass, molecular weight, and tensile strength of blend films with 50 or 75 wt% PLLA decreased more rapidly by hydrolysis than those of the non-blended PLLA, while the elongation at break of blend film with 25 wt% PLLA decreased most slowly. The results of DSC suggests that hydrolysis of PLLA was accelerated in the blend films with 50 or 75 wt% PLLA, while hydrolysis was retarded in the blend films with 25 wt% PLLA.

I. Ohkoshi *et al.* (1651, E1108) investigated miscibility of binary blends of poly[(S)-lactic acid][P(S)LA] with bacterial co-polyesters of (R)-3-hydroxybutyric acid with (R)-3-hydroxyvaleric acid (3-HV) of various molecular weights. Glass transition temperature of blend polymers depended on molecular weights of the co-polyesters. The misciblity of the blends decreased with increasing 3-HV unit in bacterial co-polyesters.

Although poly(vinyl alcohol) (PVA) is water-soluble and biodegradable, the rate of degradation is very low. K. Aoi *et al.* (1661, E1110) investigated the accelerated degradation of PVA by the use of biodegradable additives. They chose chitin-*g*-poly(2-methyl-2-oxazoline) (**1**) and chitin-*g*-poly(2-ethyl-2-oxazoline) (**2**) as degradable additives. Miscibility of **1** with PVA was higher than that of **2**. After soil burial for 150 days, weight losses of control PVA, PVA/**1** (20 wt%) blends, and PVA/**2** (20 wt%) blends were 5%, 32%, and 50%, respectively.

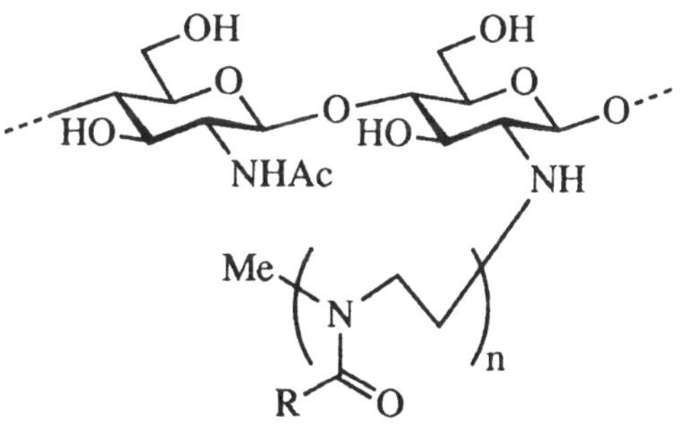

1(R=Me)
2(R=Et)

Biodegradability of PVA/DNA blends was investigated by K. Aoi *et al.* (1663, E1110). DNA was compatible with PVA in the wide range of compositions. Intercalation behavior of ethidium bromide and CD measurement revealed that DNA formed double helical strands in the blend. The weight-loss of PVA/DNA (10 wt%) and PVA/DNA (30 wt%) blends films after soil burial for 150 days were 69% and 82%, respectively. FT-IR analysis suggested that oxidation rate of PVA in the soil was accelerated by blending DNA compared with the PVA films as a control.

Structure, Properties, and Functions of Thermoresponsive Polymer Gels

TAKAHIRO SATO

Department of Macromolecular Science, Osaka University, 1-1 Machikaneyama-cho, Toyonaka, Osaka 560-0043, Japan

KEYWORDS: gel, volume phase transition, poly(*N*-isopropyl acrylamide), lower critical solution temperature, network structure, swelling, molecular recognition.

Since Tanaka[1,2] found the discontinuous *volume phase transition* of crosslinked and partially ionized polyacrylamide (polyAm) gels upon heating or cooling; thermoresponsive (or thermosensitive) polymer gels has attracted much attention by polymer scientists. Poly(*N*-isopropyl acrylamide) (polyNIPAm) hydrogel undergoes the volume phase transition in pure water without ionization,[3] and is now the most common and most extensively studied example among thermoresponsive gels. The volume phase transition of polymer gels itself is of academic interest. In addition, applications to drag derivative systems, actuators, chemical valves, and artificial muscle further stimulates the interest in thermoresponsive polymer gels. A large number of papers concerned with those gels were reported in the section of 'Polymer Gels' of the SPSJ meetings held in 1997.

In the following argument, the word "lower critical solution temperature (LCST)" will be used less accurately. Strictly speaking, the LCST can be identified with the temperature of the cloud point (or of the phase separation) only at the critical concentration of a polymer solution, we will not discriminate between both for aqueous polyNIPAm solutions in what follows. The binodal curve for this system is known to be square-well-like,[4] so that the LCST is a good approximation to the phase separation temperature at almost any concentrations of this system.

1 STRUCTURAL STUDIES

The structure and volume phase transition behavior of crosslinked polyNIPAm or poly(*N*,*N*-diethylacrylamide) (polyDEAm) gels strongly depends on the polymerization temperature. When the temperature is higher than the LCST, the growing polymer chains tend to form a separated phase and then the concentration heterogeneity (or aggregated polymer domains) is embedded in the resulting gel after the crosslinking. The degree of the heterogeneity (or the aggregated polymer domain size) is determined by competition between the rates of the chemical reaction and phase separation, the latter is affected by the temperature. Taking

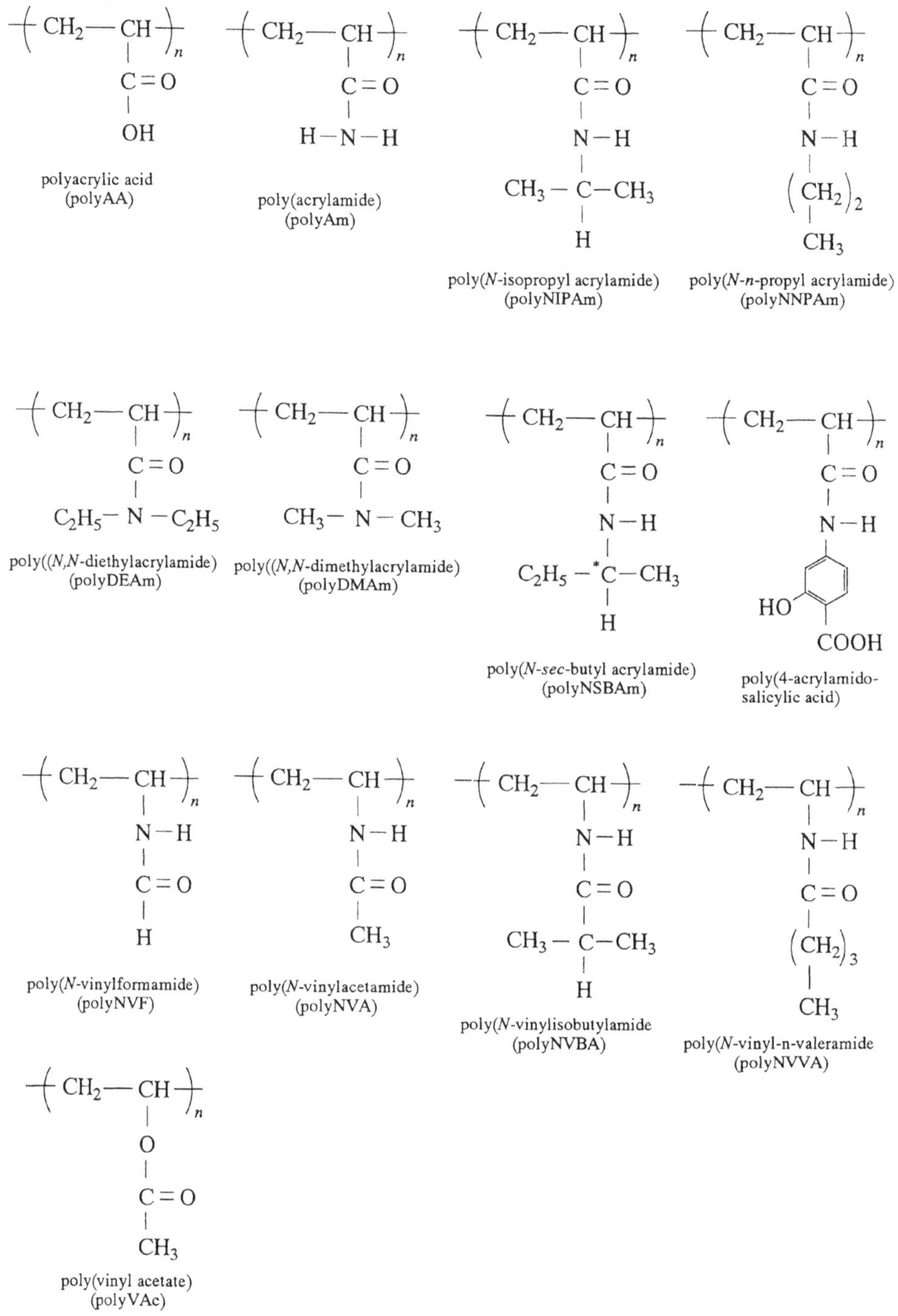

Figure 1 Chemical structures and abbreviations of polymers appearing in this review.

advantage of this structural heterogeneity, Y. Nakatani *et al.* (1976, E696) prepared porous gels by polymerizing NIPAm or DEAm with a crosslinker above the LCST (37–50°C). The resulting porous gels exhibit thermoresponsive volume changes much more rapidly than homogeneous gels. The rate of the volume change of the gels is important to apply as superabsorvent polymers.

The heterogeneity of crosslinked polyNIPAm gels were investigated by confocal laser scanning microscopy and light and small-angle neutron scattering. By confocal laser scanning microscopy, a bicontinuous domain structure was observed in polyNIPAm gels polymerized at temperatures near and higher than the LCST (25–38°C) (Y. Hirokawa *et al.*, 1918, E687). This bicontinuous structure consists of hydrophobic and hydrophilic domains, and the former is the polyNIPAm rich domain. The volume fraction of the hydrophobic domain does not change with the swelling ratio for a gel prepared at 27°C, but do for a gel prepared at 38°C. This indicates that the hydrophobic domain in the latter gel is not necessarily formed by chemically crosslinked polyNIPAm chains.

The static scattering function for a polyNIPAm gel prepared at 25°C, obtained by light and small-angle neutron scattering measurements, has a peak at a small magnitude of the scattering vector q, and also exhibits a q^{-4} dependence in a large q region (the Porod law) (T. Okamoto *et al.*, 1920, E687). The peak at small q corresponds to the interdomain distance ($\approx 12\,\mu$m) of the bicontineous structure, while the q^{-4} dependence at large q indicates a sharp interface between the bicontinuous domains with a thickness of *ca.* 50 nm.

In order to examine the effect of the heterogeneity in the gel network structure on the swelling-deswelling behavior, A. Suzuki *et al.* (1946, E691) synthesized polyNIPAm gels by polymerizing NIPAm monomers, a crosslinker, and guest microparticles of highly crosslinked polyNIPAm with a radius of $100\,\mu$m in the dry state. After the polymerization, the microparticles are regarded as highly crosslinked domains in the network. If the amount of the guest particles exceeds a critical concentration, the volume phase transition of the gel becomes continuous, and the swelling ratio in the swollen state is sharply increased. This phase transition behavior is similar to those of inhomogeneous polyNIPAm gels polymerized above the LCST without guest microparticles.

K. Ito *et al.* (1944, E691) studied the microstructure of the supporting liquid (acetone water mixture) in a partially ionized poly(acrylamide) (polyAm) gel by means of the positron annihilation lifetime measurement. This measurement gives us information about the size distribution of the free volume in liquids. The average size of the free volume of the liquid in the gel abruptly decreases, when the gel transforms from the swollen state to the collapsed state. Furthermore, the size distribution of the free volume becomes broad around the volume phase transition. These results demonstrate that the microscopic environment in polymer gels can be monitored by the positron annihilation lifetime technique.

2 VOLUME PHASE TRANSITION BEHAVIOR

H. Inomata (1928, E688) systematically investigated the swelling–deswelling behavior of *N*-substituted acrylamide hydrogels by changing the crosslink density,

N-substitutents, and the osmotic pressure of the solvent outside the gel. The crosslink density of gels changes the equilibrium swelling ratio but not the volume phase transition temperature. On the other hand, the replacement of *N*-substitutents remarkably changes both the equilibrium swelling ratio and transition temperature. When a polyNIPAm gel is immersed in aqueous poly(ethylene glycol) solutions with the osmotic pressure from 0 to 6000 Pa, the swelling ratio is appreciably changed, but the transition temperature shifts only 2 K. The original author compared these experimental results with the lattice theory of Prange *et al.*[5]

In 1992, Annaka and Tanaka[6] found the multiple volume phase transition occurring among more than two swelling states or phases in a polyampholyte gel, a random copolymer gel of acrylic acid and methyl-amido-propyl-trimethyl ammonium chloride. Afterwards, Tokita *et al.*[7] found a similar phenomenon in the *nonionic* poly(*N*-*n*-propyl acrylamide) (polyNNPAm) gel immersed in mixtures of water and various alcohol. In order to investigate this multiple volume phase transition from a microscopic point of view, H. Noda *et al.* (1926, E688) undertook fluorescence measurements for a DMAm–methacrylic acid copolymer gel with dansyl groups attached to the network. This gel undergoes the transition among three distinct swelling states with swelling ratios of 0.54, 3.9, and 4.4 by increasing pH. The fluorescence spectra for the phases 0.54 and 3.9 show two peaks at 460 and 530 nm. This demonstrates that there are two microenvironments around the dansyl probe in those two phases, indicating that the hydrogen bonding is partially maintained even in the swollen phase 3.9. On the other hand, in the most swollen phase 4.4 the spectra show a single peak at 530 nm, which indicate that all the hydrogen bonds are broken in this phase.

M. Annaka *et al.* (1958, E693) also examined a poly(4-acrylamidosalicylic acid) gel, and found four distinct phases with different degrees of swelling (swelling ratios of 0.81, 1.3, 3.4, 4.9). By changing the temperature and pH, this gel exhibits a complex swelling and deswelling behavior. The final phase of the gel depends on whether the gel has experienced the most swollen phase or the most collapsed phase in course of the swelling–deswelling process. Thus by taking advantage of this hysteresis, information can be stored and reversibly erased in the gel by changing the temperature or pH.

K. Matsuda *et al.* (2006, E701) introduced ionic groups into polyNIPAm gels by polymerizing NIPAm monomers in the presence of polyacrylic acid (polyAA) and a crosslinker, and studied the thermally-induced swelling–deswelling behavior of this gel. In a buffer solution of pH 10, where carboxyl groups in polyAA are ionized, the swelling curve shifts towards larger swelling ratio region with increasing the polyAA content. On the other hand, in a buffer solution of pH 3, where carboxylic groups are not ionized, the swelling curve shifts to the opposite direction. If higher molecular weight polyAA chains are entrapped in the polyNIPAm gel, the above effect on the swelling curve is enhanced. Matsuda *et al.* studied the same effect of entrapped polymers on the swelling behavior also using polyNIPAm gels entrapping poly(vinylpyrrolidone) and poly(ethylene oxide).

K. Suwa *et al.* (1968, E695) studied the phase separation behavior of aqueous solutions of poly(*N*-vinylacrylamides). Poly(*N*-vinylisobutylamide) (polyNVBA) has a chemical structure very similar to polyNIPAm (cf. Figure 1) and the phase behavior of their aqueous solutions is also similar to each other. Both systems possess the

LCST and the temperature is slightly higher for polyNVBA. Aqueous solutions of copolymers of NVBA and *N*-vinylvaleramide or *N*-vinylisovaleramide also exhibits similar phase behavior and the LCST can be controlled from 0°C to 100°C by changing the monomer content. They also observed an abrupt volume change in crosslinked polyNVBA gels near the LCST. Although aqueous solutions of poly(*N*-vinylformamide) (polyNVF), poly(*N*-vinylacetamide) (polyNVA), and poly(vinyl acetate) (polyVAc) do not possess the LCST, their random copolymer gels exhibit thermosensitive volume changes (K. Yamamoto *et al.*, 1970, E695). Here, NVF and NVA are hydrophilic monomers, while VAc is a hydrophobic monomer. The thermosensitivity of the copolymer gels may arise from hydrophilic–hydrophobic interactions among the comonomers.

H. Hirose *et al.* (1954, E693) studied in detail the kinetics of the swelling and shrinking processes of a cylindrical polyNIPAm gel (initial diameter of 0.47 mm) immersed in water after abrupt temperature changes. When the temperature is changed from 20°C to 40°C, the gel first shrinks rapidly up to *ca.* 100 min, then stops shrinking up to *ca.* 500 min, and finally shrinks again gradually. On the other hand, when the gel is quenched from 40°C to 20°C, it swells monotonically. By fitting the first shrinking process and the swell process of the gel to the Tanaka–Fillmore equation,[8] the relaxation times were obtained for those processes. The relaxation time of the swelling process is almost independent of the initial temperature before quenching, but that of the first shrinking process becomes faster with increasing the final temperature after the jump.

3 NEWLY DESIGNED POLYMER GELS

In order to introduce functions into polymer gels, various novel gels were designed. R. Kishi *et al.* (1978, E697; 1980, E697) synthesized copolymers of NIPAm and an acrylamide monomer carrying L-lysine group at the side chain end and their crosslinked gels. Aqueous solutions of the copolymers containing copper ions and various amino acids undergo a phase separation upon heating, and the LCST depends not only on the kinds of amino acids but also on stereo-isomers of an amino acid. Their hydrogels exhibit rather sharp volume change by changing the temperature, which is parallel to the phase separation of the corresponding aqueous solutions. Such chiral gels may be applicable to the optical resolution of amino acids. T. Aoki *et al.* (1982, E697) synthesized copolymers composed of optical active *sec*-butyl acrylamide (SBAm) and NIPAm, and found that the LCST of their aqueous solutions depends on the chirality of tryptophan added to the solutions. Therefore, this polymer gel may be also utilized to chiral recognition of amino acids.

Another attempt of the molecular recognition by the polymer gel was reported by T. Akahoshi *et al.* (1972, E696). They utilized the molecular imprinting method[9] to prepare lightly crosslinked polyNIPAm gels in the presence of norephedrine or adrenaline as guest molecules. The gel prepared is swollen and then shrunken upon heating in an aqueous solution of norephedrine or adrenaline. The gel prepared in the presence of norephedrine shrinks much more in the aqueous norephedrine solution than in the aqueous adrenaline solution, and gel prepared in the presence of adrenaline shrinks in the opposite way. Therefore, it can be said that the gel prepared by the molecular imprinting method can recognize the guest molecule.

R. Yoshida *et al.* (2010, E702) synthesized a random copolymer gel of NIPAm in which ruthenium(II) tris-(2,2′-bipyridine) ($Ru(bpy)_3^{2+}$) is covalently bonded in part to the polymer chain. Here, $Ru(bpy)_3^{2+}$ is a catalyst for the Belousov–Zhabotinsky reaction to oxidize organic substrates like malonic acid. This gel can convert the chemical oscillation induced by the Belousov–Zhabotinsky reaction to a mechanical one, and may be utilized as an intelligent material imitating self-oscillating life systems like heartbeat. The mechanism is as follows. The volume of the swelling gel with $Ru(bpy)_3$ changes sensitively with redox changes of Ru between Ru(II) and Ru(III). When this gel is immersed in an aqueous solution containing malonic acid (0.0625 M), sodium bromide (0.084 M), and nitric acid (0.3 M), the Belousov–Zhabotinsky reaction generates the periodic redox changes of $Ru(bpy)_3$ propagator in the gel, which is followed by the swelling–deswelling change of the gel. Yoshida *et al.* argued that the chemical and mechanical waves in the gel and their phase difference are connected.

A concentrated solution of linear polyNIPAm chains can form a thermoresponsive gel without any chemical crosslinking. S. Ito *et al.* (1960, E694) found the physical gelation in concentrated aqueous solutions of linear polyNIPAm (and also NIPAm and *N-t*-butyl acrylamide copolymer) upon heating above the LCST. This physical gel shrinks and exhibits syneresis by heating. Interestingly, the shrunken gel keeps the shape of the container where the gelation took place. By quenching the gel below the LCST, it transforms to the original solution with fluidity.

Y. Kaneko *et al.* (1988, E698) synthesized polyNIPAm network having comb-type polyNIPAm grafts. When its hydrogel is suddenly heated from 10°C to 40°C, the shrinkage takes place much faster than the normal polyNIPAm hydrogel without grafts. Furthermore, the rate of the shrinkage increases with increasing the molecular weight of the grafted polyNIPAm chain. When the grafted gel soaked in sodium salicylate solution is deswelled upon heating, an oscillating release of sodium salicylate from the gel was observed. This oscillating release is much more remarkable for the grafted gel than for the normal one. This phenomenon may come from the surface impermeable skin layer, which is more easily formed on the grafted gel surface. S. Nakamura *et al.* (1990, E699) further synthesized the polyNIPAm network grafted NIPAm and dimethyl acrylamide (MDAm) copolymer, and also the NIPAm–MDAm copolymer network grafted polyNIPAm. Since the LCST for NIPAm–MDAm copolymer (*ca.* 37°C) is higher than that for polyNIPAm (*ca.* 32°C), these two grafted network gels exhibit different shrinking behavior from each other and also from polyNIPAm and NIPAm-MDAm copolymer gels without grafts, after the temperature jump. For the polyNIPAm network grafted the NIPAm–MDAm copolymer, the shrinking is accelerated when jumped to temperatures higher than the LCST for the graft (37°C). This may be because the gel is prevented from forming the skin layer on its surface due to a fast squeezing of water out of the gel by hydrophobicity of the grafted chains. On the other hand, for the NIPAm–MDAm copolymer network grafted polyNIPAm, the shrinking behavior does not change as much below and above the LCST for the grafted chain.

REFERENCES

1. T. Tanaka, *Phys. Rev. Lett.*, 1978, **40**, p. 820.
2. T. Tanaka, *Sci. Am.*, 1981, **244**, p. 110.
3. Y. Hirokawa and T. Tanaka, *J. Chem. Phys.*, 1984, **81**, p. 6379.
4. M. Heskins and J. E. Guillet, *J. Macromol. Sci.-Chem.*, 1968, **A2**, p. 1441.
5. M. M. Prange, H. H. Hooper and J. M. Prausnitz, *AIChe. J.*, 1989, **35**, p. 803.
6. M. Annaka and T. Tanaka, *Nature*, 1992, **355**, p. 430.
7. H. Kawasaki, T. Nakamura, K. Miyamoto, M. Tokita and T. Komai, *J. Chem. Phys.*, 1995, **103**, p. 6241.
8. T. Tanaka and D. J. Fillmore, *J. Chem. Phys.*, 1973, **70**, p. 1214.
9. G. Wulff, *Angew. Chem. Int. Ed. Eng.*, 1995, **34**, p. 1812.

Functional Membrane, Separation Membrane and Organic Thin Films

AKON HIGUCHI

Department of Industrial Chemistry, Seikei University 3-1 Kichijoji, Kitamachi 3, Musashino, Tokyo 180-8633, Japan, TEL: +81-422-37-3748, FAX: +81-422-37-3871, E-mail: higuchi@ch.seikei.ac.jp

At the SPSJ 46th Symposium on Macromolecules, held on October 1–3, 1997, in Nagoya, 36 papers were presented in the poster session on "Functional Membranes, Separation Membranes and Organic Thin Films". This review summarizes some of the topics concerning functional membranes, separation membranes and organic thin films presented in the session.

KEYWORDS: Membrane, Film, Separation, Polymer.

OPTICAL RESOLUTION OF ISOMERS BY POLYMERIC MEMBRANES

Enantiometric discrimination of chiral organic molecules has attracted considerable attention in the field of medicine and agricultural chemicals, because the use of pure optical isomers of medicines are known to reduce and avoid harmful side effects. Preferential crystallization and column chromatography have been used for the optical resolution of racemates, but several potential advantages such as large-scale operation, energy-savings and easy operation exist with the use of membrane processes.

T. Aoki *et al.* (2157, E952) reported the optical resolution of racemic mandelic acid and R,S-2-butanol through phenylacetylene membranes having chiral oligopinanylsiloxane chains. The macromonomer used in their membrane composition was prepared by living polymerization as shown in scheme 1. The graft copolymer membranes prepared from the copolymerization of the macromonomer and *p*-(isopropylcarbonyl)phenylacetylene showed a perm selectivity of the R-isomer of mandelic acid up to 84% ee when 35 Kg/cm^2 was applied to the feed solution of racemic mandelic acid as the driving force. The membranes preferentially adsorbed R-mandelic acid and R-2-butanol. The membranes also showed the perm selectivity of R-2-butanol up to 83% ee in pervaporation when R,S-2-butanol was used as the feed solution. They discussed the effect of its chemical structure on the enantioselective permeation and separation mechanism in the graft copolymer membranes having chiral oligopinanylsiloxane grafts and three types of main chains.

K. Inoue *et al.* (2163, E953) reported the enantioselective permeation of amino acids across membranes prepared from 3α-helix bundle polyglutamates with

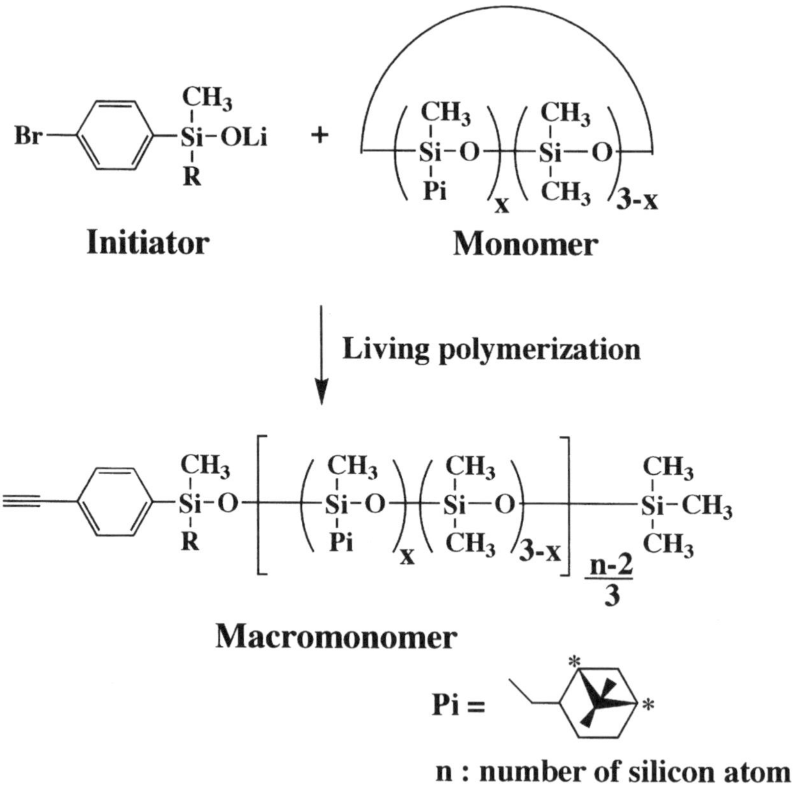

Macromonomer	R from initiator	x from monomer
APSn	CH_3	1
CPSn	Pi	1
AP_2Sn	CH_3	2

Scheme 1

oxyethylene chains.[1] A hexaarmed poly(γ-benzyl-L-glutamate) with a phosphazene core was prepared by ring-opening polymerization of the *N*-carboxyanhydride of γ-benzyl-L-glutamate. The displacement of the benzyl groups with triethylene glycol monomethyl ethers was carried out in the presence of *p*-toluensulfonic acid. The scheme of the final product in the form of membranes is shown in scheme 2. The short oxyethylene chains around the hexaarmed polyglutamate were expected to assemble side-by-side to form a relatively narrow channel along the α-helical structure. It was found that only the *D*-isomer of tryptophan permeated through the membranes. They suggested that the α-helical structure was essential for the chiral recognition of the amino acids and transportation of the substrate. It was concluded that the hexaarmed star polyglutamates carrying short oxyethylene chains functioned

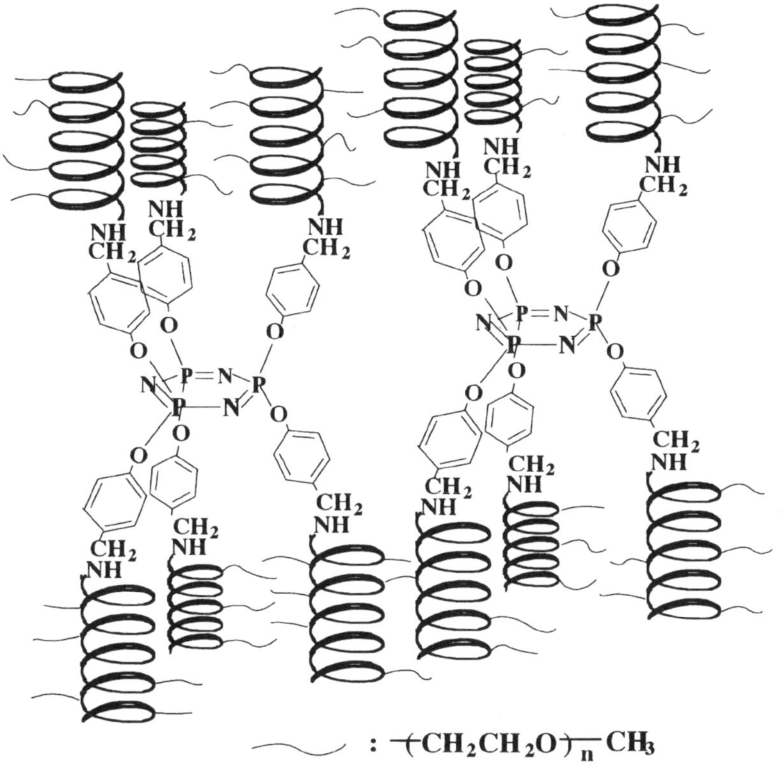

s-PBLG-EG

Scheme 2

as excellent enantioselective membranes for the tryptophan, phenylalanine and tyrosine, and that the star-shaped polymers improved the functionality for the molecular recognition.

PERVAPORATION

Pervaporation, which is one of the membrane separation processes, has been investigated for alcohol dehydration, organic solvent separation from dilute aqueous solution and recovery of useful aromatic compounds. T. Nakagawa and M. Hoshi *et al.* (2209, E984) studied the influence of diol compounds of polyurethane on the separation of aqueous phenol solution by pervaporation, which was produced as waste water in the industrial processes involved in the synthesis of phenolic resins and bisphenol-A. They prepared the polyurethane membranes by polyaddition with the polytetramethyleneglycol (PTMG) and the hexamethylenediisocyanate (HMDI). These membranes showed phenol perm selectivity. The molecular weight of the PTMG was varied in the range from 650 to 2900, and the effect of the PTMG molecular weight on the phenol separation property was investigated. Table 1 shows

TABLE 1
Pervaporation data for 1 wt% phenol–water mixture through the polyurethane membranes at 60°C[a]

Diol component	MW of diol	Flux (g/m^2hr)			Separation factor α^{Phenol}
		Total	Phenol	Water	
PTMG650	650	112	25	87	28.2
PTMG1000	1000	149	37	112	33.2
PTMG2000	2000	186	57	129	43.8
PTMG2900	2900	206	69	137	49.7

[a] Diol component is hexamethylenediisocyanate.

the flux and separation factor for a 1 wt% phenol water mixture through the polyurethane membranes having various lengths of PTMG at 60°C during pervaporation. The flux and the separation factor of the phenol increased with increasing molecular weight of the PTMG. This was due to the fact that the flux of phenol increased more rapidly than that of water with the increase in the molecular weight of PTMG, because the polymer matrix significantly swelled with the phenol-water mixture and became much flexible as the PTMG moiety and the swelling of the polymer enhanced the diffusion of the phenol molecules in the membranes.

T. Nakagawa *et al.* (2201, E983) also reported the use of poly(1-trimethylsilyl-1-propyne) membranes modified with dioctylphthalate for the removal of trichloroethylene from aqueous solution. The total flux and separation factor of the trichloroethylene were studied with increasing dioctylphthalate content in the membranes. These results were explained by the fact that the dioctylphthalate has a high affinity for trichloroethane and inhibited the permeation of water.

The separation of the benzene/cyclohexane mixtures is one of the important topics in the petrochemical industry. It is known that it is difficult to directly remove one component from benzene/cyclohexane mixtures by distillation because of the close boiling points between benzene and cyclohexane.[2] T. Uragami and T. Miyata *et al.* (2187, E981) reported the separation of a benzene/cyclohexane mixture through benzoylchitosan membranes during pervaporation (see scheme 3). The benzoylchitosan membranes showed a high benzene perm selectivity for a benzene/cyclohexane

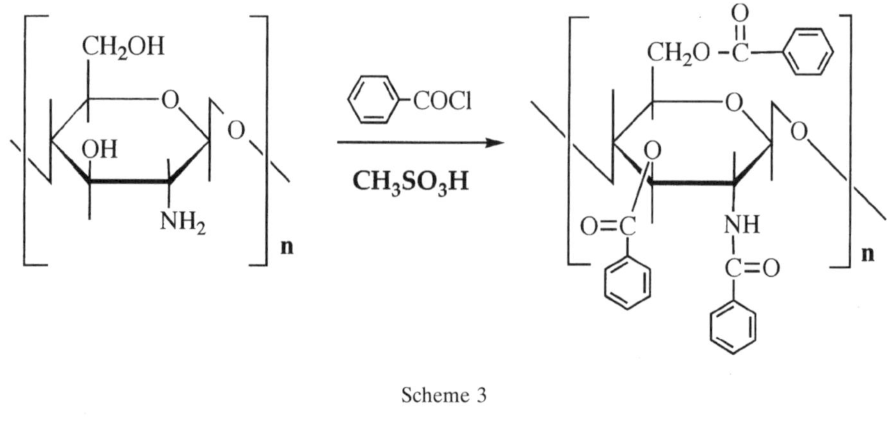

Scheme 3

mixture in their experiments. The high permeability of benzene was attributed to the strong affinity of the benzoylchitosan membranes for benzene. The high selectivity originated from the decrease in swelling of the membranes with the hard chitosan segment.

SEPARATION OF OLEFIN/PARAFFIN

Membrane separation of olefin and paraffin gases is one of the most important future projects in the membrane technology and petrochemical industries,[3] because membrane technology is an attractive energy-saving process which induces no phase transformation steps.

H. Kita and K. Okamoto (2199, E983) studied hydrocarbon gas separation using carbonized membranes prepared from polyimide precursors. The polyimide precursors were prepared from 4,4′-(hexafluoroisopropylidene)diphtalic anhydride (6FDA) and diaminobenzidine (mPD) or 6FDA and diaminobenzidine (DABZ). The performance of the carbonized membranes was found to be much higher than the precursor membranes. The 6FDA-DABZ membranes carbonized at 500°C showed high C_3H_6 permeability such as 170 barrer and an ideal selectivity of 78 which was the permeability ratio of gases between C_3H_6 and C_3H_8 in single gas permeation measurements. The permeability coefficients of both gases in mixed gas permeation measurements, however, this decreased when they were compared to those of single permeation measurements and the selectivity was observed to be 44. This was explained by the mutual interaction between the membranes and both gases.

Many papers have been already been published about the facilitated transport of olefins in liquid membranes or ion exchange membranes containing silver ions as a complexing agent. These membranes have high selectivity and high permeability, although the process must be carried out under saturated water vapor.

Mizoguchi *et al.* reported the gas permeation of C_2H_4 and C_2H_6 in Ag-exchanged Nafion membranes. The Ag-exchanged membrane in a dry form showed a high separation factor of C_2H_4 to C_2H_6 of 7.3 in their preparation method.

A. Tanioka *et al.* (2195, E982) also reported the permeation of *n*-butane, 1-butene and 1,3-butadiene through anhydrated Ag^+-doped (exchanged) polyperfluorosulfonate membranes. The Ag^+-doped membranes exhibited a relatively high permeability for 1-butene compared with *n*-butane and 1,3-butadiene. The ideal separation factor of 1-butene/*n*-butane, which was the permeability coefficient ratio of 1-butene to *n*-butane, was about 5400 in the membranes doped with $AgNO_3$ solution at 25°C. It was observed that both the permeability of 1-butene and selectivity of 1-butene/*n*-butane increased with a decrease in temperature. On the other hand, the highest ideal separation factor of 1-butene/1,3-butadiene was only 12 at 65°C in their experiments and the separation factor decreased with a decrease in temperature.

OSCILLATION OF MEMBRANE POTENTIAL

Several kinds of artificial membranes, which induce the oscillation of membrane potential, have been developed as simple models of cells and living membranes in recent years, because bio-oscillation is of vital importance in biophysics and physical chemistry. A. Higuchi and M. Hara (2233, E988) reported ion-complex membranes of DNA and hexanediaminated poly(γ-methyl-L-glutamate) and observed oscillations in the membrane potential under a concentration gradient of several salts (i.e., LiCl, NaCl, KCl, CsCl, $MgCl_2$, $CaCl_2$, $SrCl_2$, $BaCl_2$) at frequencies between 0 and 5 Hertz at pH 7.0.[4] Figure 1 shows the change with time of the membrane potential across the immobilized DNA membranes between 1 mM and 0.1 M salt solutions at pH 7.0. These rhythmic and synchronized oscillations were regarded as a simple model of nonlinear phenomena observed in organs and cells. The amplitude of the oscillation was influenced by the salts used, and the high amplitude of the oscillation was observed when KCl or salts containing a divalent cation were used in their study. Fast Fourier transport analysis revealed that the oscillation of the membrane potential was not chaotic but had specific frequencies. It was possible that a particular salt presented in the solution was identified from the amplitude and/or the power spectrum of the fast Fourier transport during the oscillation of the membrane potential.

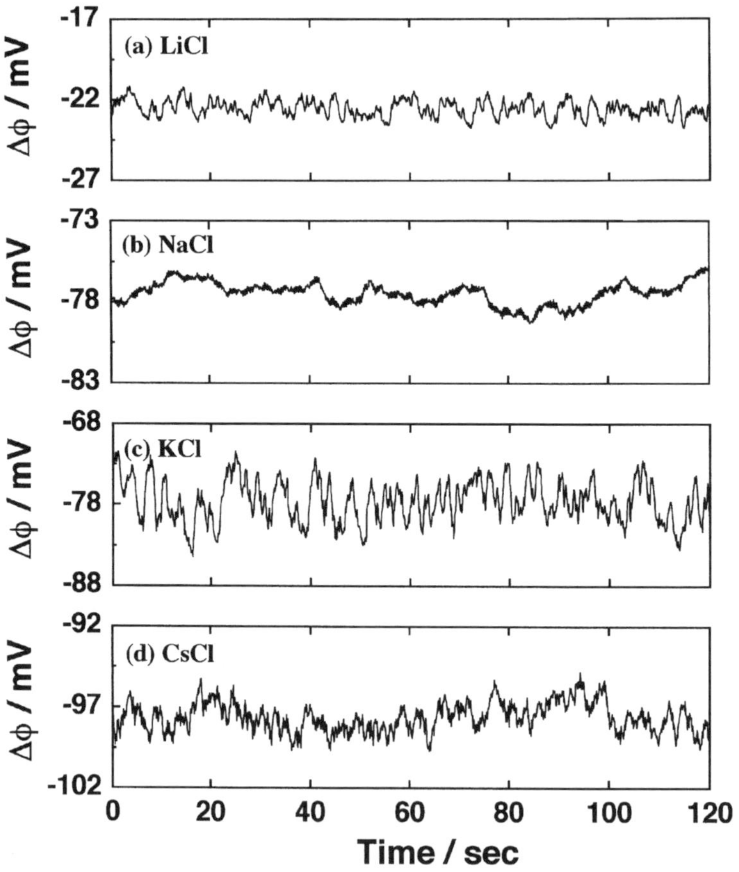

Figure 1 Time course of membrane potential across the immobilized DNA membranes between 1 mM and 0.1 M salt solutions at pH 7.0.

PHOTO-INDUCED MEMBRANE POTENTIAL

T. Hirai and H. Hayashi (2223, E987) reported a photo-induced membrane potential by plasticized poly(vinyl chloride) and poly(methylmethacrylate) membranes containing spirobenzopyran. The spirobenzopyrane, which was a photochromic dye, generated photoinduced isomerization accompanying a cationic form under acidic conditions as shown in scheme 4. Therefore, the plasticized poly(methylmethacrylate) membranes containing spirobenzopyran and acidic phosphoric ester showed a photo-induced membrane potential not only by ultraviolet light (360 nm) irradiation but also by visual light irradiation (540 nm). The visual light-induced membrane potential was generated by a decrease in protonated merocyanine in the spirobenzopyran of the membranes. On the other hand, the protonated merocyanine in the membranes caused an increase in the membrane potential during irradiation by ultraviolet light. They confirmed that the cationic form of the merocyanine was

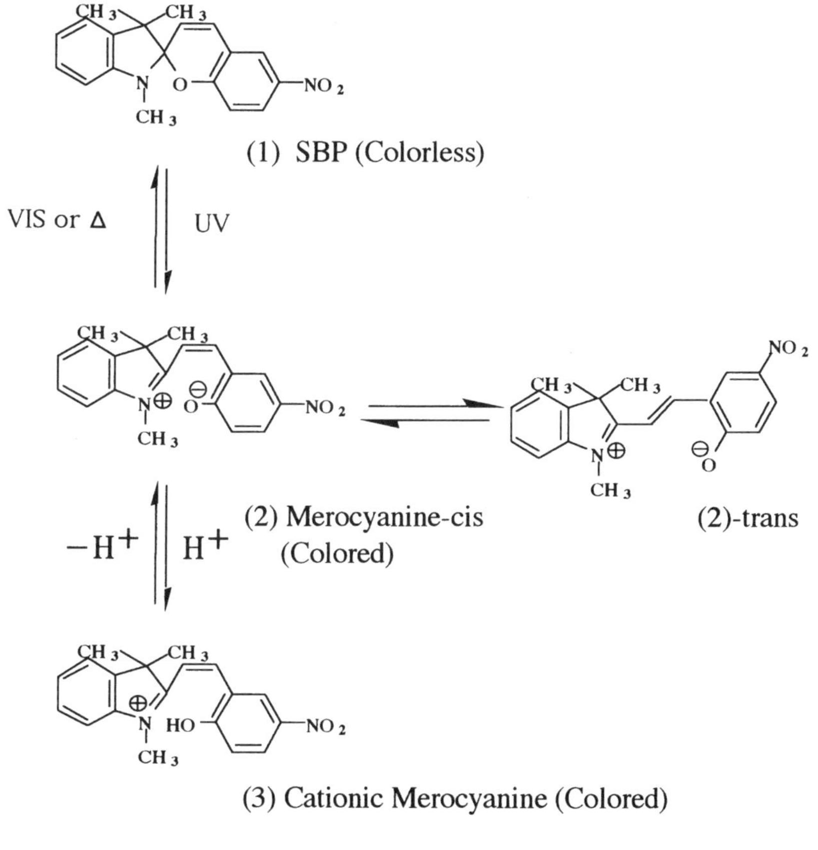

1,3,3-trimethyl-6'-nitorospiro indoline-2-2' benzopiran

Scheme 4

generated by the protons supplied from acidic species such as the acidic phosphoric ester in the membranes.

ARTIFICIAL SKIN-MODEL MEMBRANE

Transdermal drug delivery systems (TDDSs) are known to have various advantages over conventional oral dosage forms and injections such as simple dosage and improved compliance.[5] The permeability of drug candidates through the skin is an important factor for the development of a transdermal drug delivery system. Permeability data using cadaver human skin in vitro would be the most desirable method,[5] although there have been found individual variations in the skin samples during inter-laboratory reproducibility. There is a tendency that the use of animal and human skin should be restricted in the experiments to reduce animal sacrifices. Therefore, the establishment of an *in vitro* method using a human skin-alternative membrane is desired.

Nagase *et al.* reported the drug permeability of the poly(2-hydroxyethyl methacrylate) (PHEMA)/polydimethylsiloxane (PDMS) crosslinked membrane, which closely resembled the permeability of human skin. The membranes were prepared from 2-trimethylsilyloxyethyl methacrylate (HEMA-TMS) and PDMS macromonomers containing one or two methacrylonyl end groups by visible or UV light irradiation between the two glass plates, followed by hydrolysis with acetic acid to remove the trimethylsilyl group of the HEMA-TMA unit as shown in scheme 5. It was found that the permeabilities of a series of drugs with different polarities were greatly influenced by the content of the PHEMA component. It was found that the permeability coefficients of the drugs through the artificial membrane (PHEMA/PDMS = 50/50–60/40 wt%) were in good agreement with the permeability coefficients through human skin.

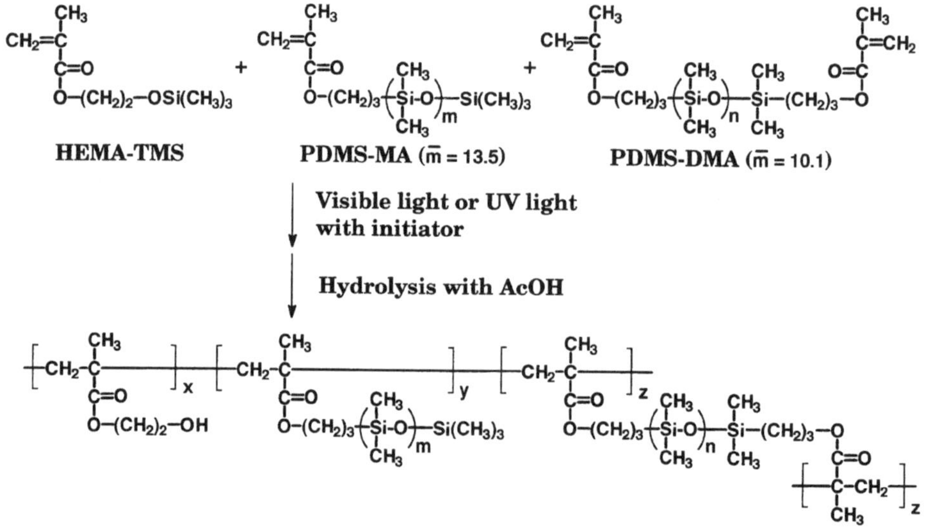

Scheme 5

LANGMUIR–BLODGETT FILMS

Self-assembled thin films have attracted a great deal of attention for their possible application in opto-electronic devices. The fabrication of thin films by a self-assembly strategy enables us to control the molecular structure at a nanoscale level. These advantages are especially useful for fabrication of non-linear optical (NLO) materials which require molecular alignment and a controlled thickness.

K. Sanui and W. Ogata *et al.* (2177, E979) fabricated electrostatic self-assembled thin films prepared with poly(thiophene-3-acetic acid) as a polyanion and a positively-charged second-order NLO chromophore as a cation. The UV-V is spectra of these films indicated that poly(thiophene-3-acetic acid) and the NLO chromophore formed a bilayer structure.

Seo *et al.* reported the synthesis of a C_{60}-containing polyimide and the preparation of a monolayer using the Langmuir–Blodgett (LB) technique. LB films of the C_{60}-containing polyimide were prepared via LB films of the corresponding polyamic acid alkyl amine salt using the precursor method. Absorption bands in both the precursor and polyimide LB films deposited on a quartz plate indicated the absorption bands at 208, 261 and 340 nm, which were typical absorption bands of C_{60}.

Kinoshita *et al.* reported the control of the molecular orientation in the monolayer consisting of a peptide-based surfactant. The molecular orientation of the poly(L-leucine)/poly(ethylene glycol) block copolymer at the air-water interface was characterized by a surface-area (π-A) isotherm of the monolayer and circular dichroism spectra of the LB film. They estimated two values of limiting area (A_L, A_s) from the π-A isotherm of the monolayer. The larger limiting area (A_L; 447 Å/molecule) was found to be much smaller than the calculated value (948 Å/molecule) when the α-helical rods lay parallel on the water surface. It was, therefore, suggested that the α-helical rod stood perpendicular to the air–water interface.

REFERENCES

1. K. Inoue, A. Miyahara and T. Itaya, *J. Am. Chem. Soc.*, 1997, **119**, p. 6191.
2. K. Inui, K. Tsukamoto, T. Miyata and T. Uragami, *J. Membrane Sci.*, 1998, **138**, p. 67.
3. K. Tanaka, A. Taguchi, J. Hao and K. Okamoto, *J. Membrane Sci.*, 1996, **121**, p. 197.
4. A. Higuchi and M. Hara, *J. Phys. Chem.*, 1996, **100**, p. 2183.
5. Y. Yamaguchi, T. Usami, H. Natsume, T. Aoyagi, Y. Nagase, K. Sugibayashi and Y. Morimoto, *Chem. Pharm. Bull.*, 1997, **45**, p. 537.

Biopolymers

KENICHI HATANAKA

Department of Biomolecular Engineering, Faculty of Bioscience and Biotechnology, Tokyo Institute of Technology, Nagatsutta-cho, Midori-ku, Yokohama 226, Japan

Special symposium session "Glycopolymers" was held in 1998. This session consisted of (1) preparation of novel saccharide chain, (2) synthesis of carbohydrate-containing polymer and its function, (3) synthesis of high-functionalized polysaccharide derivative, and (4) biochemical reaction of glycopolymers.

SYNTHESIS OF BIOACTIVE POLYMERS CARRYING OLIGOSACCHARIDES DERIVED FROM REGIOSELECTIVELY MODIFIED LACTOSES

Glycoconjugate polymers are expected as functional materials which incorporate specific virus and toxin. H. Dohi and K. Kobayashi *et al.* (2848, E750) reported an efficient synthesis of pNP-2,3,6,2′,6′-penta-*O*-acetyl-*β*-D-lactoside, which is a key intermediate to modify 3′ and 4′ hydroxyl groups regioselectively. Two bioactive

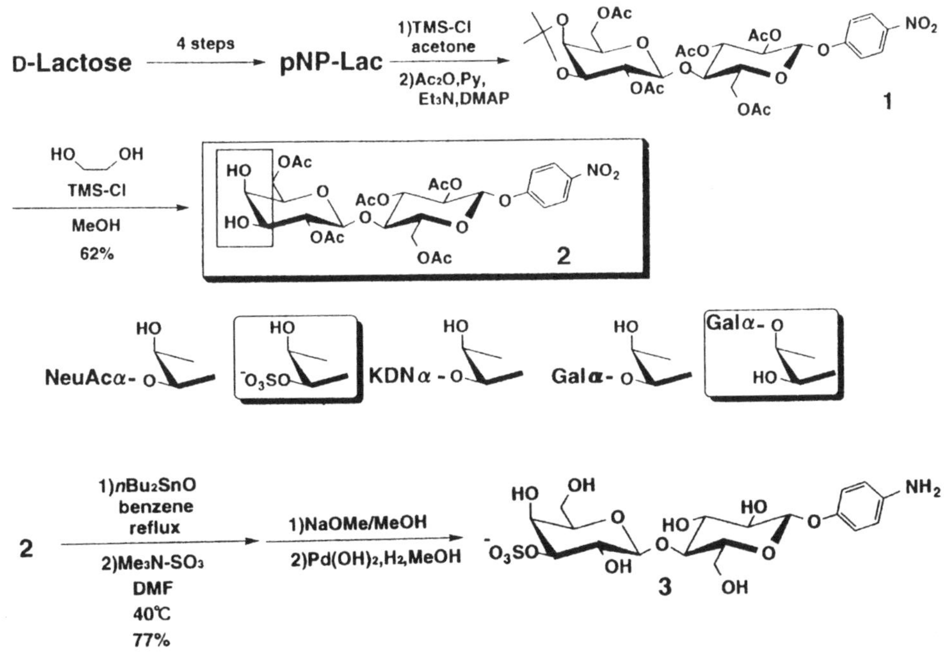

oligosaccharides were designed. One is 3′-sulfonated lactose as a mimic of sialyllactose which have high binding ability to influenza virus. Another is Galα(1→4) Galβ(1→4)Glc trisaccharide as a derivative of globotriaosylceramide (Gb3) which binds to verotoxin produced by pathogenic *E.coli* O-157. In order to develop highly functional materials which can trap microorganisms, these oligosaccharides are converted to acrylamide derivatives and then glycopolymers.

SYNTHESIS OF AMINOPOLYSACCHARIDES BY GLYCOSYLATION OF OXAZOLINE-TYPE SACCHARIDE COMPOUNDS HAVING HYDROXYL GROUPS

Aminopolysaccharides can be synthesized by ring-opening polymerization (chain reaction) of anhydrosugar derivatives having amino group precursors such as azide and phthalimide. On the other hand, J. Kadokawa *et al.* reported (2856, E751) the synthesis of aminopolysaccharides by glycosylation (stepwise reaction). Aminopolysaccharides were synthesized by acid-catalyzed polymerization of oxazoline-type saccharide monomers. Monomer having a hydroxyl group at position 6 polymerized involving stereoregular glycosylation to give a non-natural type aminopolysaccharide. The molecular weights of polymers obtained were about 12,000. Polymerization of the other monomers having two hydroxyl groups gave a hyperbranched aminopolysaccharide.

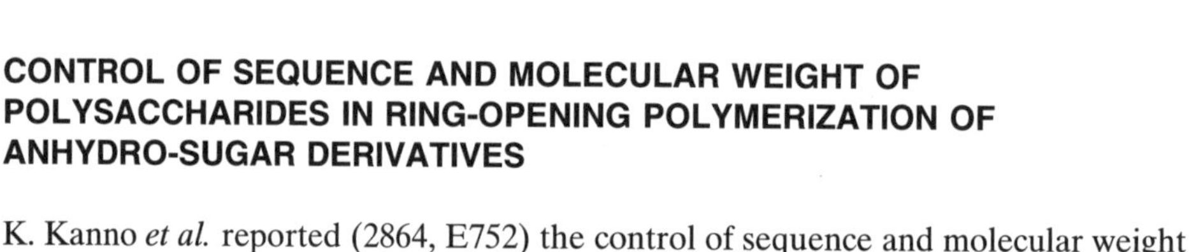

CONTROL OF SEQUENCE AND MOLECULAR WEIGHT OF POLYSACCHARIDES IN RING-OPENING POLYMERIZATION OF ANHYDRO-SUGAR DERIVATIVES

K. Kanno *et al.* reported (2864, E752) the control of sequence and molecular weight of synthetic polysaccharide. Glycosaminoglycans (GAGs), in which glucosamine and uronic acid units alternate along the chain, play various important roles *in vivo*. The relationship between chemical structures and biological activities of GAGs has been revealed by using GAG derivatives which were prepared by the modification reactions such as de-*O*-sulfation, de-*N*-sulfation, over-sulfation, degradation, and etc. In some cases, biological reactions of artificial polysaccharides or artificial oligosaccharides have revealed the structure–function relationship of the polysaccharides. However, artificial polysaccharides have been rarely used in biological investigations, because strictly designed polysaccharides with high molecular weights are difficult to synthesize. Polysaccharides consisting of disaccharide repeating units, such as GAGs have never been synthesized by polymerization reaction. Ring-opening copolymerizations of 1,6-anhydro-2-deoxy-3,4-di-*O*-benzyl-2-phthalimido-β-D-glucopyranose (1) with 1,6-anhydro-2,4-di-*O*-benzyl-3-*O*-1-(methoxycarbonyl)ethyl-β-D-glucopyranose (2) was carried in order to synthesize glucosaminoglycan-like copolysaccharide with different linkage from natural polysaccharide. The monomer reactivity ratios evaluated by the Kelen-Tüdös method were $r_1 = 0.08$ and $r_2 = 0.58$, respectively. It was indicated that the obtained copolysaccharide derivative having the same amount of each monomeric unit was rather alternating.

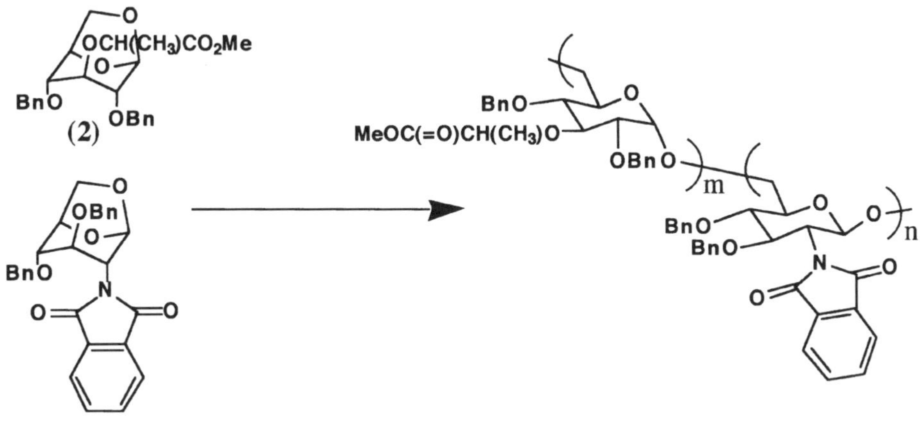

(1)

The cationic ring-opening polymerization of 1,6-anhydro-2,3,4-tri-*O*-benzyl-β-D-mannopyranose was applied to the synthesis of α-(1→6)-linked manno-oligosaccharide which is a part of natural, high-mannose-type oligosaccharides. Dimethoxymethane was added into the reaction system as a transfer reagent in order to diminish the molecular weight of the products. It was confirmed by gel permeation chromatography measurements that additional dimethoxymethane distinctly lowered the molecular weight of the oligomerization products. The presence of the —OCH_3 group, which was transferred from dimethoxymethane, at the reducing terminal of the obtained oligosaccharide derivatives was confirmed by ^{13}C-NMR measurements. In addition, methyl 2,3,4-tri-*O*-benzyl-6-*O*-methoxymethyl-α-D-mannopyranoside was synthesized as a model compound. From a comparison of the ^{13}C-NMR spectrum of the reaction product with that of the model compound; —O—CH_2—O—CH_3 group binding to the non-reducing end was found to be present. These results indicated the mechanism of the transfer reaction. Since another product was detected using ^{13}C-NMR spectroscopy, isolation of the products was carried out by silica-gel column chromatography. It was shown by ^{1}H- and ^{13}C-NMR spectroscopies, COSY, HMQC and HMBC that a 4,6-methylidene structure was also formed at the non-reducing end of the oligosaccharide derivatives.

FUNCTIONS OF CYCLODEXTRIN

Cyclic malto-oligosaccharide "cyclodextrin" shows a lot of functions. It is known that cyclodextrin (CD) binds alkyl moieties of the copolymers of acrylamide and alkyl methacrylates efficiently and selectively. A. Harada *et al.* reported (2880, E755) the interactions of CDs with guest moities of the copolymers of acrylamide with benzylmethyl acrylate and naphthylmethyl methacrylates. β-CD binds the insoluble copolymers of 2-naphylmethyl methacrylate and acrylamide to solubilize into water, although it did not solubilize the copolymer of 1-naphthylmethyl methacrylate. On the addition of β-CD the emission of the soluble copolymers of 2-naphthylmethyl methacrylate and acrylamide was remarkably enhanced, although the emission spectra of the soluble copolymers of 1-naphthylmethyl methacrylate and acrylamide remained unchanged. These results indicate that β-CD binds the 2-naphthylmethyl group selectively.

T. Nishiyama *et al.* reported (2882, E755) the hydrolysis of aliphatic polyesters by CDs. Hydrolysis was carried out in aqueous alkaline solutions at a fixed temperature. α-CD-poly(ε-caprolactone) complex was hydrolyzed much faster than poly(ε-caprolactone) only. The acceleration was also observed in α-CD-poly(alkyl adipate) hydrolysis. Hydrolysis of α-CD-poly(ε-caprolactone) was much faster at 37°C than 50°C in 5% NaOH aqueous solution indicating that there is the optimum temperature in the hydrolysis of α-CD-poly(ε-caprolactone).

MACROMOLECULES HAVING ACIDIC SACCHARIDE MOIETIES

D-Glucuronic acid exists widely as a component of polysaccharides in animals and plants and is known to have an important role in a xenobiotics metabolism system which is called the glucuronate pathway in a living body. Since its lactone was

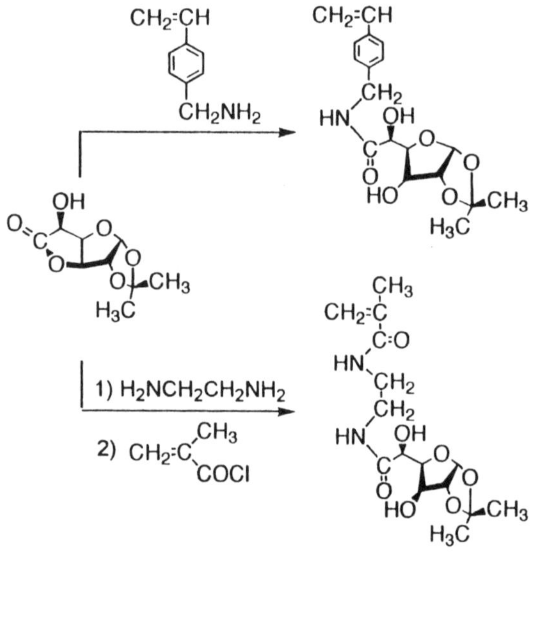

commercially available, it was used as a starting material for the synthesis of a novel amphiphilic polymer having D-glycuronyl pendants. K. Hashimoto *et al.* reported (2884, E756) the preparation of two kinds of new monomers which contain D-glucuronyl group and styryl and methacryloyl groups as a polymerizable functional group. Radical polymerization of styryl-type and methacryloyl-type monomers in dimethyl sulfoxide proceeded in a homogeneous phase at 60°C and gave a colorless powdery polymer in high yield. Through the deprotection in a mixture of trifluoroacetic acid with water (2/1, v/v), the glucofuranosyl moiety in the resulting polymer was converted to that having a pyranose ring. Solubility of deprotected polymers was found to be different from that of protected polymers in various solvents.

One of the saccharic acids, D-glucaric acid, and its derivatives are well known as competitive inhibitors of β-glucuronidase. K. Hashimoto *et al.* reported (2886, E756) the polymerization of a novel vinyl monomer having D-glucaric derivative, potassium *N-p*-vinylbenzyl-6-D-glucaramid-1-ate, which was synthesized by the reaction of D-glucaro-6,3-lactone with *p*-vinylbenzylamine, and subsequent treatment with KOH solution. Radical copolymerization of *N-p*-vinylbenzyl-6-D-glucaramid-1-ate with acrylamide in various feed ratios gave novel water-soluble glycopolymers. The resulting copolymers inhibited β-glucuronidase. The effect of the copolymer concentration in the inhibition of β-glucuronidase was examined by using the copolymers having various contents of the glucaric moiety.

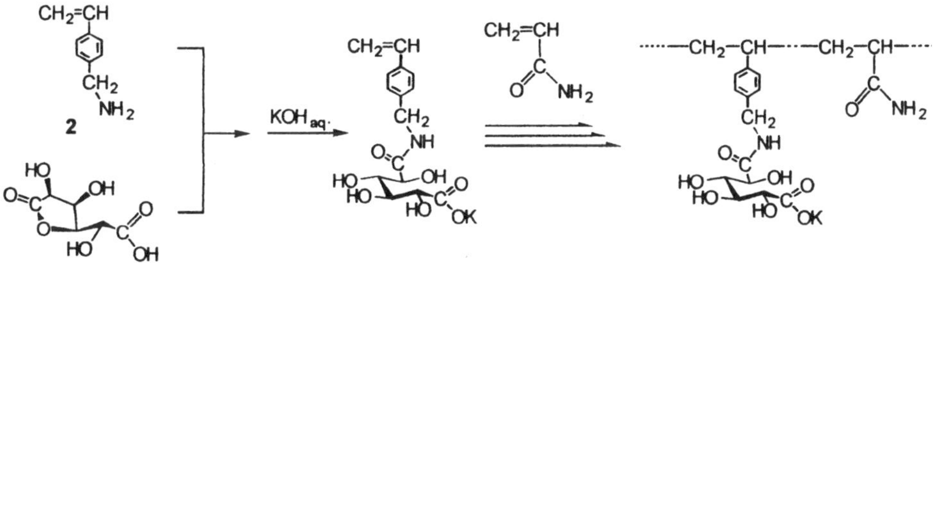

Polymer Alloys

HIDEKI YAMANE

Department of Polymer Science and Engineering, Kyoto Institute of Technology, Matsugasaki, Kyoto 606, Japan

In the SPSJ 46th Symposium of Macromolecules, Nagoya, Japan, a wide variety of topics were presented in the sessions related to the "Basic Science of Polymer Alloys" and "Enhancement of Performance of Polymer Alloys by Structure Control". Four topics were chosen for review from these sessions. Those are "Non-linear rheology of block copolymer systems", "Observation of deformation and recovery of droplet in immiscible polymer blend", "Phase Separated Structure of Immiscible Polymer Blends under Shear Flow", and "Structure control of super olefin polymers".

1 NON-LINEAR RHEOLOGY OF BLOCK COPOLYMER SYSTEMS

Block copolymers in which immiscible polymer chains are connected by the covalent bonding exhibit peculiar rheological behavior depending on the composition and the molecular weight of the components. The relationships between the nonlinear rheological behavior and structure of di- and tri-block copolymer systems were examined by H. Watanabe *et al.* (2546, E705, 2548, E705).

Anionically polymerized styrene-isoprene diblock copolymer (SI) in a low molecular weight homo-polyisoprene matrix forms spherical micelles with glassy styrene cores and soft isoprene corona. The viscosity η of this micellar dispersion exhibited a two-step shear-thinning behavior. They (2546, E705) examined the molecular origin of this behavior in relation to the relaxational features of the SI micelles. The micelles exhibited both fast and slow relaxation processes in stress relaxation experiments. The fast process, exhibiting modest damping of the relaxation modulus, and the slow process, exhibiting strong damping, have been attributed to the relaxation of individual corona and to the relaxation of anisotropy in the spatial distribution of the micelles via their diffusion, respectively.[1] They utilized these relaxational data in a BKZ constitutive equation to calculate the viscosity η_{BKZ} and showed that η_{BKZ} agreed well with the η data. This indicates that the shear-thinning behavior of the SI micelles had molecular origins identical to those for the nonlinear damping for the fast and slow processes.

Situation in the triblock copolymer solutions is quite complicated. H. Watanabe *et al.* (2548, E705) anionically polymerized styrene-isoprene-styrene tri-block copolymers with dipole-inverted isoprene block at the center of the chain (SIIS). The SIIS solutions exhibited rubbery, plastic and viscous behavior at low, intermediate, and high temperatures, respectively, in an isoprene-selective solvent. In the rubbery and plastic regimes, the styrene blocks were segregated to form spherical domains, and the isoprene blocks took either the loop- or bridge-conformation. They estimated the loop fraction in these regimes to be 60% by comparing the motion of free chain ends of I block in the SI di-block copolymer and that of the center of I block in SIIS tri-block copolymer. These loops have osmotically constrained conformation. At a low temperature, interdigitated loops and bridge play a significant role. In the high-T side in the plastic regime where the S/I immiscibility is rather small, this constraint resulted in the yield stress σ_y being dominated by dangling (non-interdigitated) loops.

2 OBSERVATION OF DEFORMATION AND RECOVERY OF DROPLET IN IMMISCIBLE POLYMER BLEND

In immiscible polymer blends, the minor component is generally present as the dispersed phase (droplets) in a continuous phase of the major component. Such multiphase polymer systems show pronounced elastic properties and very long relaxation time processes. It has been considered that this very long relaxation time process corresponds to the process in which deformed droplet recovers from the deformed state to its original spherical shape.

R. Hayashi *et al.* (2550, E705) directly observed the shape recovery of poly (isobutylene) (PIB) droplet embedded in an immiscible poly(dimethylsiloxane) (PDMS) matrix after application of various magnitudes of large step shear strain. The applied strain is large enough that the blend system is expected to show nonlinear viscoelastic behavior, but small enough that the droplet does not break up. During an earlier stage of shape recovery, the initial flat (leaf-like) ellipsoid changes its shape without reducing the droplet strain mostly in the shear direction. During

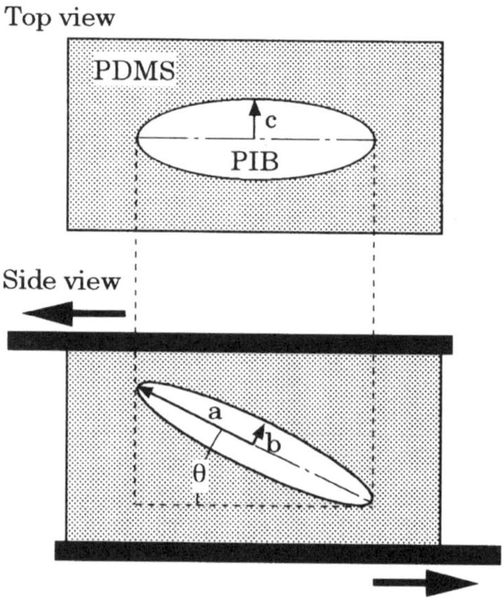

Figure 1 Semi axes a, b, and c and orientation angle θ of a deformed droplet.

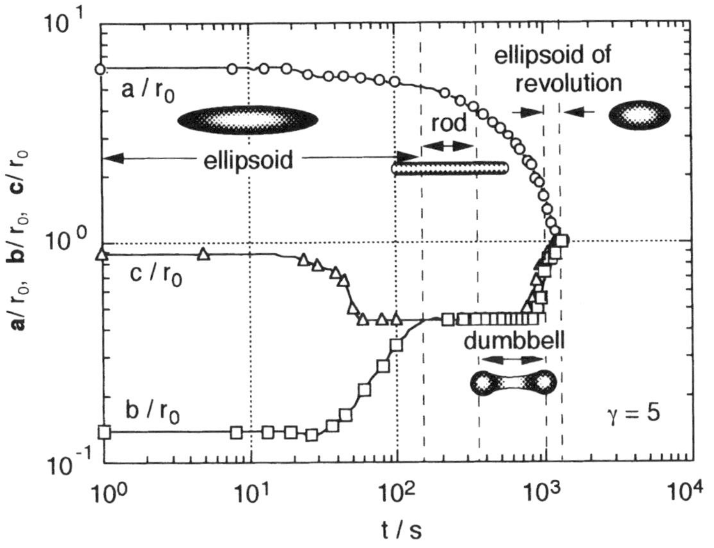

Figure 2 Time dependences of the normalized semi axes a/r_0, b/r_0 and c/r_0 after application of shear strain of $\gamma = 5$ with droplet shapes. r_0 is a radius of original sphere.

the final stage of the recovery, where the droplet shape is an ellipsoid of revolution, reduction of the interfacial area is accomplished by reducing the droplet stretch. They obtained a unique time constant which expresses the reduction of the droplet strain during the final stage (ellipsoid of revolution to sphere). This unique time constant does not depend on the magnitude of the applied strain and is nearly equal to the relaxation time of the dispersed phase in the blend for linear viscoelasticity predicted by the emulsion model of Palierne.[2] They explained the changes in shape during the recovery processes by a model calculation for the relation between the interfacial area and the stretch ratio of the droplet.

3 PHASE SEPARATED STRUCTURE OF IMMISCIBLE POLYMER BLENDS UNDER SHEAR FLOW

An elementary step in the mixing process of multi-component polymeric materials is the deformation of dispersed droplets in the flow fields, yielding an increase in the interfacial area between the two components accompanied by a decrease in the local dimensions (break up) perpendicular to the flow direction. Such change in the domain structure strongly affect the viscoelastic properties of the polymer blends. Doi and Ohta have proposed a constitutive equation for the immiscible blend of equiviscous Newtonian fluids.[3] Their equation predicts that the shear stress in steady shear flow is proportional to the shear rate γ, a scaling relation exists between the stress growth after shear jump and the shear strain, and the domain size regulated by the flow is inversely proportional to the shear rate.

K. Matsuzaka *et al.* (2554, E706) studied the changes in the domain structure and the viscosity of polystyrene/polybutadiene dioctylphthalate solution in shear flow field after jumping the shear rate from γ_0 to γ_1 (shear jump, $\gamma_0 < \gamma_1$). They showed that the viscosity gradually increases and the domain deforms within the shear strain γ_1 of 2. After showing a maximum at a shear strain γ_1 of 2, the viscosity gradually decreases. During this period, the domain deforms to be a string like structure in the flow direction without being destroyed up to several tens of shear strain. In these two regions, the growth in shear stress is described by the shear strain $\gamma_0 t$. Then the viscosity again increases to some constant value at a higher shear strain. In this region, the domain breaks into small fragments and the growth in shear stress is regulated by the shear strain $\gamma_1 t$.

4 STRUCTURE CONTROL OF SUPER OLEFIN POLYMERS

Super olefin polymer (SOP) is composed of the blend of highly stereoregular low molecular weight polypropylene and ethylene-α-olefin elastomer filled with inorganic particles such as talc. This blend/composite material is widely utilized for the automobile parts recently.

It has been reported that the olefinic elastomer is dissolved selectively in the amorphous region of polypropylene in SOP resulted in the pillar shaped polypropylene crystalline domain dispersed in a elastomer matrix. K. Yamada *et al.* (2673, E726) reported the spherulitic morphology of isotactic polypropylene with various degree of isotacticity. They showed the degree of cross-hatching composed of radial and tangential lamellae, which deteriorates the mechanical properties, decreased with increase of isotacticity and the crystallization temperature. This spherulitic structure changes to b-axis oriented pillar shaped structure when olefinic elastomer and talc are mixed. In injection molded parts, leaf-like talc tends to align its surface parallel to the parts surface and the crystalline domain of polypropylene grown on this talc surface is highly ordered perpendicular to the parts surface. The importance of the talc orientation induced by the flow to the b-axis orientation of the crystalline domain of polypropylene was demonstrated by S. Moriya *et al.* (2681, E727), who analyzed the isothermal crystallization behavior of polypropylene in SOP under steady shear flow. M. Naiki *et al.* (2679, E727) observed the structure of transcrystallized polypropylene grown isothermally on the talc surface by optical and transmission electron microscope. Y. Obata *et al.* (2677, E726) showed this structure and orientation of the pillar shaped crystalline domain are strongly dependent on the amount, size, and purity of talc filled in SOP as well as the degree of streoregularity of the isotactic polypropylene.

REFERENCES

1. T. Sato, H. Watanabe and K. Osaki, *Macromolecules*, 1996, **29**, p. 3881.
2. J.F. Palierne, *Rheol. Acta*, 1990, **29**, p. 204; 1991, **30**, p. 497 (E).
3. M. Doi and T. Ohta, *J. Chem. Phys.*, 1991, **95**, p. 1242.

Physical Properties of Polymeric Solids

TISATO KAJIYAMA and ATSUSHI TAKAHARA

Department of Materials Physics and Chemistry, Graduate School of Engineering, Kyushu University, Hakozaki, Higashi-ku, Fukuoka 812-81, JAPAN

KEYWORDS: Mechanical properties, Thermal molecular motion, Deformation, Composites, Fatigue, Fracture, Dielectric properties, Optical properties.

1 THERMOMECHANICAL PROPERTIES

Physicochemical properties of polymeric solids strongly depend on the states of aggregation structure and thermal molecular motion. The glass transition behavior of copolymers is related to the chemical structures and sequence distributions of monomers in copolymers. The theories of diad model[1] have been applied to describe the composition dependence of T_g for random copolymers. S. Teramachi *et al.* (3217, E846) studied the relationships between the glass transition temperature, T_g and composition of styrene(St)-methacrylate random copolymers prepared by a free radical copolymerization. The relationship between T_g and diad sequence of the St/*t*-butyl methacrylate (*t* BMA) copolymers followed the diad model theory. However, in the case of St/*i*-butylmethacrylate (*i*BMA) and St/*n*-butyl methacrylate (*n*BMA) copolymers, the diad model could not be applied.

Positron annihilation technique has been applied for the nondestructive detection of nanoscale defects in metals and semiconductors. This technique can be used as one of the methods to detect free volume in polymeric solids. M. Ban, A. Uedono *et al.* (3191, E841) discussed the glass transition temperature, T_g and the relaxation process in polypropylene (PP), polyethylene (PE), and polystyrene (PS) by positron annihilation technique. The lifetime of pick-off annihilation of orthopositronium, τ_3 and its intensity, I_3 were measured in the vicinity of T_g. It has been known that the magnitude of τ_3 is proportional to the size of free volume and I_3 is proportional to the concentration of free volume. T_g was determined as an onset of an increase in the temperature coefficient of I_3. The values of the temperature coefficients of τ_3 for these polymers were almost same below T_g. The T_g determined from τ_3 corresponded to the T_g measured by other procedures. The temperature coefficients of I_3 for these samples decreased with increasing temperature between 100 and 250 K, and increased again with increasing temperature above 250 K.

2 STRUCTURE AND PROPERTY RELATIONSHIPS

Various polyolefin blend systems have been prepared in order to improve their mechanical properties. K. Nitta *et al.* (3195, E842) studied the morphology and mechanical properties of [PP/ethylene-α-olefin copolymer] blends. It was found that the blends of PP with ethylene-rich copolymers showed a phase separation. Dynamic viscoelastic measurement revealed that the blend of PP with olefin-rich ethylene/α-olefin copolymer showed α_a-absorption which located between T_{α_a}'s of PP and ethylene-α-olefin copolymer. The small angle X-ray scattering (SAXS) of the [PP/olefin-rich ethylene-α-olefin copolymer] blend showed the increase in long period compared with that of PP since the α-olefin rich copolymers were incorporated into the amorphous region of PP. The [PP/olefin-rich ethylene-α-olefin copolymer] miscible blend showed a remarkable improvement on ductile behavior. Also, it has been concluded from the small angle light scattering (SALS) measurement that the spherulites in miscible blends is deformed even in the higher elongation. On the other hand, the [PP/ethylene-rich ethylene-α-olefin copolymer] immiscible blends showed brittle behavior with stress-whitening upon elongation.

K. Nitta, M. Terano *et al.* (3197, E842) studied the effect of addition of polypropylene-b-poly(ethylene-co-propylene) (PP-b-EPR) block copolymer in order to improve mechanical properties of PP and EPR blend systems. The novel PP-b-EPR with the PP weight fraction of 0.5 was prepared with a short period polymerization method. The temperature dependence of dynamic viscoelasticity of PP-b-EPR showed the α_c-relaxation of crystalline phase as well as the α_a-relaxation of amorphous phase. In the case of the (PP/EPR/PP-b-EPR) ternary blend, the α_a-relaxation of PP shifted to the lower temperature side compared with that of the (PP/EPR) blends. This indicates that PP-b-EPR is dissolved in the amorphous PP phase. Simultaneous measurements of infrared spectra (IR) and stress-strain behavior revealed that the chain orientation of PP in the PP/EPR blends hardly occurred during elongation. On the other hand, (PP/EPR/PP-b-EPR) ternary blend showed the chain orientation of PP and distinct yielding upon elongation.

Epoxy resins have been used for various technological applications. S. Nakamura *et al.* (3231, E848) studied the effect of ester residues of active esters on their mechanical properties. Bisphenol A diglycidylether (DGE) was cured with various esters such as trialkyloxybenzene, tripivaloxyloxybenzene, tribenzyloxybenzene. The α_a-absorption temperature, T_{α_a} of the epoxy resin cured with various esters was evaluated on the basis of dynamic viscoelastic measurement. The T_{α_a} became lower with increasing the length of linear alkyl residues. The crosslink density decreased and the molecular weight between crosslinks increased with increasing length of linear alkylchains. These results indicate that the crosslink structure of epoxy resins cured with active esters becomes looser by the introduction of linear alkyl ester groups. The linear alkyl chain might also act as an internal plasticizer. On the other hand, the branched alkyl and phenyl groups of active ester restricted internal rotation of the main chains resulting in an increase of T_{α_a}.

Ochi *et al.* (3233, E848) studied the thermal and mechanical properties of mesogenic biphenol-DGE epoxy resins cured with phenol novolaks. The effects of stereo structure of curing agents on the thermal and mechanical properties of the cured epoxy resin were investigated on the basis of dynamic viscoelastic measurement. The mesogenic epoxy resin cured with catechol novolak which has neighboring active hydrogens had the very low and broad α_a-absorption peak and fairly high rubbery modulus. However, the same resin cured with novolaks which has methyl or phenyl branches showed the distinct α_a-absorption peak and lower rubbery modulus. Moreover, in the case of the former system, a well-defined Schlieren texture being characteristics of nematic liquid crystal was observed under polarizing optical microscopy (POM). Therefore it is apparent that the orientation of mesogenic group in the former system makes the thermal molecular motion of network chain is suppressed even in the high temperature region. The change of mesogenic texture with curing time was observed under POM. The Schlieren texture was appeared at the gelation point. This result indicated that the orientation of mesogenic group was proceeded with the formation of network structure.

T. Konishi, T. Itoh *et al.* (3187, E841) studied the phase transition behavior of solution-grown or as-synthesized even-even nylons with hexamethylenediamine moiety (nylons 62, 64, 68, 610, 612) as well as nylons 6, 46, and 69. The change in crystalline structure with temperature was studied on the basis of wide angle X-ray diffraction (WAXD). The specific heat, *Cp* was measured with DSC. Any anomaly in *Cp* was not observed in the nylon 6 and 46 crystals, while the first order phase transition was detected for the nylon 62 crystal. Although such a phase-transition aspect generally tends to be ambiguous with increasing Y in nylon 6Y, the *Cp* anomaly in the nylon 69 crystal, in which the amide groups form the hydrogen bonds only partly, was less remarkable than that of nylon 612. These results indicate that the hexamethylene moiety plays an intrinsic role on the phase transition in the nylon crystals. Also, a high degree of freedom for molecular motion made symmetry of the intermolecular interaction potential high so as to disturb the appearance of phase-transition in nylon crystals.

S. Koda, H. Nomura *et al.* (3203, E843) proposed a novel method to estimate the partial specific adiabatic compressibility on the basis of the three phase model for EPR. The magnitude of partial specific adiabatic compressibility reflects not only the stiffness of amorphous phase but also the state of interphase. The partial specific adiabatic compressibility of EPR was estimated from the measurement of sound velocity and density. Sound velocity was obtained from the measurement of the transmission time t through the specimen with the thickness, at 303 K. The time-to-amplitude converter method employing a double transducer system was used to determine the magnitude of t. The sound velocity of EPR decreased with an increase of the amorphous phase fraction. The limiting partial specific volume and compressibility were $1.52\,\mathrm{cm}^3\,\mathrm{g}^{-1}$ and $0.97 \times 10^{-10}\,\mathrm{Pa}^{-1}$, respectively. This method might be applicable for the evaluation of interphase stiffness or interphase thickness of polymer composites.

3 DEFORMATION AND ORIENTATION

Brody *et al.* proposed that tensile characteristics of fibers depend on the inherent network draw ratio.[2] H. Shirataki, K. Okajima *et al.* (3229, E848) studied the relationship between tensile properties and network draw ratio for poly(ethylene-terephthalate) (PET) fibers. The network draw ratio is defined as an extension of unique intrinsic network structure. PET fibers with the wide ranges of molecular orientation and crystallinity were prepared by the cold drawing of melt spun yarns in a temperature-controlled water bath and their subsequent annealing for these samples. The true stress-strain curves for all samples could be principally superimposed to a master curve which corresponded to the stress–strain curve for the original non-oriented amorphous yarn. Then this indicates that the original (intrinsic) network structure is not significantly affected by molecular orientation and crystallinity. Tensile properties of these fibers were studied systematically in terms of network draw ratio which was determined from the magnitude of shift factor for superimposing the true stress-strain curves to the master curve. It was concluded from the tensile drawing behavior that mechanical properties including the yielding and breaking behaviors of PETwere directly correlated with the network draw ratio.

Since an aromatic main chain liquid crystalline polymer (LCP) has anisotropic diamagnetism of the main chain, a magnetic field might induce an orientation of the LCPs, E. Ito *et al.* (3221, E846) prepared the oriented films of thermotropic liquid crystalline polyester, Xydar under applying a magnetic field. The hot-pressed film of Xydar was heat-treated in a magnetic field of 6 T at 753 K for 10 min. The magnetically oriented sample showed the similar degree of orientation to that of the uniaxially stretched film. The linear thermal expansion coefficient of the oriented films was measured in the directions parallel and perpendicular to the orientation direction. Up to Tg, the thermal expansion coefficients were comparable for the uniaxially stretched and the magnetically oriented film in both parallel and perpendicular directions. At elevated temperature, the magnetically oriented films exhibited lower thermal expansion in both parallel and perpendicular directions than the uniaxially stretched film. Also, the magnetically oriented film had higher melting enthalpy and density than those of mechanically oriented ones. POM observation showed the presence of the texture corresponding to nonuniform orientation for the magnetically oriented film. The origin of the difference in thermal expansion behavior might arise from different thermal histories of the sample, as well as the difference in the oriented structures.

M. Matsuo *et al.* (3227, E847) analyzed the aggregation structure of polyethylene and (polyethylene/starch) composite films prepared by simultaneous biaxial stretching. The gel films of ultrahigh molecular weight PE(UHMWPE) and (UHMWPE/starch) composite were obtained from their decalin solutions. The maximum biaxial draw ratio of 3×3 was attained for the films prepared from the solutions with the concentration of $0.45\,g\,dl^{-1}$. On the other hand, the maximum biaxial draw ratio of 8.7×8.7 could be realized at the concentration of $0.9\,g\,dl^{-1}$. In the case of the film prepared from the $0.45\,g\,dl^{-1}$ solution, decreases in melting temperature and crystallite size were observed with biaxial stretching. The WAXD of edge view showing six diffraction arcs of the (110) plane, indicated the presence of two types of crystallite orientation. The storage modulus of the film was sensitive to the concentration of the solution for preparation of gel. The magnitude of modulus for the film prepared from the $0.6\,g\,dl^{-1}$ solution at the maximum draw ratio of 6×6 was much lower than that of the film prepared from $0.7\,g\,dl^{-1}$ solution at the same draw ratio (maximum draw ratio of 7.3×7.3). This indicated that most of tie molecules and microfibrils in the biaxially stretched film prepared from the

0.6 g dl^{-1} solution were teared by the elongation up to the maximum draw ratio. The (UHMWPE/starch) composite is expected to show biodegradability. (UHMWPE/starch) composite film was prepared and elongated up to 4.5×4.5. Morphological observation revealed that the starch particles were embedded among the fibrillar networks.

The mechanical properties of Nylon 6 strongly depend on the crystalline forms. M. Ito, T. Kanamoto *et al.* (3185, E840) studied the effects of polymorphism on the deformation behavior of nylon 6. A solid-state extrusion was carried out to prepare the samples with different crystalline forms and different pre-drawn morphologies. The effects of polymorphism on the deformation behavior of nylon 6 were investigated. The samples used were solution grown crystal mats (SGC mats) and melt-crystallized films (MGC). As-grown crystal forms of these samples were α-form. These were treated by I_2-KI aqueous solution followed by the treatment with aqueous solution of $Na_2S_2O_3$. The crystalline form in both samples were completely changed into γ-form by these treatments. The achievable extrusion ratio for the treated samples was considerably higher than those for the original untreated samples. That is, the deformability of the sample with the γ-form crystal was higher than that with α-form crystal. On the other hand, the structural analysis of these samples revealed that there was large difference in the noncrystalline structure between the two samples. The high deformability for the samples with the γ-form crystal might be closely related to a specific noncrystalline structure developed in the samples with γ-form.

4 POLYMER COMPOSITES

Nonconductive polymer composites can be applied for the container of superconductivity magnet. The properties of composites at cryogenic temperature has been paid great attention these days. It has been reported that the heat conductivity of amorphous polymers is remarkably smaller than that of metals and ceramics.[3] On the other hand, the relatively high heat conductivity of crystalline polymer has been reported.[4] T. Kashima *et al.* (3225, E847) studied the thermal conductivity of the poly(*p*-benzobisoxazole) (PBO) fiber and the (PBO-fiber/epoxy resin) composites (PBOFRP). The thermal conductivity (κ) and the thermal diffusivity (α) parallel (=) and perpendicular ($\perp$) to the fiber direction of these materials were measured at cryogenic temperature. The magnitude of $\kappa_=$ of the PBO fiber was remarkably high, that is, 1.4 and 60 $Wm^{-1}K^{-1}$ at 20 and 273 K, respectively. Therefore, it may be expected that the mechanism of heat conduction in PBOFRP is governed by phonon conduction along the direction of a molecular chain. The magnitude of $\kappa_=$ of the PBOFRP with the fiber volume fraction of 60% was also as large as 20 $W m^{-1}K^{-1}$ at 273 K, of which the value was higher than that of steel. On the other hand, $\kappa_\perp$ of PBOFRP was as small as epoxy resin. An anisotropy of κ ($\kappa_=/\kappa_\perp$-) was as large as 28.6 at 273 K and 7 at 20 K. The mean free path *l* of phonon in PBO calculated from α was 11.5 nm and its relaxation time, τ was 4.0×10^{-12} sec at 200 K.

M. Matsuo *et al.* (3223, E847) studied mechanical and thermal properties of (carbon black(CB)/ultra-high molecular weight polyethylene (UHMWPE)) composites. The (CB/UHMWPE) composites were crosslinked by dicumyl peroxide

(DCP). The DCP was introduced into PE gels prepared by crystallization from a dilute solution and the gel was dried at 323 K. The compositions of (CB/UHMWPE) films were 1/1, 3/1, 5/1, 9/1. The film was crosslinked at 423–433 K. The crosslinked (CB/UHMWPE) films with 1/1 and 9/1 compositions maintained their external shapes up to 573 and 473 K, respectively. The crystallinity of the crosslinked films became lower with increasing the content of CB. The electron conductivity increased with the CB content but was hardly affected by the crosslink density. This indicates that the formation of crosslink plays an important role to prepare (CB/UHMWPE) electrical conductive composite material with high-heat resistance.

5 FRACTURE AND FATIGUE

Craze formation process is closely related to the fracture behavior of polymeric solids. H. Hayashi *et al.* (3205, E844) studied the molecular mechanism of brittle fracture in PP on the basis of transmission electron microscopy (TEM) and electron diffraction (ED). When the craze propagated along the spherulite boundary, the craze opening width was large and the craze/bulk interface was smooth. However, when the craze propagates through spherulite, the craze opening width was small and the craze/bulk interface was rough. The fibrils were oriented primarily along the load direction in the crazes and ED pattern in the small angle region was similar to that from the craze fibril of PS. The ED pattern from the undeformed region was partially oriented ring. On the other hand, the ED pattern from the fibrils in the craze was clear diffraction spots, indicating the assembly of highly oriented crystallites along the loading direction. The fibril extension ratio for the craze was estimated to be 2.0 from the volume fraction of the fibrils in the craze.

The presence of solvent plays an important role in the fracture behavior of glassy polymeric solids. M. Kawagoe *et al.* (3379, E845) studied the arrest and healing of a surface crack in PMMA due to the Case II diffusion of methanol. The effect of compressive stress indued by the Case II diffusion of methanol on the preexisting crack in a surface swollen layer of PMMA was investigated. The induced stress was analyzed by a finite element method (FEM) based on the continuum elastic mechanics. The growth of crack in the surface swollen layer under static tension in methanol at 293 K was arrested for a long time at a position where the internal compressive stress along the loading direction took the maximum magnitude near the boundary between swollen layer and glassy core. The crack arrested under internal compressive stress in the swollen layer completely disappeared in methanol for 3 min after unloading at 313 K. Such a crack healing, however, was not observed both in methanol at 293 K and in the overall swollen specimen even at 313 K. Therefore, it seems reasonable to conclude that both higher temperature above T_g of swollen PMMA(304 K swollen at 313 K) and the significant internal compressive stress are necessary for the crack healing.

Fatigue strength and lifetime of polymeric materials are important characteristics for practical performance. The most of fatigue studies have been done based on fracture mechanical analyses which were initially applied to metals. Little attention has been paid on the relationship between viscoelastic behavior of polymeric materials and fatigue behaviors.[5] K. Takeda *et al.* (3213, E845) studied fatigue behavior of engineering plastics such as poly(phenylene ether) (PPE), PS and (PPE/PS) blends. Fatigue lifetime of the specimen decreased with an increase in number of cyclic straining. It was observed that the weight average molecular weight of the specimen decreased by 20% from the initial value after fatigue test. The dynamic viscoelasticity and surface temperature of the specimen were monitored during the cyclic fatigue. The hysteresis energy was evaluated from the dynamic loss modulus. The total hysteresis energy loss was divided into the heating energy and the energy required for an irreversible structural change. The fraction of energy appeared as heat increased with PPE content in the blend system. T. Kajiyama, A. Takahara *et al.* (3215, E845) studied fatigue behaviors of polymeric fibers with different polymer chain rigidities on the basis of nonlinear dynamic viscoelastic measurement under cyclic fatigue. The zone nonlinear dynamic viscoelastic analysis was proposed as a new method for analysis of nonlinear dynamic viscoelastic behaviors under cyclic straining.[6] Each cyclic deformation was divided into twelve zones: six tensile and six recovery zones. Poly(vinyl alcohol), Nylon 6(poly(ε-caprolactam)), poly(ethylene terephthalate), poly(*p*-phenylene terephtalamide) and Vectran (a copolyester of *p*-hydroxy benzoate (HBA) and 2-hydroxy-6-naphthoic acid (HNA)) fibers were used as specimens. Nonlinear dynamic viscoelasticity and fatigue performance of polymeric fibers strongly depended on the chain rigidity of polymeric fibers. The polymeric fibers with rigid molecular chains showed pronounced nonlinear viscoelastic characteristics compared with those with flexible ones. Also, based on the zone nonlinear dynamic viscoelastic analyses, it was found that the nonlinear viscoelastic behaviors of polymeric fibers was predominantly induced in the recovery process rather than in the tensile process during a single period of cyclic deformation, and also, the more remarkable nonlinear viscoelastic behavior was exhibited in the zone with higher strain rate. The polymeric fiber which exhibited remarkable nonlinear dynamic viscoelasticity showed extremely poor fatigue performance.

6 DIELECTRIC AND FERROELECTRIC PROPERTIES

The application of polymeric materials in a radio frequency (RF) region has been paid great attention these days due to the development of mobile communication systems. N. Amaya, T. Yamada *et al.* (3169, E838) proposed an advanced cavity perturbation method as an improved technique for evaluating the complex permittivity of RF-use polymeric materials. Considerable improvements have been made for an accurate evaluation, such as the resonance curve area method, the active resonance curve area method and the periodic least square method. Major problems in the conventional cursor function method currently installed in network analyzers, were improved at least five times as accurate as the conventional one. The complex permittivity of various polymeric materials in a pseudo-microwave range was evaluated by using the improved method. The dispersion of resonance frequency and Q-factor evaluated by the resonance curve method are less than that evaluated from the cursor function method. This advanced cavity perturbation method is extremely useful for reliable evaluation of polymeric materials in a RF range.

K. Adachi, K. Nishikawa (3173, E838: 3175, E839) prepared piezoelectric elastomer with space charge. The effect of an electric field on the morphology and polarization of telechelic polydimethylsiloxane (PDMS) dispersed with poly(propylene oxide) (PPO) [PDMS/PPO elastomer] was investigated. The PDMS was crosslinked above 350 K and turned into a transparent elastomer. As reported by several authors, a droplet of PPO deformed into an ellipsoid when an electric field was weak but burst under a strong electric field.[7] Under the condition that the polarized drops were broken into smaller droplets, they were charged either positively or negatively and then, migrated along the direction of an electric field, resulting in a generation of an electric polarization. Therefore, if the system is crosslinked under an electric field, the polarization may be frozen in and a space-charge type electret can be formed. The piezoelectric constant. d_{11} of the (PDMS/PPO) elastomer was measured under stepwise compression. When the stepwise compression was applied to the (PDMS/PPO) elastomer, a negative voltage was always observed indicating that the polarization decreased by compression. The change of polarization was proportional to the magnitude of deformation. The magnitude of d_{11} was almost the same as d_{31} of the β-form of poly(vinylidene fluoride). On the other hand, in the case of impact loading, the resulting signal showed damping oscillation. This indicates that the sample elastomer oscillated by impact deformation and at the same time, it generates the piezoelectric voltage. From the frequency of oscillation, the Young's modulus of elastomer was evaluated.

7 OPTICAL PROPERTIES

The fluctuation theory predicts that an isotropic light scattering loss of optical amorphous polymer glasses decreases with a decrease in isothermal compressibility and refractive index.[8] N. Tanio, Y. Koike (3235, E849) estimated a light scattering loss of optical amorphous polymer based on its molecular structure. In order to prepare polymer glasses with low light scattering loss, the isothermal compressibility of polymers should be evaluated. However, the magnitudes of β for most polymers have not been measured precisely by direct mechanical measurement. The β was estimated from the relationships among intrinsic molar volume, molecular weight between entanglements, cross section of polymer chain and isothermal compressibility at the liquid–liquid phase transition temperature. Then, the magnitude of isotropic scattering was estimated from the magnitudes of isothermal compressibility and refractive index. The estimated isotropic light scattering loss of PMMA was in good agreement with the experimental β value. It was confirmed that the isotropic light scattering loss of the amorphous polymer can be estimated from its molecular structure assuming a frozen model at around glass transition temperature.

N. Tanio, Y. Koike *et al.* (3237, E849) studied the relationship between physical aging and light scattering loss of optical amorphous polymer glasses. Isothermal aging was carried out for the low-loss PMMA glass at temperature below the glass transition temperature. The light scattering loss of the PMMA glasses depended on the polymerization and heat-treatment conditions. When the PMMA was polymerized or heat-treated above T_g, the excess scattering intensity disappeared and the isotropic light scattering loss was reduced to the value calculated from the thermally induced fluctuation theory. The effect of enthalpy relaxation on the light scattering loss of the PMMA glass with no excess scattering was investigated by DSC and light scattering measurements. The light scattering intensity of the PMMA glass did not increase with increasing aging time. This indicate that the light scattering loss of the PMMA glass is not affected by physical aging.

It has been well known that the birefiringence of PMMA could be reduced by blending an optically anisotropic low molecular weight component such as trans-stilbene (*t*SB). This is a conventional method to control residual birefringence of polymers. In order to utilize this technique, the orientational relaxation of a low molecular weight component in a polymer should be clarified. K. Osaki, T. Inoue *et al.* (3239, E849) studied the reorientation of small molecules in the polymer matrix in the vicinity of glass transition region. The dynamic birefringence and dynamic viscoelasticity of (PMMA/*t*SB) blends were measured at around a glass-to-rubber transition region to clarify the reorientation relaxation mechanism. The blend system was transparent up to the addition of 20 wt% stilbene. The creep measurement revealed that the negative orientation birefringence of PMMA at room temperature was well canceled by blending 3 wt% *t*SB. The complex Young's modulus, E* of the (PMMA/*t*SB) blends showed a relaxation behavior similar to that of neat PMMA except that the T_g decreased with increasing *t*SB content. The frequency dependence of the complex strain optical coefficient, O*, remarkably changed with the *t*SB content. For the (PMMA/*t*SB) blends with the *t*SB content above 10 wt%, the magnitude of O* was proportional to that of E* at a high frequency range, following the ordinary stress-optical rule. Since O* reflected mostly the reorientation of *t*SB in a high *t*SB contents, this result indicate the cooperative reorientation of the two components.

REFERENCES

1. H. Suzuki and V.B.F. Mathod, *Macromolecules*, 1989, **22**, p. 1380.
2. H. Brody and J. Macromol, *Sci.-Phys.*, 1983, **B22**, 19, p. 407.
3. T. Bhowmick and S. Pattanyak, *Cryogenics*, 1990, **30**, p. 116, 122, 795.
4. C.L. Choy, S.P. Wang, K. Young and J. Polym, *Sci., Polym. Phys. Ed.*, 1985, **23**, p. 1495.
5. A. Takahara, K. Yamada, T. Kajiyama and M. Takayanagi, *J. Appl. Polym. Sci.*, 1980, **25**, p. 597.
6. T. Liang, K. Saito, A. Takahara and T. Kajiyama, *Polym. J.*, 1996, **29**, p. 801.
7. C.G. Garton and Z. Krauski, *Proc. Roy. Soc.*, London, 1964, **A280**, p. 211.
8. A. Einstein, *Ann. Phys.*, 1910, **33**, p. 1275.

Current Awareness

DISSERTATION ABSTRACTS

The following titles have been selected from Dissertation Abstacts International by University Microfilms International. The titles have been organized under a series of key-word headings. The full abstract may be found in the referenced issue of Dissertation Abstracts or Masters Abstracts (designated source). The last entry (DAXXXXXXX, BRDXXXX, MAXXXXX OR XX/XXXXXC) gives the identification code that may be used to order a copy of the full text when available from University Microfilms International, 300 North Zeeb Road, P.O. Box 1764, Ann Arbor, Michigan 48106, U.S.A. or by telephoning (toll-free) 800-521-3042 in the US. Dissertation titles are published with the permission of the University Microfilms International, publishers of Dissertation Abstracts International.

Subject-Area-Keyword	Name	Thesis/Year/University	Source
Adhesion	J. Wohlgenannt	Technische Universitaet Graz, Austria, In German (1996) 208pp.	58/819c
	W.L. Dechent	University of Missouri-Rolla (1996) 103pp.	729-B DA9722423
Adhesive systems	J.L. King, II	The University of Akron (1996) 109pp.	6964-B DA9712825
	X. Li	The University of Akron (1996) 220pp.	6964-B DA9711893
Adsorption studies	D.S. Grzegorczyk	University of Virginia (1997) 150pp.	6400-B DA9708637
	P.C. Dreux	University of Pennsylvania (1997) 280pp.	1402-B DA9727213
Anionic polymerization	J. Lee	The University of Akron (1996) 214pp.	6964-B DA9712826
	J.R. Warmkessel	The University of Akron (1997) 122pp.	735-B DA9723601
Associative polymers	K. Persson	Kungliga Tekniska Hogskolan, Sweden (1995) 147pp.	58/793c
Batteries	Y. Ma.	University of California, Berkeley (1996) 146pp.	908-B DA9723092
Biodegradable materials	C. Yu	The State University of New Jersey-New Brunswick (1997) 149pp.	7539-B DA9717469
	G.H. Crotts, III	Temple University (1997) 122pp.	1298-B DA9724226
	S.L. Ishaug-Riley	Rice University (1997) 161pp.	1392-B DA9727567
	R.C. Thomson	Rice University (1997) 108pp.	1396-B DA9727617
Biodegradation	T.M. Scherer	University of Massachusetts (1996) 310pp.	6289-B DA9709649
	G. Renner	Technische Universitaet Graz, Austria (1996) 150pp.	58/986c
	D.R. Confer	The University of Arizona (1996) 248pp.	892-B DA9720659
	C.A. Murphy	The University of Connecticut (1997) 98pp.	1674-B DA9730893
Biomaterials	M.A.B. Kruft	Technische Universiteit Eindhoven, The Netherlands (1997)	58/3801c

Biomedical materials	G. Hanff	Lunds Universitet, Sweden (1996) 112pp.	58/549c
	C.B. Brink	Goteborgs Universitet, Sweden (1995) 57pp.	58/778c
	G.B. Cornwall	Queen's University at Kingston, Canada (1996) 222pp.	381-B DANN15262
	P.V. Joshi	University of Massachusetts-Lowell (1997) 73pp. p1059	MA1384177
Biopolymers	M.H. Orroy	Norges Tekniske Hogskole, Norway (1996) 65pp.	58/975c
Biosensors	T. Kaku	Polytechnic University (1996) 257pp.	1905-B DA9729115
Biosynthesis	J. Zhang	University of Massachusetts-Lowell (1996) 125pp.	6968-B DA9713787
Blends	R.R. Shinde	University of Kentucky (1996) 187pp.	6409-B DA9709200
	K. Eersels	Katholieke Universiteit Leuven, Belgium (1996) 157pp.	58/807c
	D. Li	Universite Laval, Canada (1996) 213pp.	7555-B DANN14213
	F. Lin	The University of Akron (1996) 140pp.	6965-B DA9712827
	K. Mimura	The University of Michigan (1996) 244pp.	7175-B DA9712041
	D. Winoto	Northwestern University (1994) 176pp.	7181-B DA9714709
	Y. Yan	Universite Laval, Canada (1996) 133pp. p. 823	MAMM14353
	J.A. McNally	Queen's University of Belfast, Northern Ireland (1996) 335pp.	58/2464c
	A. Van der Wal	Universiteit Twente, The Netherlands (1996) 139pp.	58/2713c
	K.M. Kit	University of Delaware (1996) 182pp.	372-B DA9718757
	K.A. Schult	The University of Texas at Austin (1996) 310pp.	309-B DA9719488
	R.J. Gavlik	University of Massachusetts-Lowell (1996) 86pp. p. 1054	MA1383702
	A.G. Damani	University of Massachusetts-Lowell (1997) 105pp. p. 1058	MA1383701
	Y. Ghebremeskel	The University of Connecticut (1996) 202pp.	729-B DA9723466
	J.K. Maranas	Princeton University (1997) 302pp.	1407-B DA9724771
	K.W. Foreman	The University of Chicago (1997) 264pp.	1905-B DA9729808
	D. Vroom	San Jose State University (1997) 64pp. 1460	MA1384728
Block copolymer	T.J. Martin	The University of Texas at Austin (1996) 108pp.	227-B DA9719282
Blood compatibility	J.P. Lens	Universiteit Twente, The Netherlands (1996) 232pp.	58/2463c
Capillary electrophoresis	A. Fridstrom	Uppsala Universitet, Sweden (1996) 43pp.	58/3674c
Carbon fibre reinforced plastic	A.Z.Y.H. Fam	The University of Manitoba, Canada (1996) 241pp. p. 557	MAMM13115
Cationic polymers	M.X. Tang	University of California, San Francisco (1996) 130pp.	1396-B DA9726635
Cationic processes	M.R. Clark	The University of North Carolina at Chapel Hill (1997) 217pp.	1881-B DA9730503
Cellulose	K. Lindell	Lunds Universitet, Sweden (1996) 67pp.	58/788c
	L. Mao	Universite Laval, Canada (1996) 186pp.	7555-B DANN14228

Cellulose	T.D. Reynolds	University of Cincinnati (1996) 283pp.	6870-B DA9713132
	T.C.O. Gren	Uppsala Universitet, Sweden (1996) 59pp.	53/3628c
	G. Wang	Lunds Universitet, Sweden (1997)	58/3792c
Characterization	K. Khougaz	McGill University, Canada (1996) 320pp.	6285-B DANN12402
	M.A. Olshavsky	The Pennsylvania State University (1996) 209pp.	7556-B DA9716283
	C.S. Reed	The Pennsylvania State University (1996) 172pp.	7556-B DA9716300
	Y.C. Liang	Cornell University (1997) 149pp.	7556-B DA9716153
	A. Park	Massachusetts Institute of Technology (1996) 1p.	7631-B
	B. Narasimhan	Purdue University (1996) 340pp.	7095-B DA9713570
	H. Chun	The University of Akron (1997) 202pp.	7166-B DA9711886
	C. Rodriguez Espinosa	Universidad de Navarra, Spain, In Spanish (1996) 230pp.	58/2456c
	S. Mawson	The University of Texas at Austin (1996) 283pp.	305-B DA9719429
	S.R. Challa	Case Western Reserve University (1996)	902-B DA9723504
	H. Moaddel	Case Western Reserve University (1996) 136pp.	731-B DA9720438
	H.S. Tamber	State University of New York College of Envornmental Science & Forestry (1997) 229pp.	DA9724784
	B. Tan	Virginia Polytechnic Institute and State University (1997) 260pp.	1313-B DA9726308
	S. Venkataramani	University of Massachusetts-Lowell (1997) 111pp.	1313-B DA9726278
	A.R. Kannurpatti	University of Colorado at Boulder (1997) 213pp.	1405-B DA9725749
	D. Li	Universite Laval, Canada (1996) 213pp.	1905-B DANN14221
	G.W. Busser	Universiteit Twente, The Netherlands (1997) 162pp.	58/3773c
	J.F. Legault	Royal Military College of Canada, Canada, In French (1995) 110pp. 1422	MAMM16598
Chemical sensors	G.O. Noonan	Michigan State University (1996) 123pp.	177-B DA9718870
Coatings	S. Zhang	Eastern Michigan University (1996) 99pp. p. 539	MA1382529
Colloids	S.F. Ahmed	Georgia Institute of Technology (1996) 236pp.	6396-B DA9709700
Composites	J.W. Littles, Jr.	Georgia Institute of Technology (1996) 114pp.	6423-B DA9709742
	Z. Zhang	Auburn University (1996) 180pp.	6508-B DA9709157
	H.K. Kung	University of Houston (1996) 248pp.	6521-B DA9710103
	N.M. Alif	Florida Atlantic University (1996) 186pp.	6548-B DA9707531
	S. Govindarajan	The State University of New Jersey-New Brunswick (1997) 114pp.	7692-B DA9717436
	H.B. Su	Kansas State University (1996) 254pp.	7100-B DA9714360
	A.A. Al-Ostaz	Michigan State University (1996) 279pp.	DA9718803
	R. Belardinelli	The University of Texas at Arlington (1996) 263pp.	369-B DA9718531
	M.S. Bhalerao	The University of Texas at Austin (1996) 227pp.	378-B DA9719303

Composites	X. Wang	State University of New York at Buffalo (1997) 271pp.	394-B DA9719188
	D.D. Hartranft	University of Delaware (1997) 272pp.	406-B DA9718753
	J.K. Farooqi	King Fahd University of Petroleum and Minerals, Saudi Arabia (1996) p. 149pp.	MA1384114
	Y. Liu	The University of Michigan (1997) 219pp.	908-B DA9722032
	J.L. Lombardi	The University of Arizona (1996) 170pp.	908-B DA9720652
	S.W. Hsiao	The University of Michigan (1997) 160pp.	927-B DA9722000
	C. Park	The University of Michigan (1997) 199pp.	732-B DA9722058
	S.E. Campbell	Clarkson University (1997) 132pp.	833-B DA9723493
	N.A.F. Al-Rawashdeh	Georgetown University (1997) 268pp.	715-B DA9720760
	J. Kim	The University of Michigan (1997) 137pp.	730-B DA9722016
	J.M. Barr	University of Missouri-Rolla (1997) 135pp.	1469-B DA9726335
	M.J. Creedon	Alfred University (1996) 193pp.	1471-B DA9724082
	H. Guan	Wayne State University (1997) 193pp.	1486-B DA9725829
	H. Zhao	Wayne State University (1997) 140pp.	1499-B DA9725885
	S.D. Burnside	Cornell University (1997) 182pp.	1873-B DA9727892
	R.J. Gehr	The University of Rochester (1997) 174pp.	1952-B DA9728442
	I.J. Beyerlein	Cornell University (1997) 284pp.	1962-B DA9727887
	S.S. Daggett	Wichita State University (1997) 240pp.	1963-B DA9730250
	A.A. Bent	Massachusetts Institute of Technology (1997) 1p.	1987-B
	C.D. Chapman	Texas A&M University (1997) 169pp.	1987-B DA9729171
	E.L. Poole	University of Washington (1997) 165pp.	1989-B DA9730065
	P.I. Rodriguez	The University of Mississippi (1997) 270pp.	2072-B DA9729789
	M. Alonso Rodrigo	Universidad de Valladolid, Spain, In Spanish (1994) 193pp.	58/3794c
	Q. Liu	Universiteit Twente, The Netherlands (1997) 160pp.	58/3803c
	D.C. Shah	University of Alberta, Canada (1996) 269pp. 1460	MAMM18323
	R. Chaarani	University du Quebec a Chicoutimi, Canada In French (1996) 141pp. 1477	MAMM16751
Computer simulation	Y. Liu	The University of Southern Mississippi (1996) 129pp.	6369-B DA9708980
Conducting polymer	K.C. Park	Polytechnic University (1997) 112pp.	6288-B DA9709162
	Z. Qi	McGill University, Canada (1996) 310pp.	6289-B DANN12460
	F. Deng	Georgia Institute of Technology (1996) 253pp.	6261-B DA9709715
	S.V. Frolov	The University of Utah (1996) 302pp.	6320-B DA9709681
	M.E. Ahlskog	Helsinki University of Technology, Finland (1996) 44pp.	58/862c
	R.V. Parthasarathy	Colarado State University (1996) 204pp.	227-B DA9719601

Conformational analysis	L. Zhang	Wayne State University (1996) 137pp.	7687-B DA9715945
Conjugated polymers	M.E. Chandross	The University of Arizona (1996) 169pp.	6999-B DA9713418
	J.F. Partee	Iowa State University (1997) 108pp.	1343-B DA9725448
Copolymers	D.E. Carranza	California State University, Fullerton (1997) 69pp. p. 536	MA1382410
	V. Tanrattanakul	Case Western Reserve University (1996) 188pp.	960-B DA9720453
	Y. Kim	The University of Akron (1997) 175pp.	730-B DA9723590
Crystallization	E.B. Orler	The University of Southern Mississippi (1996) 181pp.	6288-B DA9708969
Cure	Y.E. Xu	The University of Connecticut (1997) 146pp.	1907-B DA9730902
	J. Xavier Ramis	Universitat Politecnica de Catalunya, Spain, In Spanish (1994) 338pp.	58/3808c
Degradation	X. Xiao	The University of Utah (1996) 146pp.	6412-B DA9708434
	D.A. Sodergard	Abo Akademi, Finland (1996) 68pp.	58/815c
	B.H. Cumpston	Massachusetts Institute of Technology (1996) 1p.	7625-B
	D.I. Kim	University of California, Los Angeles (1996) 171pp.	7090-B DA9711589
	C.P. Martin	University of Southern California (1996) 58pp. p. 848	MA1383537
	J.S. Goldmeer	Case Western Reserve University (1996) 228pp.	925-B DA9723507
Design of superstructures	J.A. Pickering	The University of Connecticut (1996) 340pp.	228-B DA9718502
Deuterium NMR	W.Y. Lin	University of Missouri-Rolla (1997) 167pp.	176-B DA9719988
Drag reduction	R. Sureshkumar	University of Delaware (1996) 249pp.	228-B DA9718778
Drug delivery	H. Ghandehari	The University of Utah (1996) 187pp.	6202-B DA9709114
	A.J. Lee	University of Nottingham, UK (1996) 207pp.	58/2321c
	R.Z. Salem	Massachusetts College of Pharmacy and Allied Health Sciences (1997) 241pp.	DA9725960
Electrical Properties	S.L. Wu	The State University of New Jersey-New Brunswich (1997) 189pp.	7687-B DA9717467
	B.T. McCuistian	Texas Tech University (1996) 132pp.	7011-B DA9711301
Electrically conducting polymer	F. Gubbels	Universite de l'Etat a Liege, Belgium, In French (1995) 176pp.	58/3799c
Electrically conductive composites	M.E. Weber	McGill University, Canada (1996) 312pp.	6411-B DANN12508
Electron beam-initiated heterogeneous grafting	A. Wirsen	Kungliga Tekniska Hogskolan, Sweden (1995) 160pp.	58/818c
Emulsion particles	G.T.D. Shouldice	University of Waterloo, Canada (1996) 223pp.	734-B DANN15343
Emulsion polymerization	H.C.J. Chou	University of Missouri-Rolla (1996) 167pp.	6284-B DA9707970
	H. Guo	McMaster University, Canada (1996) 284pp.	6401-B DANN13652

Emulsion polymerization	S. Mohammed	Lehigh University (1997) 197pp.	7094-B DA9715040
	Q. Li	University of Southern California (1996) 336pp.	304-B DA9720254
	X. Li	University of Southern California (1997) 139pp. 1422	MA1384904
	E. Ozdeger	Lehigh University (1997) 300pp.	1906-B DA9730308
Extrusion	A.J. Harlin	Helsinki University of Technology, Finland (1996)	58/2760c
Extrusion blow molding	M.E. Duffett	University of Massachusetts-Lowell (1997) 205pp. p. 586	MA1382640
	S.L. Dumont	University of Massachusetts-Lowell (1996) 80pp. p. 897	MA1382641
Fatigue	Z. Zhang	University of Illinois at Urbana-Champaign (1997) 210pp.	7687-B DA9717352
Fiber coatings	I.C. Finegan	Wayne State University (1997) 359pp.	1485-B DA9725825
Fiber reinforced plastics	D.D. Arola	University of Washington (1996) 410pp.	7689-B DA9716809
Fiber-reinforced composite materials	S.M. Toffoli	The State University of New Jersey-New Brunswick (1996) 155pp.	7180-B DA9711143
Filament-winding	D.R. Kokan	Georgia Institute of Technology (1997) 151pp.	1383-B DA9725177
Finite element method	Z.M. Lin	The University of Manitoba, Canada (1995) 122pp.	6423-B DANN13300
FTIR	A. Singhal	The State University of New Jersey-New Brunswick (1996) 117pp.	6896-B DA9711133
Fuel cells	M. Ottoy	Norges Tekniske Hogskole, Norway (1996) 194pp.	58/792c
	J. Wang	Case Western Reserve University (1996) 200pp.	DA9720458
Gas chromatography	Y. Kim	University of Massachusetts-Lowell (1996) 242pp.	6893-B DA9713784
Gas diffusion	M.L. Greenfield	University of California, Berkeley (1996) 270pp.	836-B DA9723000
Gas separation	J.M. Levasalmi	University of Massachusetts (1996) 138pp.	6286-B DA9709619
Gels	S. Achanta	Purdue University (1995) 287pp.	1398-B DA9725672
Glass Fibre Reinforced Plastic	F. Farahmand	The University of Manitoba, Canada (1996) 154pp. p. 557	MAMM13116
	C.R. Michaluk	The University of Manitoba, Canada (1996) 199pp. p. 559	MAMM13373
	R.R. Kudrathaya	University of Massachusetts-Lowell (1996) 86pp. p. 587	MA1382644
Health and Safety	I.M. Andersson	Kungliga Tekniska Hogskolan, Sweden (1995) 107pp.	58/604c
Hydrogels	M.J. Lesho	The Johns Hopkins University (1997) 218pp.	293-B DA9718988
Injection molding	C.J. Beard	University of Massachusetts-Lowell (1996) 109pp. p. 586	MA1382628
	M.J. Janczyk	University of Massachusetts-Lowell (1996) 89pp. p. 587	MA1382643
	B. Xie	University of Maryland College Park (1996) 225pp.	406B DA9719851
A.A. Khare	University of Massachusetts-Lowell	(1996) 101pp. p. 1054	MA1384179

Injection molding	G.R. Saraiya	University of Massachusetts-Lowell (1997) 110pp. p. 1059	MA1384186
Interpenetrating polymer networks	F.E. Du Prez	Rijksuniversiteit te Gent, Belgium, In Dutch (1996) 164pp.	58/3797c
Ion-selective electrodes	M.S. Espadas-Torre	The University of Michigan (1996) 145pp.	6891-B DA9711960
Ionic transport	S. Chintapalli	The University of Oklahoma (1996) 283pp.	6276-B DA9710982
Isocyanates	H. Tinnerberg	Lunds Universitet, Sweden (1996) 140pp.	58/2231c
Latex	J. Xu	Lehigh University (1996) 219pp.	6968-B DA9715043
Light scattering	S. Sadasivan	Clarkson University (1997) 125pp.	7632-B DA9717496
Living polymerization	J. Zhuang	University of Maryland College Park (1996) 168pp.	262-B DA9719859
Macromolecular assemblies	L.M. Dupray	The University of North Carolina at Chapel Hill (1996) 227pp.	7520-B DA9715691
Mechanical behavior	D.J. Macon	University of Massachusetts (1997) 161pp.	909-B DA9721477
	H.F. Hsiao	The Ohio State University (1997) 124pp.	837-B DA9721108
Mechanical properties	J. Wang	State University of New York College of Environmental Science & Forestry (1996) 150pp.	6291-B DA9708414
	G.V. Laverde	University of Massachusetts-Lowell (1997) 66pp. p. 1054	MA1384182
Melt viscosities	D.M. Burke	University of Massachusetts-Lowell (1996) 186pp.	6284-B DA9708444
Membrane permeation	N. Zhu	New Jersey Institute of Technology (1997) 161pp.	1856-B DA9730393
Membrane polymers	H.C. Shen	North Carolina State University (1996) 309pp.	6408-B DA9708345
Membranes	I. Genne	Katholieke Universiteit Leuven, Belgium (1996) 139pp.	58/809c
	S. Moller-Holst	Norges Tekniske Hogskole, Norway (1996) 132pp.	58/985c
	R. Garcia i Valls	Universitat Autonoma de Barcelona, Spain, In Spanish (1995) 256pp.	58/2363c
	J.M.M. Peeters	Universiteit Twente, The Netherlands (1997) 160pp.	58/3668c
Metathesis polymerisation	C.D. Chad	The University of North Carolina at Chapel Hill (1996) 167pp.	7555-B DA9715746
	M. Ungerank	Technische Universitaet Graz, Austria, In German (1996) 161pp.	58/817c
Microemulsions	K.L. Harrison	The University of Texas at Austin (1996) 286pp.	300-B DA9719372
	H. Bagger-Jorgensen	Lunds Universitet, Sweden (1997) 198pp.	58/3795c
Microstructure	M.G. Pigeon	University of Waterloo, Canada (1996) 332pp.	732-B DANN15334
Modelling	B.H. Brouwer	Queen's University at Kingston, Canada (1996) 126pp. p. 823	MAMM15113
	P.Y. Vuillaume	Universite Laval, Canada, In French (1996) 165pp. p. 824	MAMM14350
	R.S. Mirviss	California State University, Long Beach (1996) 86pp. p. 888	MA1383272

Modelling	R.A.W. Mee	Queen's University of Belfast, Northern Ireland (1996)	58/2465c
	S.J. Barsky	Simon Fraser University, Canada (1996) 124pp.	1946-B DANN16786
	Z.H. Duan	The Florida State University (1997) 81pp.	1910-B DA9729698
	M.R. Gownder	Texas A&M University (1996) 174pp.	370-B DA9718351
Molecular composites	J.M. Briner	University of Cincinnati (1996) 132pp.	6276-B DA9707712
Molecular recognition	C. Wang	Massachusetts Institute of Technology (1997) 1p.	1907-B
Monte Carlo simulations	R.H.C. Janssen	Technische Universiteit Eindhoven, The Netherlands (1996)	58/812c
Morphology	K.L. Singfield	McGill University, Canada (1996) 260pp.	6290-B DANN12487
	P.M. Cham	Virginia Polytechnic Institute and State University (1996) 214pp.	6337-B DA9710942
	C. Kvarnstrom	Abo Akademi, Finland	58/691c
	R. De Cooman	Katholieke Universiteit Leuven, Belgium, In Dutch (1994) 172pp.	58/805c
	M.S. Hedenqvist	Kungliga Tekniska Hogskolan, Sweden (1995) 330pp.	58/811c
	Y. Sjonell	Kungliga Tekniska Hogskolan, Sweden (1995) 115pp.	58/1131c
	L.A. Zook	The University of Iowa (1996) 134pp.	7635-B DA9715277
	J.M. Dieitzel	The University of Akron (1996) 110pp.	6961-B DA9712821
	T.P. Vainio	Helsinki University of Technology, Finland (1996) 56pp.	58/2466c
	K. Wegsten	Katholieke Universiteit Leuven, Belgium, In Dutch (1996) 158pp.	58/2467c
	H.S. Jeon	Polytechnic University (1997) 224pp.	302-B DA9718682
	S.C. Han	The University of Akron (1997) 174pp.	926-B DA9723585
	S. Balijepalli	University of Delaware (1997) 197pp.	728-B DA9722688
	J.P. Armistead	The Johns Hopkins University (1997) 197pp.	1904-B DA9730657
	L. Levitt	University of Minnesota (1997) 179pp.	2010-B DA9728967
	P.A. Bentley	University of Southampton, UK (1995)	58/3672c
	O.J. Karlsson	Lunds Universitet, Sweden (1997) 163pp.	58/3800c
	L. Quintanilla Sierra	Universidad de Valladolid, Spain, In Spanish (1993) 158pp.	58/4257c
	S. Moffatt	Universite Laval, Canada, In French (1996) 168pp. 1423	MAMM17472
	D. Tessier	Universite Laval, Canada, In French (1996) 102pp. 1423	MAMM17537
Nanocomposites	J.G. Gu	Michigan State University (1997) 115pp. 1518	MA1385046
Nanoparticles	A.B.R. Mayer	University of Cincinnati (1996) 141pp.	6287-B DA9707727
	E.S. Rodgers	Queen's University of Belfast, Northern Ireland (1996)	58/3635c
	M.J. Shephard	Queen's University of Belfast, Northern Ireland (1996)	58/3637c
Network formation	X. Zeng	Michigan Technological University (1996) 193pp.	6291-B DA9710099
Neutron scattering	B.D. Ermi	University of Southern California (1996) 257pp.	216-B DA9720219

NMR	V.E. Litman	The University of Akron (1995) 110pp.	671-B DA9723593
	L.E. Stephans	Lehigh University (1997) 135pp.	1855-B DA9730312
NMR imaging	Z. Mei	The University of British Columbia, Canada (1996) 274pp.	220-B DANN14799
NMR spectroscopy	V.M. Russell	Case Western Reserve University (1996) 211pp.	960-B DA9723525
Nonlinear optical studies	X. Zhuang	University of California, Berkeley (1996) 142pp.	771-B DA9723254
PEEK's	E.A. Cetin	University of Massachusetts (1996) 285pp.	6260-B DA9709580
	R.H. Mehta	University of Kentucky (1996) 202pp.	7094-B DA9713765
Peptides	M.A. Schuerman	The University of North Carolina at Chapel Hill (1996) 157pp.	6271-B DA9708173
Permeability	Y.Y. Chang	Michigan State University (1996) 88pp. p. 885	MA1383340
	H. Lee	Michigan State University (1996) 165pp. p. 885	MA1383375
Photo-degradation	D.V. Trinh	University of Missouri-Rolla (1997) 110pp.	735-B DA9722418
Photophysics	X.L. Jiang	University of Massachusetts-Lowell (1997) 94pp.	1354-B DA9726263
Photo-polymerization	J.J. Colman	University of California, San Diego (1996) 162pp.	7520-B DA9714817
Physical aging	M.D. Shelby	Virginia Polytechnic Institute and State University (1997) 290pp.	406-B DA9719929
Physical properties	C.K. Smith	University of Calgary (Canada) (1996) 190pp.	6290-B DANN12804
	M. Rooney	The Johns Hopkins University (1996) 200pp.	374-B DA9719020
	V.C. Long	The University of North Carolina at Chapel Hill (1996) 196pp.	7580-B DA9715740
	B.L. Volodin	The University of Arizona (1996) 158pp.	7024-B DA9713438
	J.R. Paterson	Queen's University at Kingston, Canada (1996) 154pp. p. 832	MAMM15183
Poly(amide-imides)	Q. Hu	Virginia Polytechnic Institute and State University (1996) 214pp.	301-B DA9719916
Poly(ethylene terephthalate)	J.S. Raghavan	North Carolina State University (1997) 160pp.	1511-B DA9726088
Poly(ethylene)	R. Lin	The University of Oklahoma (1997) 224pp.	1406-B DA9724431
Poly(imino-methylene)	J.T. Huang	University of Rhode Island (1996) 89pp.	
	M. Kim	University of Rhode Island (1996) 171pp.	
Polyacetylene	B.W. Davis	Rice University (1997) 73pp. p. 1026	MA1384354
Polyamides	M.J. Winningham	Cornell University (1997) 249pp.	7557-B DA9716131
Poly carbodiimides	A.A. Goodwin	University of California, Berkeley (1996) 304pp.	730-B DA9722995
Polydiacetylene	B.L. Lawrence	University of Central Florida (1997) 216pp.	876-B DA9723890
Polyelectrolyte	E.L. Sokolov	State University of New York at Stony Brook (1996) 170pp.	734-B DA9722196
	F.J. Yeh	State University of New York at Stony Brook (1996) 138pp.	736-B DA9720923
	G. Schultz	Polytechnic University (1997) 148pp.	1906-B DA9729116

Polyelectrolyte	D.C. Boris	The University of Rochester (1997) 220pp.	259-B DA9719938
	J. Sudor	Indiana University (1997) 303pp.	1260-B DA9727978
	L.B. Eriksson	Lunds Universitet, Sweden (1997) 180pp.	58/3777c
Polyesters	D.J. Frich	University of Illinois at Urbana-Champaign (1996) 181pp.	6962-B
	P.A. Hubbard	The University of Akron (1996) 112pp.	6963-B DA9712823
Polyethylene	V. Thomas	Texas A&M University (1996) 117pp.	375-B DA9718470
	W. Ding	The University of Utah (1997) 143pp.	299-B DA9718738
	J.P. Van Buskirk	Texas A&M University-Kingsville (1997) 79pp. p. 1045	MA1383972
	J.F. Wilson	University of Houston (1997) 112pp.	1356-B DA9728740
	P. Venugopalan	Massachusetts Institute of Technology (1997) 1p.	2014-B
	X. Zhang	Queen's University of Kingston, Canada (1997) 113pp. 1423	MAMM17873
Polyimidazole	H. Nie	University of Louisville (1996) 263pp.	6241-B DA9709450
Polyimide	K.C. Sheth	University of Massachusetts (1996) 154pp.	6290-B DA9709653
	N.R. Tu	The University of Manitoba, Canada (1995) 102pp. p. 571	MAMM13538
	Y.S. Kang	The University of Texas at Austin (1996) 146pp.	372-B DA9719399
Polyketones	M.I. Wagner	The University of North Carolina at Chapel Hill (1996) 145pp.	6272-B DA9708183
Polymer coatings	Y. Mao	The University of Oklahoma (1996) 158pp.	6225-B DA9710980
Polymer dynamics	M. Melchior	Eidgenossische Technische Hochschule Zurich, Switzerland (1997)	58/4032c
Polymer electrolyte batteries	J.P. Fellner	The University of Dayton (1997) 94pp.	2068-B DA9730410
Polymer electrolytes	A. Ferry	Umea Universitet, Sweden (1996) 114pp.	58/2449c
	D. Weng	Case Western Reserve University (1996) 165pp.	845-B DA9720459
Polymer foams	J.A. Kweeder	Clarkson University (1997) 94pp.	839-B DA9723494
Polymer fracture	T.N. Krupenkin	Case Western Reserve University (1996) 111pp.	766-B DA9723514
Polymer interfaces	U. Sawhney	Columbia University (1997) 129pp.	841-B DA9723846
Polymer melts	Y. Liu	The University of Connecticut (1996) 194pp.	6965-B DA9711617
	T.M. Rundqvist	Lunds Universitet, Sweden (1997) 116pp.	58/4258c
Polymer membranes	A. Bos	Universiteit Twente, The Netherlands (1996) 160pp.	58/2690c
Polymer relaxation	K.E. Hamilton	Northwestern University (1996) 373pp.	7089-B DA9714598
Polymer solutions	K.J. Zhang	University of Maryland College Park (1996) 220pp.	6344-B DA9707690
	M.A. Johnson	The University of Wisconsin-Madison (1996) 189pp.	7554-B DA9708276
	M.T. Kezirian	Massachusetts Institute of Technology (1996) 1p.	7629-B

Polymer solutions	M.B. Wisnudel	Northwestern University (1996) 411pp.	7101-B DA9714710
	R. Levicky	University of Minnesota (1996) 269pp.	7173-B DA9711425
	N. Wu	Lehigh University (1997) 134pp.	1907-B DA9730313
	K.E. Martel	Universite Laval, Canada, In French (1995) 136pp. 1499	MAMM17463
Polymer supported reagents	D.H.J. Miller	The University of Tennessee (1996) 194pp.	6287-B DA9709042
Polymer supports	M.J. Sundell	Abo Akademi, Finland (1994) 160pp.	58/816c
Polymerization	C.M. Killian	The University of North Carolina at Chapel Hill (1996) 177pp.	7554-B DA9715725
	N.J. Rodak	Cornell University (1997) 245pp.	7556-B DA9714908
	J. Kim	The University of Akron (1996) 136pp.	6964-B DA9712824
	J.D.A. Cid	Case Western Reserve University (1996) 170pp.	959-B DA9720405
Polypeptide	C.G. Worley	The University of North Carolina at Chapel Hill (1996) 212pp.	6283-B DA9708188
Polypropylenes	N.J. Macauley	Queen's University of Belfast, Northern Ireland (1996) 296pp.	58/4256c
Polysilanes	L. Heisler	Marquette University (1996) 167pp.	217-B DA9719077
Polyurethane	V. Bollaert	Katholieke Universiteit Leuven, Belgium, In Dutch (1996)	58/804c
	S.D.Y. Tse	University of California, Berkeley (1996) 179pp.	940-B DA9723223
	M.A. Schubert	Case Western Reserve University (1996) 159pp.	733-B DA9723527
	P.O. Ukpabi	Cornell University (1997) 98pp.	2104-B DA9727883
Polyurethane foam	R.J. Werbowesky	The University of Manitoba, Canada (1995) 113pp. p. 534	MAMM13556
Polyurethanes	S. Sapatnekar	Case Western Reserve University (Health Sciences) (1996) 140pp.	7467-B DA9714991
	J.D. van Heumen	University of Guelph, Canada (1996) 249pp.	7557-B DANN14478
Raman spectroscopy	N.H. Fontaine	Colorado School of Mines (1997) 1p.	1951-B
	J.C. Rodriguez Cabello	Universidad de Valladolid, Spain, In Spanish (1994) 193pp.	58/3884c
	C.M. Child	The University of Texas at Austin (1996) 128pp.	214-B DA9719324
Reaction injection molding	J.Y.R. Duh	University of Minnesota (1996) 162pp.	6514-B DA9709343
Reaction kinetics	K.A. Wolske	University of Minnesota (1996) 141pp.	7182-B DA9711459
Relaxation processes	R.Y. Jin	The University of Utah (1997) 172pp.	7678-B DA9717361
	J.C. Hooker	Northwestern University (1996) 261pp.	7169-B DA9714608
	M. Mours	University of Massachusetts (1997) 225pp.	840-B DA9721481
Rheology	M.L. Sentmanat	McGill University, Canada (1995) 256pp.	6408-B DANN12480
	A.M. van der Vorst	Universiteit Twente, The Netherlands (1996) 140pp.	58/908c
	J. Bonilla-Rios	Texas A&M University (1996) 331pp.	7624-B DA9718301
	C. Dubois	Universite Laval, Canada, In French (1996) 280pp.	7626-B DANN14130

Rheology	D.M. Shemo	The State University of New Jersey-New Brunswick (1997) 266pp.	7685-B DA9717457
	S. Chang	The University of Akron (1997) 260pp.	6960-B DA9712819
	J.M. Forbes	Northern Illinois University (1996) 156pp.	7494-B DA9716539
	B.M. Sheth	University of Massachusetts-Lowell (1997) 123pp. p. 1055	MA1384188
	M.A. Stroup-Gardiner	University of Minnesota (1997) 138pp.	853-B DA9721645
	Y.W. Inn	Case Western Reserve University (1996) 119pp.	775-B DA9720417
	L. Kasehagen	University of Minnesota (1997) 184pp.	838-B DA9721626
	M.J. MacDonald	University of California, Berkeley (1996) 183pp.	839-B DA9723096
Ring-opening polymerization	W.M. Stevels	Universiteit Twente, The Netherlands (1997) 109pp.	58/3806c
Rotationally moulded products	J.M. Butterfield	Queen's University of Belfast, Northern Ireland (1996) 269pp.	58/4255c
Screw extruders	M.H. Hong	The University of Akron (1997) 259pp.	959-B DA9723586
Second harmonic nonlinear optical properties	S.K. Lor	Hong Kong University of Science and Technology (UK) (1996) 165pp.	6287-B DA9709096
		Universiteit Twente, The Netherlands (1996) 140pp.	58/908c
	A.C. Kowalczyk	Case Western Reserve University (1996) 172pp.	781-B DA9720427
	M. Heylen	Katholieke Universiteit Leuven, Belgium, In Dutch, 199pp.	58/2461c
Secondary lithium-ion batteries	R.L. Nafshun	Oregon State University (1996) 206pp.	6924-B DA9711840
Self Assembly	K. Verstraeten	Katholieke Universiteit Leuven, Belgium, In Dutch (1995) 239pp.	58/800c
Self-assembled monolayers	L. Xing	The University of Akron (1996) 128pp.	6967-B DA9712835
Self-assembly	C.Y. Huang	University of Massachusetts (1997) 118pp.	837-B DA9721461
	N. Koneripalli	University of Minnesota (1997) 220pp.	1905-B DA9728965
Sensors	H. Zhao	The State University of New Jersey-New Brunswich (1997) 120pp.	7634-B DA9717472
	D. Keyvani	University of Illinois at Chicago (1996) 117pp.	7129-B DA9713264
	B.G. Healey	Tufts University (1997) 134pp.	1256-B DA9726588
Separation	C.A. Vandervoorde	Massachusetts Institute of Technology (1996) 1p.	7633-B
Solution behaviour	A.L. Ogden	University of Illinois at Urbana-Champaign (1997) 141pp.	7682-B DA9717319
	S. Mallapragada	Purdue University (1996) 226pp.	7093-B DA9713551
	H.C. Yun	Polytechnic University (1997) 140pp.	1313-B DA9726326
Spectroscopy analysis	H. Zhuang	State University of New York at Buffalo (1997) 275pp.	178-B DA9719199
	T.S. Kaniganq	McGill University, Canada (1996) 240pp.	6285-B DANN12398

Structure property relationships	D.P. Ching	San Jose State University (1997) 85pp. 1505	MA1384676
	S. Bensason	Case Western Reserve University (1996) 156pp.	728-B DA9723501
	P.J. Harney	State University of New York at Stony Brook (1996) 182pp.	730-B DA9722778
	W. Chinsirikul	The Pennsylvania State University (1996) 190pp.	7675-B DA9716208
Supercritical fluid CO_2	Y. Zhang	The University of Toledo (1996) 206pp.	845-B DA9721038
	M.F. Vincent	Georgia Institute of Technology (1997) 173pp.	1313-B DA9725197
	J.J. Watkins	University of Massachusetts (1997) 177pp.	735-B DA9725197
Supramolecular networks	G.D. Storrier	University of New South Wales, Australia (1996) 1p.	1312-B
Surface active polymers	D.V. Patwardhan	University of Cincinnati (1996) 104pp.	6966-B DA9713130
Syntheses	S.E. Wali-Alami	Universite Laval, Canada, In French (1996) 264pp.	7557-B DANN14351
	H.J. Paulussen	Limburgs Universitair Centrum, Belgium, In Dutch (1996) 146pp.	6966-B DA9714210
	X. Lin	State University of New York College of Environmental Science & Forestry (1996) 245pp.	6287-B DA9708413
	C. Martinez	McGill University, Canada (1995) 274pp.	6287-B DANN12432
	D. Bi	Renssalaer Polytechnic Institute (1996) 195pp.	6284-B DA9708902
	P.J. Hocking	McGill University, Canada (1996) 301pp.	6285-B DANN12383
	C.F. Laub	The University of Connecticut (1996) 146pp.	6286-B DA9707840
	J.L. Lee	Polytechnic University (1996) 100pp.	6286-B DA9709897
	C.J. Neef	The University of Oklahoma (1996) 202pp.	6288-B DA9709871
	L.D. Peeters	Universitaire Instelling Antwerpen, Belgium, In Dutch (1996) 169pp.	6289-B DA9708706
	B. Wu	University of Massachusetts (1996) 127pp.	6291-B DA9709668
	Y. Yang	City University of New York (1996) 122pp.	6291-B DA9707167
	X. Xu	Tulane University (1996) 246pp.	6413-B DA9708733
	F. Malik	Open University, UK (1993)	58/771c
	H. Andersson	Kungliga Tekniska Hogskolan, Sweden (1995) 131pp.	58/803c
	D.R.E. Devroey	Katholieke Universiteit Leuven, Belgium, In Dutch (1996) 227pp.	58/806c
	G.K. Dudley	The Pennsylvania State University (1996) 149pp.	7554-B DA9716215
	D.P. Schrum	Purdue University (1996) 195pp.	6895-B DA9713596
	W. Wei	University of Pennsylvania (1996) 224pp.	6928-B DA9713027
	Y. Chen	University of Illinois at Urbana-Champaign (1996) 185pp.	6961-B DA9712230
	D.L. Compton	University of Illinois at Urbana-Champaign (1996) 169pp.	6961-B DA9712237

Syntheses	H. Dixon	The University of Akron (1996) 135pp.	6962-B DA9711892
	T. Jang	The University of Michigan (1996) 128pp.	6963-B DA9711995
	T.M. Marsalko	The University of Akron (1996) 205pp.	6966-B DA9712829
	Z. Pi	The University of Akron (1996) 129pp.	6967-B DA9711895
	J. Sang	The University of Akron (1996) 179pp.	6967-B DA9711901
	G.E. Spilman	The University of Michigan (1996) 249pp.	6967-B DA9712095
	G.M. Kloster	Northwestern University (1996) 130pp.	7171-B DA9714629
	C. Yue	The University of Alabama in Huntsville (1996) 153pp.	7182-B DA9713832
	S.L. Penner	The University of Western Ontario, Canada (1996) 97pp.	MAMM15015
	X. Xu	Florida Atlantic University (1997) 112pp. p. 824	MA1383084
	E.E. Law	Queen's University of Belfast, Northern Ireland (1996) 147pp.	58/2462c
	J.C. Mastrangelo	The University of Rochester (1996) 203pp.	227-B DA9719947
	T.T. Trial	The University of Southern Mississippi (1996)	229-B DA971898
	D. Yu	The University of Chicago (1997) 235pp.	229-B DA9720065
	V.P. Menon	Colorado State University (1996) 215pp.	176-B DA9719592
	M. Hu	York University, Canada (1996) 282pp.	204-B DANN14601
	D.K. Deak	University of Massachusetts (1997) 194pp.	959-B DA9721441
	D.E. Hutchens	The University of Southern Mississippi (1986) 138pp.	959-B DA9722681
	L.A. Prexta	The University of Akron (1997) 154pp.	732-B DA9723598
	Z. Pu	University of Cincinnati (1997) 140pp.	733-B DA9722374
	A. Sellinger	The University of Michigan (1997) 243pp.	733-B DA9722088
	S.S. Sun	University of Southern California (1996) 133pp.	734-B DA9720297
	T.I. Wallow	University of California, Berkeley (1996) 360pp.	735-B DA9723238
	G.R. Ehteshami	The University of Arizona (1996) 307pp.	836-B DA9720585
	H. Ndayikengur-ukiye	Universitaire Instelling Antwerpen, Belgium (1997) 230pp.	706-B DA9724077
	L.S. Boffa	University of California, Berkeley (1996) 301pp.	729-B DA9722871
	S. Corona-Galvan	The University of Akron (1997) 220pp.	729-B DA9723581
	L.M. Lu	The University of Akron (1997) 184pp.	731-B DA9723594
	C.J. Dunlap	University of Minnesota (1997) 169pp.	1254-B DA9724166
	R. MacD. Hands	University of Colorado at Boulder (1997) 188pp.	1281-B DA9725737
	K.G. Marra	University of Pittsburgh (1996) 194pp.	1293-B DA9726865
	W. Chen	Iowa State University (1997) 148pp.	1311-B DA9725401
	X. Hu	Georgia Institute of Technology (1997) 194pp.	1311-B DA9725173
	S.R. Schricker	University of California, Santa Barbara (1997) 146pp.	1312-B DA9727728
	B.E. Fru	Green State University (1996) 130pp.	1314-B DA9726229

Syntheses	L.A. Ahlberg Randall	University of California, Davis (1997) 192pp.	1880-B DA9728630
	P.M. Swoboda	Technische Universitaet Graz, Austria, In German (1997) 202pp.	58/3807c
	C. Howley	Dalhousie University, Canada (1996) 172pp. 1422	MAMM16022
	M. Almassi	Ecole Polytechnique, Canada (1996) 163pp. 1454	MAMM17702
Thermal degradation	J. Xue	Marquette University (1996) 164pp.	229-B DA9719078
Thermodynamic properties	B.L. Neal	University of Delaware (1997) 252pp.	306-B DA9718767
	O. Sommelius	Lunds Universitet, Sweden (1997) 15pp.	58/3906c
Thermoset	J. Lange	Kungliga Tekniska Hogskolan, Sweden (1995) 99pp.	58/813c
Thin film structures	J.S. McElvain	University of California, Santa Barbara (1996) 169pp.	261-B DA9718605
Thin films	Z. Li	State University of New York at Stony Brook (1996) 141pp.	6965-B DA9712810
	Y. Du	University of New York at Buffalo (1997) 259pp.	173-B DA9719119
	J.B. Dion	Cornell University (1997) 228pp.	7167-B DA9714926
Thin-film electrodes	S.G. Yan	Northwestern University (1997) 201pp.	1879-B DA9731367
Transport properties	T. Radiotis	McGill University, Canada (1996) 277pp.	6289-B DANN12463
Ultrafiltration	S. Inguva	Wayne State University (1996) 118pp.	7627-B DA9715852
Viscoelastic properties	F.I. Braid	The University of Wisconsin-Madison (1996) 367pp.	6284-B DA9707908
	R. Hagen	Kungliga Tekniska Hogskolan, Sweden (1995) 135pp.	58/810c
	L. Lunderg	Kungliga Tekniska Hogskolan, Sweden (1995) 131pp.	58/814c
	S.J. Huang	Columbia University (1997) 135pp.	2007-B DA9728221
	H. Gao	University of South Florida (1996) 170pp.	6962-B DA9710785
Water-soluble polymers	L. Jarnstrom	Kungliga Tekniska Hogskolan, Sweden (1995) 220pp.	58/292c

INDEX